Natural Product Genomics and Metabolomics of Marine Bacteria

Natural Product Genomics and Metabolomics of Marine Bacteria

Editor

Max Crüsemann

MDPI • Basel • Beijing • Wuhan • Barcelona • Belgrade • Manchester • Tokyo • Cluj • Tianjin

Editor
Max Crüsemann
Universität Bonn
Germany

Editorial Office
MDPI
St. Alban-Anlage 66
4052 Basel, Switzerland

This is a reprint of articles from the Special Issue published online in the open access journal *Marine Drugs* (ISSN 1660-3397) (available at: https://www.mdpi.com/journal/marinedrugs/special_issues/Natural_Product_Genomics_Metabolomics_Marine_Bacteria).

For citation purposes, cite each article independently as indicated on the article page online and as indicated below:

LastName, A.A.; LastName, B.B.; LastName, C.C. Article Title. *Journal Name* **Year**, *Volume Number*, Page Range.

ISBN 978-3-0365-3299-8 (Hbk)
ISBN 978-3-0365-3300-1 (PDF)

Contents

About the Editor . . . . **vii**

Preface to "Natural Product Genomics and Metabolomics of Marine Bacteria" . . . . **ix**

Max Crüsemann
Coupling Mass Spectral and Genomic Information to Improve Bacterial Natural Product Discovery Workflows
Reprinted from: *Mar. Drugs* **2021**, *19*, 142, doi:10.3390/md19030142 . . . . **1**

Sylvia Soldatou, Grímur Hjörleifsson Eldjárn, Andrew Ramsay, Justin J. J. van der Hooft, Alison H. Hughes, Simon Rogers and Katherine R. Duncan
Comparative Metabologenomics Analysis of Polar Actinomycetes
Reprinted from: *Mar. Drugs* **2021**, *19*, 103, doi:10.3390/md19020103 . . . . **11**

Ira Handayani, Hamada Saad, Shanti Ratnakomala, Puspita Lisdiyanti, Wien Kusharyoto, Janina Krause, Andreas Kulik, Wolfgang Wohlleben, Saefuddin Aziz, Harald Gross, Athina Gavriilidou, Nadine Ziemert and Yvonne Mast
Mining Indonesian Microbial Biodiversity for Novel Natural Compounds by a Combined Genome Mining and Molecular Networking Approach
Reprinted from: *Mar. Drugs* **2021**, *19*, 316, doi:10.3390/md19060316 . . . . **33**

Christopher A. Leber, C. Benjamin Naman, Lena Keller, Jehad Almaliti, Eduardo J. E. Caro-Diaz, Evgenia Glukhov, Valsamma Joseph, T. P. Sajeevan, Andres Joshua Reyes, Jason S. Biggs, Te Li, Ye Yuan, Shan He, Xiaojun Yan and William H. Gerwick
Applying a Chemogeographic Strategy for Natural Product Discovery from the Marine Cyanobacterium *Moorena bouillonii*
Reprinted from: *Mar. Drugs* **2020**, *18*, 515, doi:10.3390/md18100515 . . . . **61**

Riyanti, Michael Marner, Christoph Hartwig, Maria A. Patras, Stevy I. M. Wodi, Frets J. Rieuwpassa, Frans G. Ijong, Walter Balansa and Till F. Schäberle
Sustainable Low-Volume Analysis of Environmental Samples by Semi-Automated Prioritization of Extracts for Natural Product Research (SeaPEPR)
Reprinted from: *Mar. Drugs* **2020**, *18*, 649, doi:10.3390/md18120649 . . . . **87**

Janira Prichula, Muriel Primon-Barros, Romeu C. Z. Luz, Ícaro M. S. Castro, Thiago G. S. Paim, Maurício Tavares, Rodrigo Ligabue-Braun, Pedro A. d'Azevedo, Jeverson Frazzon, Ana P. G. Frazzon, Adriana Seixas and Michael S. Gilmore
Genome Mining for Antimicrobial Compounds in Wild Marine Animals-Associated Enterococci
Reprinted from: *Mar. Drugs* **2021**, *19*, 328, doi:10.3390/md19060328 . . . . **103**

Despoina Konstantinou, Rafael V. Popin, David P. Fewer, Kaarina Sivonen and Spyros Gkelis
Genome Reduction and Secondary Metabolism of the Marine Sponge-Associated Cyanobacterium *Leptothoe*
Reprinted from: *Mar. Drugs* **2021**, *19*, 298, doi:10.3390/md19060298 . . . . **125**

Lijian Ding, Rinat Bar-Shalom, Dikla Aharonovich, Naoaki Kurisawa, Gaurav Patial, Shuang Li, Shan He, Xiaojun Yan, Arihiro Iwasaki, Kiyotake Suenaga, Chengcong Zhu, Haixi Luo, Fuli Tian, Fuad Fares, C. Benjamin Naman and Tal Luzzatto-Knaan
Metabolomic Characterization of a cf. *Neolyngbya* Cyanobacterium from the South China Sea Reveals Wenchangamide A, a Lipopeptide with In Vitro Apoptotic Potential in Colon Cancer Cells
Reprinted from: *Mar. Drugs* **2021**, *19*, 397, doi:10.3390/md19070397 . . . . **143**

Joko T. Wibowo, Matthias Y. Kellermann, Matthias Köck, Masteria Y. Putra, Tutik Murniasih, Kathrin I. Mohr, Joachim Wink, Dimas F. Praditya, Eike Steinmann and Peter J. Schupp
Anti-Infective and Antiviral Activity of Valinomycin and Its Analogues from a Sea Cucumber-Associated Bacterium, *Streptomyces* sp. SV 21
Reprinted from: *Mar. Drugs* **2021**, *19*, 81, doi:10.3390/md19020081 . . . . **161**

Thomas Dzeha, Michael John Hall and James Grant Burgess
Micrococcin P1 and P2 from Epibiotic Bacteria Associated with Isolates of *Moorea producens* from Kenya
Reprinted from: *Mar. Drugs* **2022**, *20*, 128, doi:10.3390/md20020128 . . . . **175**

Xiyan Wang, Thomas Isbrandt, Mikael Lenz Strube, Sara Skøtt Paulsen, Maike Wennekers Nielsen, Yannick Buijs, Erwin M. Schoof, Thomas Ostenfeld Larsen, Lone Gram and Sheng-Da Zhang
Chitin Degradation Machinery and Secondary Metabolite Profiles in the Marine Bacterium *Pseudoalteromonas rubra* S4059
Reprinted from: *Mar. Drugs* **2021**, *19*, 108, doi:10.3390/md19020108 . . . . **193**

Ricardo Valencia, Valentina González, Agustina Undabarrena, Leonardo Zamora-Leiva, Juan A. Ugalde and Beatriz Cámara
An Integrative Bioinformatic Analysis for Keratinase Detection in Marine-Derived *Streptomyces*
Reprinted from: *Mar. Drugs* **2021**, *19*, 286, doi:10.3390/md19060286 . . . . **209**

About the Editor

Max Crüsemann is currently a Junior Research Group Leader in the Institute of Pharmaceutical Biology, University of Bonn. He studied Pharmacy at the University of Marburg, and obtained his Ph.D. from the University of Bonn for biosynthetic studies on a complex bacterial natural product (advisor Prof. Jörn Piel). After post-doctoral training on bacterial natural product genomics and metabolomics in the group of Prof. Bradley Moore at the Scripps Institution of Oceanography, San Diego, he returned to Bonn to Prof. Gabriele König's group and started his independent career in 2017. He and his group are interested in omics-guided discovery and biosynthetic studies of bacterial natural products.

Preface to "Natural Product Genomics and Metabolomics of Marine Bacteria"

In the last decade, bacterial natural product research has changed. The technical advances in genome sequencing have led to an enormous increase of available sequence information. In parallel, fast, and efficient bioinformatic pipelines to mine all these sequences for natural product biosynthesis genes have emerged. These improvements now allow for the cheap and rapid estimation of an organism's biosynthetic potential, and comparing it to that of other organisms, a procedure called "genome mining".

On the other hand, the development of innovative metabolomics workflows, mostly based on high resolution tandem mass spectrometry, enables the quick identification of natural products from complex samples, the visualization of their structural relationships in molecular networks, and the rapid dereplication of known natural products from metabolomic datasets.

Currently, several innovative approaches to link metabolomic and genomic datasets are being developed and explored. These are anticipated to further improve natural product discovery workflows in the next decade.

This Special Issue on the topic contains twelve articles. In addition to a short review on recent advances in linking bacterial genomic and metabolomic information (1), a collection of original research articles, written by experts in the field has been assembled. The articles cover diverse topics, such as natural product discovery approaches from larger genomic and metabolomic datasets (2,3), the development of novel strategies for natural product discovery workflows (4,5), comparative genomic studies analyzing the natural product potential of marine organisms (6,7), the isolation and structure elucidation of bioactive specialized metabolites (8–10), as well as studies on degrading enzymes of marine bacteria (11,12).

I would like to thank all authors for their meaningful and exciting contributions to this Special Issue. Furthermore, all reviewers of the articles and the editorial team of *Marine Drugs* are acknowledged for their help in creating this diverse collection of stimulating state-of-the-art research articles in the field of marine natural products.

Max Crüsemann
Editor

marine drugs

Review

Coupling Mass Spectral and Genomic Information to Improve Bacterial Natural Product Discovery Workflows

Max Crüsemann

Institute for Pharmaceutical Biology, University of Bonn, Nussallee 6, 53115 Bonn, Germany; cruesemann@uni-bonn.de

Abstract: Bacterial natural products possess potent bioactivities and high structural diversity and are typically encoded in biosynthetic gene clusters. Traditional natural product discovery approaches rely on UV- and bioassay-guided fractionation and are limited in terms of dereplication. Recent advances in mass spectrometry, sequencing and bioinformatics have led to large-scale accumulation of genomic and mass spectral data that is increasingly used for signature-based or correlation-based mass spectrometry genome mining approaches that enable rapid linking of metabolomic and genomic information to accelerate and rationalize natural product discovery. In this mini-review, these approaches are presented, and discovery examples provided. Finally, future opportunities and challenges for paired omics-based natural products discovery workflows are discussed.

Keywords: bacterial natural products; mass spectrometry; genome mining; paired omics

Citation: Crüsemann, M. Coupling Mass Spectral and Genomic Information to Improve Bacterial Natural Product Discovery Workflows. *Mar. Drugs* **2021**, *19*, 142. https://doi.org/10.3390/md19030142

Academic Editor: Vassilios Roussis

Received: 26 January 2021
Accepted: 4 March 2021
Published: 5 March 2021

1. Introduction

Due to their impressive structural diversity and their wide range of bioactivities, natural products (NP) have been, and are still extensively used by humankind as important sources for drugs [1]. NP structures are generated by the concerted action of biosynthetic enzymes. These are encoded in genes which are, in bacteria, usually grouped to biosynthetic gene clusters (BGCs). This circumstance has facilitated bioinformatics analyses and predictions about the number and classes of natural products that can be synthesized by a bacterial strain [2]. This procedure is termed "genome mining", a rapidly growing field that has advanced NP research in the last 15 years [3,4]. Sets of closely related BGCs with similar gene content can be grouped into gene cluster families (GCF), that encode the production of identical or highly similar molecules. The recent advances in DNA sequencing have led to a massive accumulation of sequence data in the databases which, in turn, fueled the development of large-scale BGC and GCF analysis pipelines and databases such as BiG-SCAPE [5], BiG-SLICE [6] and BiG-FAM [7] by Medema and colleagues. These frameworks enable the systematic estimation and comparison of NP biosynthetic potential in increasing numbers of bacterial strains.

Biosynthetic machineries usually do not only lead to one single natural product, but may produce a suite of structurally related metabolites through relaxed substrate specificities, causing enzymatic processing of structurally different precursors and intermediates. Mass spectrometry (MS)-based workflows offer opportunities to chart the metabolic diversity that is present in a complex sample, e.g., a crude bacterial extract. The metabolic diversity in complex NP mixtures can be regarded as a collection of "molecular families", a term for structurally related compounds with related MS fragmentation (MS/MS) spectra [8]. As an outstanding example, the public community data repository and analysis platform GNPS [9,10], developed by Dorrestein, Bandeira and colleagues, offers opportunities for the detailed analysis and visualization of natural product MS/MS fragmentation data by molecular networking. The GNPS environment has also integrated several useful annotation, classification and dereplication tools [11–17] that, if used altogether, aid in obtaining the maximum amount of information from an MS/MS spectrum or dataset of interest.

One of the most important goals in natural product discovery and the basis for any state-of-the-art biosynthetic study is the direct linkage of a metabolite to its BGC. The classical and most reliable way to establish such a link is either the heterologous expression or the activation of a cryptic BGC, with subsequent detection and characterization of the target compounds in the heterologous or engineered host, or the deletion of the BGC or key biosynthetic genes thereof in the NP producer to abolish production of the natural product of interest. However, although significant advances have been made in these areas [18,19], these approaches are still relatively laborious and time consuming because only a single biosynthetic pathway can be targeted in one experimental workflow, that typically requires several, sometimes cumbersome cloning and transformation procedures. In contrast, MS-guided genome mining techniques that have been developed, enable the parallel establishment of multiple compound-BGC linkages and dereplication in a much more time-effective workflow. The acquisition and in-depth analysis of paired datasets comprising MS/MS data of culture extracts and genome sequences of their producers is thus of promise to accelerate and improve any bacterial NP discovery program.

Concepts and successful examples of linking chemical and biosynthetic space have lately been reviewed by Duncan and coworkers [20]. Another detailed application-oriented review by van der Hooft, Medema and colleagues mainly focused on the key technologies that enable making these linkages [21]. This minireview particularly intends to highlight concepts to directly link mass spectral information and BGCs by (i) signature-based approaches (peptidogenomics and glycogenomics), as well as (ii) correlation-based approaches (pattern-based genome mining, metabologenomics) and provides discovery examples. Finally, latest developments and future promises and challenges in linking biosynthetic and metabolomic data of natural products are presented and discussed.

2. Concepts and Examples for Linking Genomic and Metabolomic Data

2.1. *Experiment-Guided Genome Mining: Peptidogenomics and Glycogenomics*

These two MS-guided genome mining approaches were developed and pioneered by Kersten, Dorrestein and Moore [22,23]. Both workflows are dependent on the presence of specific signatures, i.e., mass shifts or fragmentation ions, in an MS/MS spectrum from bacterial compound mixtures. These distinctive signatures may be linked to a BGC predicted to encode the biosynthetic machinery to produce NPs with structural motifs to yield these MS/MS fragments. This procedure is particularly applicable for peptides and glycosylated molecules (Figure 1).

In peptidogenomics, the mass shifts relate to the fragmentation of peptides into their constituents, i.e., proteinogenic or modified, non-proteinogenic amino acids, a process that allows for automation [22,24]. A number of subsequent amino acid MS/MS mass shifts constitutes a "sequence tag", which is instrumental in the search for the respective BGC in the producers' genome (Figure 1A). For ribosomally synthesized and modified peptide natural products (RiPP), the sequence tag is part of a small, encoded protein, usually clustered with genes encoding posttranslationally modifying enzymes, that is queried in the producers' genome e.g., by six-frame translations. Nonribosomal peptides (NRP) are synthesized by multimodular assembly line megaenzymes. Here, a detected sequence tag relates to a BGC encoding a sequence of modules with predictable adenylation domain specificities. In glycogenomics, diagnostic mass shifts or fragments are caused by the fragmentation of bonds to sugars or, preferably, modified deoxysugars, both frequently observed features of bioactive natural products [23]. The biosynthesis of deoxysugars is typically encoded by subclusters of modifying biosynthetic genes and glycosyltransferases, clustered with genes encoding core NP biosynthetic machineries (e.g., polyketide synthases) and can be matched with the detected MS/MS deoxysugar fragment(s) (Figure 1B).

In a landmark study in 2011, the concept of peptidogenomics was introduced to the NP community and systematically used to uncover and characterize a series of novel RiPPs from well investigated *Streptomyces* strains such as *S. lividans*, *S. coelicolor* and *S. griseus*. Additionally, five novel analogs of the nonribosomal lipopeptide stendomycin were characterized from *S. hygroscopicus* and connected to their BGC (Figure 1A) [22]. In a subsequent study, *Streptomyces roseosporus* natural products were mapped with a combination of molecular networking and peptidogenomics which led to the discovery of the stenothricin BGC [25]. Another peptidogenomic study on *S. roseosporus* based on imaging MS revealed that the potent antibiotic peptide arylomycin was of nonribosomal origin [26]. Bromoalterochromides were discovered and connected to their BGC in two marine *Pseudoalteromonas* bacteria from a large scale nano-DESI MS/MS dataset of *Bacillus* and *Pseudoalteromonas* strains [8]. From the plant pathogen *Ralstonia solanacearum*, the bioactive lipopeptide ralsolamycin was also identified using the peptidogenomic approach [27].

The peptidogenomic concept was automated by Pevzner, Mohimani and colleagues, leading to the development of automated peptidogenomics tools specifically designed for RiPPs (RiPP-Quest) [28], NRPs (NRP-Quest) [29] and both (Pep2Path) [30]. Application of RiPP-Quest enabled the discovery of informatipeptin (Figure 1C), a new class III lanthipeptide from *Streptomyces viridochromogenes*. Recently, the development of MetaMiner, an advancement of the RiPP-Quest tool, designed for the query of larger datasets e.g., from metagenomes, and its application to several datasets in the GNPS database led to the discovery and annotation of seven previously unknown RiPPs [31].

The development of the glycogenomic approach and its proof-of-principle application to a set of marine actinomycete crude extracts enabled discovery and MS-guided isolation of arenimycin B (Figure 1D), a type II polyketide comprising the two characteristic deoxysugar moieties forosamine and O-methyl rhamnose from the marine actinomycete *Salinispora arenicola* CNB527 [23]. The derivative arenimycin A, containing only O-methyl rhamnose, had previously been isolated from another *S. arenicola* strain [32] by classical, UV-guided purification. However, analysis of the biosynthetic potential of CNB527 suggested that a candidate BGC for arenimycin biosynthetic machinery could be capable of adding another sugar moiety to the molecule. After its characterization, it was thus concluded that arenimycin B is actually the end product of the biosynthetic pathway, and was notably found to be more bioactive than the previously isolated arenimycin A, showing a twofold or greater increase in activity against clinically relevant, multidrug-resistant strains of *Staphylococcus aureus* [23]. Another glycogenomic example with marine origin is the discovery of five rosamicin derivatives from the marine actinomycete *Salinispora pacifica* CNS237 (Figure 1B) [33]. This group of antibiotically active, glycosylated polyketides, among them three unprecedented analogs, was discovered by their characteristic desosamine fragment from a large MS/MS dataset that was used to prioritize marine actinomycete strains by molecular networking [34]. After their dereplication and subsequent structure elucidation, it was later revealed that these compounds are actually the end product of their polyketide synthase (PKS) assembly line pathway that is, however, also responsible for the production of salinipyrone and pacificanone, linear polyketides that had previously been isolated by a classical approach [35]. Unexpectedly, both appeared to be shunt products of the PKS, as proven by mutagenesis experiments in the rosamicin assembly line [33]. Analogously to peptidogenomics, glycogenomics also holds potential for automation, although this has not yet been implemented.

2.2. Correlation-Based Approaches on Larger Paired Datasets: Pattern-Based Genome Mining, Metabologenomics

Another possibility to link genomic with metabolomic information is the application of correlation-based approaches. Here metabolite patterns, obtained from larger MS datasets of sequenced bacteria, are compared and correlated with their BGC or GCF patterns, derived from comparative analyses of a set of genomes (Figure 2). Notably, these correlations are independent of the chemical class of the detected metabolites. Talented NP producers such as actinomycetes harbor a multitude of BGCs, whereas taxonomically closely related strains characteristically possess overlapping patterns of encoded BGCs. This means that homologous BGCs are frequently encoded in more than one or several related strains, while other BGCs are unique for particular strains. An illustrative model for this phenomenon is the marine actinomycete genus *Salinispora* [36].

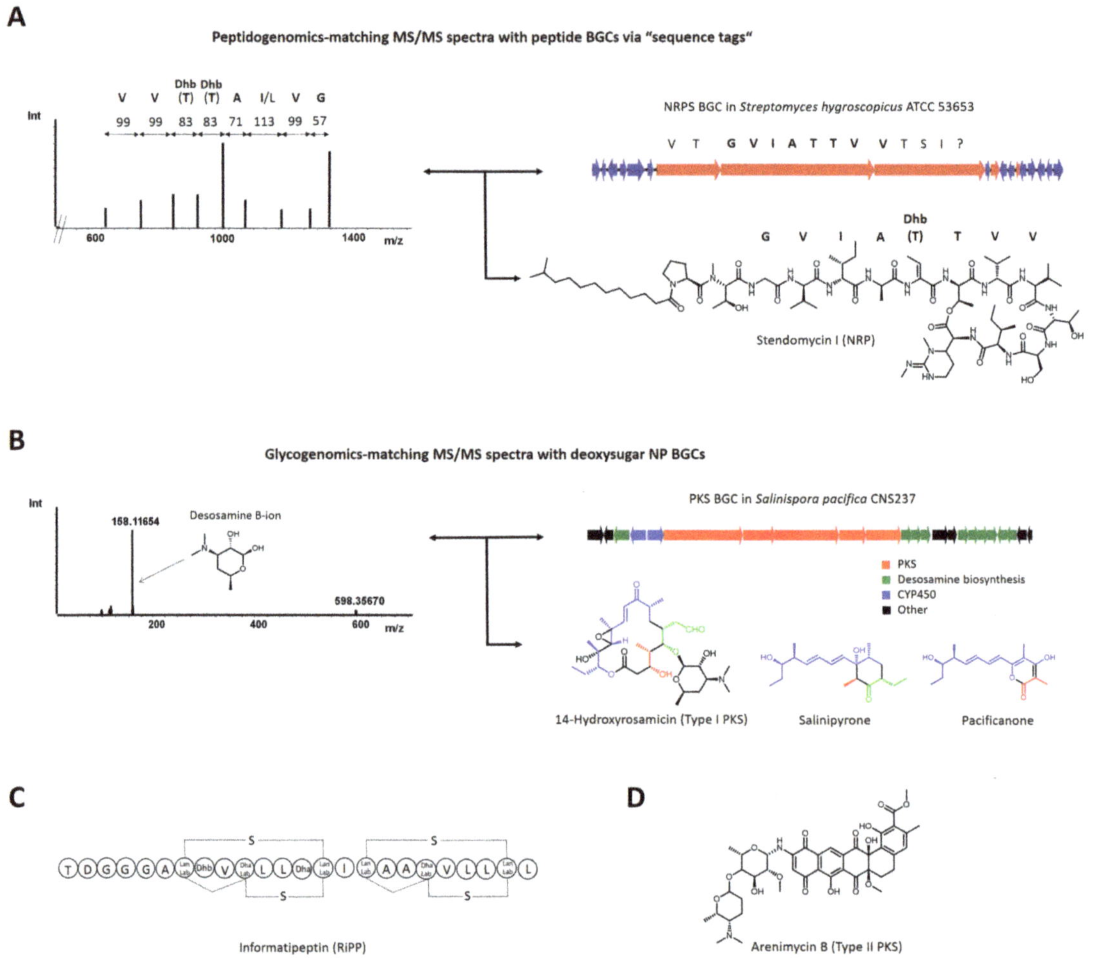

Figure 1. Concepts and discovery examples for experiment-guided genome mining. (**A**) Peptidogenomics: *Streptomyces hygroscopicus* MS/MS data yielded a sequence tag with eight amino acids, two of them dehydrated threonines (Dhb). The sequence tag matched with a sequence of adenylation domain predictions of an orphan nonribosomal peptide synthetase BGC, facilitating the targeted isolation and characterization of stendomycin lipopeptides [22]. The second threonine dehydration appeared only during MS/MS fragmentation as elimination product of the ester bond. (**B**) Glycogenomics: Matching of MS/MS spectra of *Salinispora pacifica* CNS237 with a type I polyketide synthase BGC encoding deoxysugar biosynthesis genes revealed several rosamicin derivatives and enabled their targeted isolation and further characterization. The previously isolated linear polyketides salinipyrone and pacificanone appear to be shunt products of the rosamicin PKS, revealed by mutagenesis experiments. Building blocks synthesized by the same module(s) are color-coded accordingly [33]. (**C**) Further natural products from different classes discovered by the peptidogenomic [28] and (**D**) glycogenomic approach [23]. For more details regarding these concepts, please refer to references [22,23].

Salinispora species and strains are very closely related on 16S-RNA level, but can be discriminated by the presence of species- or strain-specific patterns of encoded NP BGCs (compare Figure 2A, left). In a remarkable genome mining study led by Ziemert and Jensen, 75 *Salinispora* strains were analyzed and compared regarding their PKS and NRPS pathway variety and evolution [37]. This comprehensive analysis was later extended to 119 strains and to other pathway types such as terpenes and RiPPs [38].

In a pioneering study from the Jensen and Moore labs, the metabolomes of 35 *Salinispora* strains were visualized with GNPS molecular networking and then compared with the NRPS/PKS BGC patterns of the respective strains to establish compound-BGC links [39]. These correlative analyses enabled the linkage of an orphan BGC to the polyketide arenicolide and the targeted isolation, structure elucidation and biological characterization of the cytotoxic, echinomycin-like nonribosomal depsipeptide retimycin A, that was encoded and produced by only one strain in the collection, *S. arenicola* CNT005 (Figure 2A).

An analogous study was performed in the bacterial genera *Photorhabdus* and *Xenorhabdus*, both associated with insects and known for prolific natural product production, by the Bode group [40]. Here, a metabolomic network from HPLC-MS/MS data of 30 strains was created, annotated and compared with BGC patterns in the respective strains (Figure 2B). This study revealed the robust expression of known metabolites under laboratory conditions in a number of strains, but also led to the detection of previously unidentified metabolite classes in these bacteria, such as the novel xefoampeptides and tilivallin and connection to their BGCs. Furthermore, novel depsipeptides named fatflabets and xeneprotides were discovered from analysis of the molecular network, and their structures elucidated. However, a complete BGC for these novel compound families could not be assigned with certainty.

A similar concept to bridge metabolomic and genomic information, termed metabologenomics, was developed in the Metcalf and Kelleher labs (Figure 2C). This approach relies on the establishment of correlations between MS spectra and GCFs in a huge dataset of 830 sequenced actinomycete bacteria, of which 178 were subjected to detailed HPLC-MS metabolic profiling in different culture media [41]. Here, a correlation score between GCF and MS1 data was generated and then applied by searching for exact masses of predicted metabolites in the dataset. Subsequent mining of this extensive, paired dataset for detected metabolites encoded by biochemically interesting BGCs enabled the discovery and characterization of several natural products such as tambromycin [42], rimosamides [43] and tyrobetaines [44] and the detailed investigation of their biosynthetic pathways.

Zdouc, Sosio and colleagues recently performed a detailed metabolomic investigation of the actinobacterial genus *Planomonospora* [45]. Four of the 72 investigated strains were also genome-sequenced, which allowed for a paired omics analysis leading to the annotation of a BGC for the thiopeptide siomycin and congeners. Furthermore, two novel biaryl-linked tripeptides were isolated after network analysis and their structures elucidated. They represent the first members of a widespread novel class of small RiPPs, encoded by the smallest gene ever reported, as revealed by peptidogenomics and heterologous expression [46]. Metabologenomics was also used by the Duncan lab for the evaluation of a dataset of 25 polar actinomycetes, published in this Special Issue [47]. Their metabolomes were analyzed and correlated to genome data by using a newly developed tool, NP-linker, designed for the automated establishment of NP-BGC correlations [48].

In a recent study on the biosynthetic and metabolic diversity in the actinomycete genus *Nocardia*, metabolite-BGC correlations were analyzed based on a double-network approach by the Ziemert and Kaysser groups [49]: A metabolomic network was constructed with GNPS molecular networking [9], as well as a BGC network of all selected strains created via BiG-SCAPE [5]. Then, both networks were analyzed and compared for correlations of molecular families and gene cluster families over the same number of strains. This strategy was validated by the strain-specific discovery and annotation of a battery of unprecedented nocobactin-like siderophores.

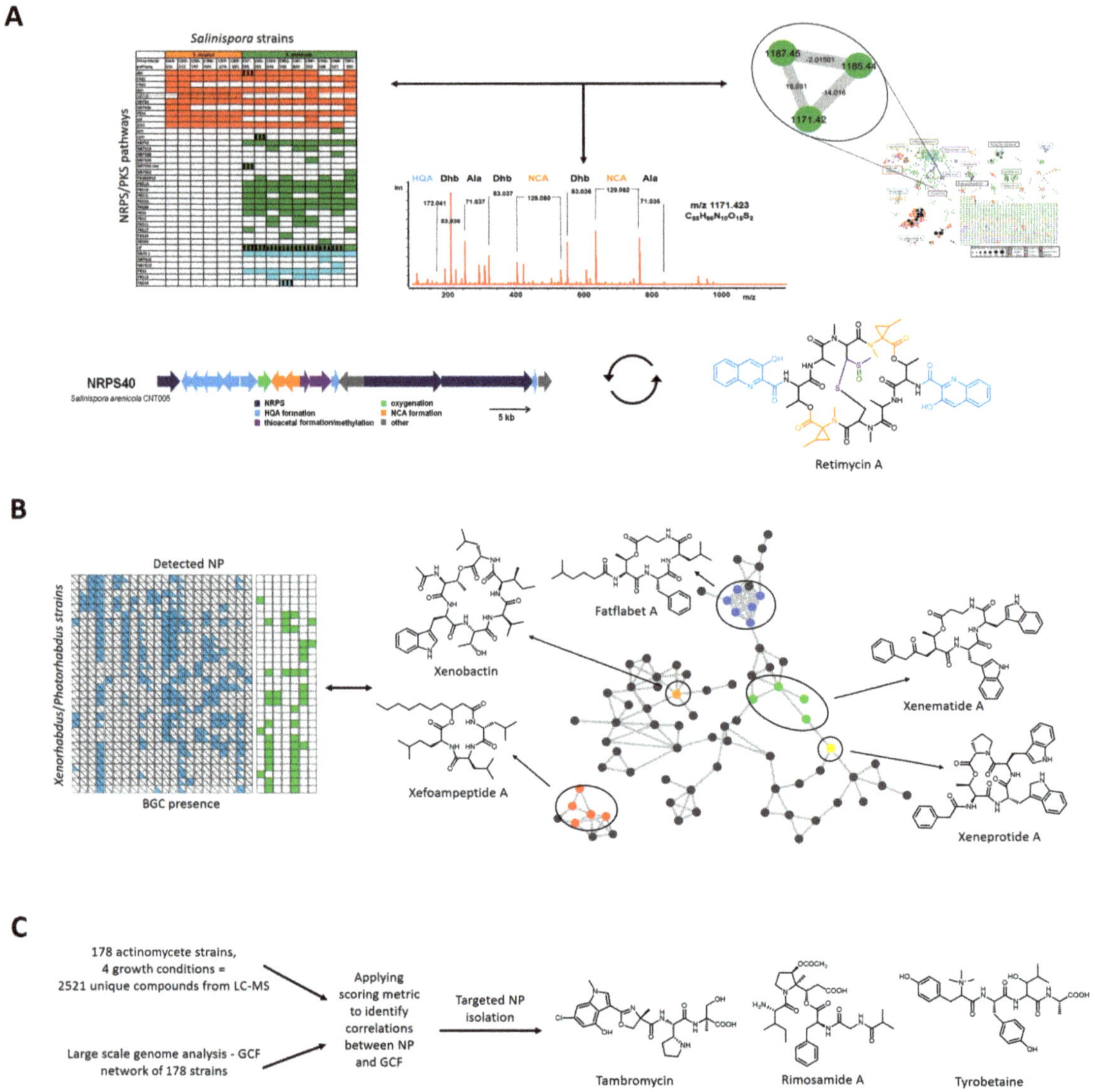

Figure 2. Discovery examples for correlation-based approaches using paired datasets. (**A**) Correlation of *Salinispora* strain BGC patterns with a molecular network of 35 strains led to the identification of a candidate peptide, encoded and produced by only one strain in the dataset. The peptide was matched to its NRPS BGC with additional help of the peptidogenomic approach. The structure of the elucidated metabolite retimycin A is depicted. Building blocks are color-coded corresponding to responsible biosynthetic genes [39]. Taken from reference 39 and rearranged with permission of Elsevier. (**B**) *Xenorhabdus* and *Photorhabdus* strains were analyzed for BGC patterns and production of encoded metabolites (left). Subsequent molecular network analysis led to the identification and discovery of several NRPS-derived cyclic depsipeptides (right) [40]. (**C**) Metabologenomic workflow of a 178 strain actinomycetes dataset [41–44]. An example for the applied scoring metric can be found in reference 21.

The generation of standardized community repositories such as MIBiG for characterized NP BGCs [50], and the GNPS database for MS/MS data of NP datasets and compounds [9], has improved and facilitated many natural products workflows. However, genome-metabolome links have not been systematically documented and are cumbersome to search for. To overcome this obstacle and to standardize NP-BGC links that can be reused by the community for further projects, recently the paired omics database has been developed and launched [51]. This platform gathers a large number of paired datasets generated by the NP community including links to MS/MS datasets on GNPS and sequence data of characterized BGCs on MIBiG and standardized metabolite-BGC links were generated. This standardized and open community database may be very useful for the application and automation of future correlative network-based approaches and prioritization of novel metabolites and BGCs that are worth investigating.

An alternative pipeline for bioinformatic analyses of BGCs and compound-cluster matching was developed by the Magarvey lab [52]: Here, a prediction engine (PRISM) identifies and predicts BGC in microbial genomes. A retrobiosynthetic algorithm (GRAPE) performs retrobiosynthetic analyses of known natural products and suggests a likely BGC for these metabolites. A matching algorithm (GARLIC) then compares PRISM and GRAPE outputs and gives matching scores. By that procedure, BGCs with unknown products can be identified with high confidence. Additionally, a "genomes to natural products" (GNP) algorithm matches LC-MS/MS data to BGCs by structure prediction, substructure analysis and in silico fragmentation prediction generating confidence scores of the NP-BGC matches [53]. Notably, this pipeline is restricted to modular PKS and NRPS pathways.

To conclude, in the last decade, several novel MS-guided genome mining workflows and global, standardized mass spectral and BGC databases have been developed and led to a significant number of natural product discoveries. For reliable NP-BGC linkages, these paired omics workflows rely on high quality MS/MS and sequence data and bioinformatic, mass spectral and biosynthetic knowledge. To further expand a paired omics NP mining workflow to other natural product classes, the integrated use of recently developed substructure annotation tools [11], classification-based methods [54] and fragmentation trees [55] together with the use of further improved automated linking approaches [48] are of great promise. Structure elucidation remains a major bottleneck in NP discovery pipelines, and is often limited by the low yields of the NP of interest. However, the development of neural network algorithms for NMR analysis [56] and novel structure elucidation methods such as MicroED [57] may, integrated into the described workflows, further brighten the future for natural product research and enable many exciting discoveries.

Funding: The author acknowledges a postdoctoral fellowship from the Deutsche Forschungsgemeinschaft (DFG), grant number CR464-1.

Conflicts of Interest: The author declares no conflict of interest.

References

1. Newman, D.J.; Cragg, G.M. Natural Products as Sources of New Drugs over the Nearly Four Decades from 01/1981 to 09/2019. *J. Nat. Prod.* **2020**, *83*, 770–803. [CrossRef] [PubMed]
2. Blin, K.; Shaw, S.; Steinke, K.; Villebro, R.; Ziemert, N.; Lee, S.Y.; Medema, M.H.; Weber, T. antiSMASH 5.0: Updates to the secondary metabolite genome mining pipeline. *Nucleic Acids Res.* **2019**, *47*, W81–W87. [PubMed]
3. Ziemert, N.; Alanjary, M.; Weber, T. The evolution of genome mining in microbes—A review. *Nat. Prod. Rep.* **2016**, *33*, 988–1005. [CrossRef] [PubMed]
4. Kenshole, E.; Herisse, M.; Michael, M.; Pidot, S.J. Natural product discovery through microbial genome mining. *Curr. Opin. Chem. Biol.* **2020**, *60*, 47–54. [CrossRef]
5. Navarro-Muñoz, J.C.; Selem-Mojica, N.; Mullowney, M.W.; Kautsar, S.A.; Tryon, J.H.; Parkinson, E.I.; De Los Santos, E.L.C.; Yeong, M.; Cruz-Morales, P.; Abubucker, S.; et al. A computational framework to explore large-scale biosynthetic diversity. *Nat. Chem. Biol.* **2020**, *16*, 60–68. [CrossRef] [PubMed]
6. Kautsar, S.A.; Van der Hooft, J.J.J.; De Ridder, D.; Medema, M.H. BiG-SLiCE: A highly scalable tool maps the diversity of 1.2 million biosynthetic gene clusters. *Gigascience* **2021**, *10*, giaa154. [CrossRef] [PubMed]

7. Kautsar, S.A.; Blin, K.; Shaw, S.; Weber, T.; Medema, M.H. BiG-FAM: The biosynthetic gene cluster families database. *Nucleic Acids Res.* **2021**, *49*, D490–D497. [CrossRef]
8. Nguyen, D.D.; Wu, C.H.; Moree, W.J.; Lamsa, A.; Medema, M.H.; Zhao, X.; Gavilan, R.G.; Aparicio, M.; Atencio, L.; Jackson, C.; et al. MS/MS networking guided analysis of molecule and gene cluster families. *Proc. Natl. Acad. Sci. USA* **2013**, *110*, 2611–2620. [CrossRef] [PubMed]
9. Wang, M.; Carver, J.J.; Phelan, V.V.; Sanchez, L.M.; Garg, N.; Peng, Y.; Nguyen, D.D.; Watrous, J.; Kapono, C.A.; Luzzatto-Knaan, T.; et al. Sharing and community curation of mass spectrometry data with Global Natural Products Social Molecular Networking. *Nat. Biotechnol.* **2016**, *34*, 828–837. [CrossRef] [PubMed]
10. Aron, A.T.; Gentry, E.C.; McPhail, K.L.; Nothias, L.F.; Nothias-Esposito, M.; Bouslimani, A.; Petras, D.; Gauglitz, J.M.; Sikora, N.; Vargas, F.; et al. Reproducible molecular networking of untargeted mass spectrometry data using GNPS. *Nat. Protoc.* **2020**, *15*, 1954–1991. [CrossRef]
11. Van der Hooft, J.J.J.; Wandy, J.; Young, F.; Padmanabhan, S.; Gerasimidis, K.; Burgess, K.E.V.; Barrett, M.P.; Rogers, S. Unsupervised Discovery and Comparison of Structural Families Across Multiple Samples in Untargeted Metabolomics. *Anal. Chem.* **2017**, *89*, 7569–7577. [CrossRef] [PubMed]
12. Da Silva, R.R.; Wang, M.; Nothias, L.F.; Van der Hooft, J.J.J.; Caraballo-Rodríguez, A.M.; Fox, E.; Balunas, M.J.; Klassen, J.L.; Lopes, N.P.; Dorrestein, P.C. Propagating annotations of molecular networks using in silico fragmentation. *PLoS Comput. Biol.* **2018**, *14*, e1006089. [CrossRef] [PubMed]
13. Ernst, M.; Kang, K.B.; Caraballo-Rodríguez, A.M.; Nothias, L.F.; Wandy, J.; Chen, C.; Wang, M.; Rogers, S.; Medema, M.H.; Dorrestein, P.C.; et al. MolNetEnhancer: Enhanced Molecular Networks by Integrating Metabolome Mining and Annotation Tools. *Metabolites* **2019**, *9*, 144. [CrossRef]
14. Jarmusch, A.K.; Wang, M.; Aceves, C.M.; Advani, R.S.; Aguirre, S.; Aksenov, A.A.; Aleti, G.; Aron, A.T.; Bauermeister, A.; Bolleddu, S.; et al. ReDU: A framework to find and reanalyze public mass spectrometry data. *Nat. Methods* **2020**, *17*, 901–904. [CrossRef] [PubMed]
15. Wang, M.; Jarmusch, A.K.; Vargas, F.; Aksenov, A.A.; Gauglitz, J.M.; Weldon, K.; Petras, D.; Da Silva, R.R.; Quinn, R.A.; Melnik, A.V.; et al. Mass spectrometry searches using MASST. *Nat. Biotechnol.* **2020**, *38*, 23–26. [CrossRef]
16. Mohimani, H.; Gurevich, A.; Mikheenko, A.; Garg, N.; Nothias, L.F.; Ninomiya, A.; Takada, K.; Dorrestein, P.C.; Pevzner, P.A. Dereplication of peptidic natural products through database search of mass spectra. *Nat. Chem. Biol.* **2017**, *13*, 30–37. [CrossRef]
17. Mohimani, H.; Gurevich, A.; Shlemov, A.; Mikheenko, A.; Korobeynikov, A.; Cao, L.; Shcherbin, E.; Nothias, L.F.; Dorrestein, P.C.; Pevzner, P.A. Dereplication of microbial metabolites through database search of mass spectra. *Nat. Commun.* **2018**, *9*, 4035. [CrossRef]
18. Zhang, J.J.; Tang, X.; Moore, B.S. Genetic platforms for heterologous expression of microbial natural products. *Nat. Prod. Rep.* **2019**, *36*, 1313–1332. [CrossRef] [PubMed]
19. Tong, Y.; Weber, T.; Lee, S.Y. CRISPR/Cas-based genome engineering in natural product discovery. *Nat. Prod. Rep.* **2019**, *36*, 1262–1280. [CrossRef] [PubMed]
20. Soldatou, S.; Eldjarn, G.H.; Huerta-Uribe, A.; Rogers, S.; Duncan, K.R. Linking biosynthetic and chemical space to accelerate microbial secondary metabolite discovery. *FEMS Microbiol. Lett.* **2019**, *366*, fnz142. [CrossRef]
21. Van der Hooft, J.J.J.; Mohimani, H.; Bauermeister, A.; Dorrestein, P.C.; Duncan, K.R.; Medema, M.H. Linking genomics and metabolomics to chart specialized metabolic diversity. *Chem Soc. Rev.* **2020**, *49*, 3297–3314. [CrossRef]
22. Kersten, R.D.; Yang, Y.L.; Xu, Y.; Cimermancic, P.; Nam, S.J.; Fenical, W.; Fischbach, M.A.; Moore, B.S.; Dorrestein, P.C. A mass spectrometry-guided genome mining approach for natural product peptidogenomics. *Nat. Chem. Biol.* **2011**, *7*, 794–802. [CrossRef]
23. Kersten, R.D.; Ziemert, N.; Gonzalez, D.J.; Duggan, B.M.; Nizet, V.; Dorrestein, P.C.; Moore, B.S. Glycogenomics as a mass spectrometry-guided genome-mining method for microbial glycosylated molecules. *Proc. Natl. Acad. Sci. USA* **2013**, *110*, E4407–E4416. [CrossRef] [PubMed]
24. Mohimani, H.; Pevzner, P.A. Dereplication, sequencing and identification of peptidic natural products: From genome mining to peptidogenomics to spectral networks. *Nat. Prod. Rep.* **2016**, *33*, 73–86. [CrossRef]
25. Liu, W.T.; Lamsa, A.; Wong, W.R.; Boudreau, P.D.; Kersten, R.D.; Peng, Y.; Moree, W.J.; Duggan, B.M.; Moore, B.S.; Gerwick, W.H.; et al. MS/MS-based networking and peptidogenomics guided genome mining revealed the stenothricin gene cluster in Streptomyces roseosporus. *J. Antibiot.* **2014**, *67*, 99–104. [CrossRef] [PubMed]
26. Liu, W.T.; Kersten, R.D.; Yang, Y.L.; Moore, B.S.; Dorrestein, P.C. Imaging mass spectrometry and genome mining via short sequence tagging identified the anti-infective agent arylomycin in Streptomyces roseosporus. *J. Am. Chem. Soc.* **2011**, *133*, 18010–18013. [CrossRef]
27. Spraker, J.E.; Sanchez, L.M.; Lowe, T.M.; Dorrestein, P.C.; Keller, N.P. Ralstonia solanacearum lipopeptide induces chlamydospore development in fungi and facilitates bacterial entry into fungal tissues. *ISME J.* **2016**, *10*, 2317–2330. [CrossRef] [PubMed]
28. Mohimani, H.; Kersten, R.D.; Liu, W.T.; Wang, M.; Purvine, S.O.; Wu, S.; Brewer, H.M.; Pasa-Tolic, L.; Bandeira, N.; Moore, B.S.; et al. Automated genome mining of ribosomal peptide natural products. *ACS Chem. Biol.* **2014**, *9*, 1545–1551. [CrossRef]
29. Mohimani, H.; Liu, W.T.; Kersten, R.D.; Moore, B.S.; Dorrestein, P.C.; Pevzner, P.A. NRPquest: Coupling Mass Spectrometry and Genome Mining for Nonribosomal Peptide Discovery. *J. Nat. Prod.* **2014**, *77*, 1902–1909. [CrossRef] [PubMed]
30. Medema, M.H.; Paalvast, Y.; Nguyen, D.D.; Melnik, A.; Dorrestein, P.C.; Takano, E.; Breitling, R. Pep2Path: Automated mass spectrometry-guided genome mining of peptidic natural products. *PLoS Comput. Biol.* **2014**, *10*, e1003822. [CrossRef]

31. Cao, L.; Gurevich, A.; Alexander, K.L.; Naman, C.B.; Leão, T.; Glukhov, E.; Luzzatto-Knaan, T.; Vargas, F.; Quinn, R.A.; Bouslimani, A.; et al. MetaMiner: A Scalable Peptidogenomics Approach for Discovery of Ribosomal Peptide Natural Products with Blind Modifications from Microbial Communities. *Cell Syst.* **2019**, *9*, 600–608.e4. [CrossRef]
32. Asolkar, R.N.; Kirkland, T.N.; Jensen, P.R.; Fenical, W. Arenimycin, an antibiotic effective against rifampin- and methicillin-resistant *Staphylococcus aureus* from the marine actinomycete *Salinispora arenicola*. *J. Antibiot.* **2010**, *63*, 37–39. [CrossRef]
33. Awakawa, T.; Crüsemann, M.; Munguia, J.; Ziemert, N.; Nizet, V.; Fenical, W.; Moore, B.S. Salinipyrone and Pacificanone Are Biosynthetic By-products of the Rosamicin Polyketide Synthase. *Chembiochem* **2015**, *16*, 1443–1447. [CrossRef] [PubMed]
34. Crüsemann, M.; O'Neill, E.C.; Larson, C.B.; Melnik, A.V.; Floros, D.J.; Da Silva, R.R.; Jensen, P.R.; Dorrestein, P.C.; Moore, B.S. Prioritizing Natural Product Diversity in a Collection of 146 Bacterial Strains Based on Growth and Extraction Protocols. *J. Nat. Prod.* **2017**, *80*, 588–597. [CrossRef]
35. Oh, D.C.; Gontang, E.A.; Kauffman, C.A.; Jensen, P.R.; Fenical, W. Salinipyrones and pacificanones, mixed-precursor polyketides from the marine actinomycete *Salinispora pacifica*. *J. Nat. Prod.* **2008**, *71*, 570–575. [CrossRef] [PubMed]
36. Jensen, P.R.; Moore, B.S.; Fenical, W. The marine actinomycete genus Salinispora: A model organism for secondary metabolite discovery. *Nat. Prod. Rep.* **2015**, *32*, 738–751. [CrossRef] [PubMed]
37. Ziemert, N.; Lechner, A.; Wietz, M.; Millán-Aguiñaga, N.; Chavarria, K.L.; Jensen, P.R. Diversity and evolution of secondary metabolism in the marine actinomycete genus *Salinispora*. *Proc. Natl. Acad. Sci. USA* **2014**, *111*, E1130–E1139. [CrossRef] [PubMed]
38. Letzel, A.C.; Li, J.; Amos, G.C.A.; Millán-Aguiñaga, N.; Ginigini, J.; Abdelmohsen, U.R.; Gaudêncio, S.P.; Ziemert, N.; Moore, B.S.; Jensen, P.R. Genomic insights into specialized metabolism in the marine actinomycete *Salinispora*. *Environ. Microbiol.* **2017**, *19*, 3660–3673. [CrossRef]
39. Duncan, K.R.; Crüsemann, M.; Lechner, A.; Sarkar, A.; Li, J.; Ziemert, N.; Wang, M.; Bandeira, N.; Moore, B.S.; Dorrestein, P.C.; et al. Molecular networking and pattern-based genome mining improves discovery of biosynthetic gene clusters and their products from *Salinispora* species. *Chem. Biol.* **2015**, *22*, 460–471. [CrossRef] [PubMed]
40. Tobias, N.J.; Wolff, H.; Djahanschiri, B.; Grundmann, F.; Kronenwerth, M.; Shi, Y.M.; Simonyi, S.; Grün, P.; Shapiro-Ilan, D.; Pidot, S.J.; et al. Natural product diversity associated with the nematode symbionts *Photorhabdus* and *Xenorhabdus*. *Nat. Microbiol.* **2017**, *2*, 1676–1685. [CrossRef] [PubMed]
41. Doroghazi, J.R.; Albright, J.C.; Goering, A.W.; Ju, K.S.; Haines, R.R.; Tchalukov, K.A.; Labeda, D.P.; Kelleher, N.L.; Metcalf, W.W. A roadmap for natural product discovery based on large-scale genomics and metabolomics. *Nat. Chem. Biol.* **2014**, *10*, 963–968. [CrossRef]
42. Goering, A.W.; McClure, R.A.; Doroghazi, J.R.; Albright, J.C.; Haverland, N.A.; Zhang, Y.; Ju, K.S.; Thomson, R.J.; Metcalf, W.W.; Kelleher, N.L. Metabologenomics: Correlation of microbial gene clusters with metabolites drives discovery of a nonribosomal peptide with an unusual amino acid monomer. *ACS Cent. Sci.* **2016**, *2*, 99–108. [CrossRef] [PubMed]
43. McClure, R.A.; Goering, A.W.; Ju, K.S.; Baccile, J.A.; Schroeder, F.C.; Metcalf, W.W.; Thomson, R.J.; Kelleher, N.L. Elucidating the Rimosamide-Detoxin Natural Product Families and Their Biosynthesis Using Metabolite/Gene Cluster Correlations. *ACS Chem. Biol.* **2016**, *11*, 3452–3460. [CrossRef]
44. Parkinson, E.I.; Tryon, J.H.; Goering, A.W.; Ju, K.S.; McClure, R.A.; Kemball, J.D.; Zhukovsky, S.; Labeda, D.P.; Thomson, R.J.; Kelleher, N.L.; et al. Discovery of the Tyrobetaine Natural Products and Their Biosynthetic Gene Cluster via Metabologenomics. *ACS Chem. Biol.* **2018**, *13*, 1029–1037. [CrossRef]
45. Zdouc, M.M.; Iorio, M.; Maffioli, S.I.; Crüsemann, M.; Donadio, S.; Sosio, M. Planomonospora: A Metabolomics Perspective on an Underexplored Actinobacteria Genus. *J. Nat. Prod.* **2021**, *84*, 204–219. [CrossRef]
46. Zdouc, M.M.; Alanjary, M.M.; Zarazúa, G.S.; Maffioli, S.I.; Crüsemann, M.; Medema, M.H.; Donadio, S.; Sosio, M. A biaryl-linked tripeptide from *Planomonospora* reveals a widespread class of minimal RiPP gene clusters. *Cell Chem. Biol.* **2020**. [CrossRef]
47. Soldatou, S.; Eldjárn, G.H.; Ramsey, A.; Van der Hooft, J.J.J.; Hughes, A.H.; Rogers, S.; Duncan, K.R. Comparative Metabologenomics Analysis of Polar Actinomycetes. *Marine Drugs* **2021**, *19*, 103. [CrossRef] [PubMed]
48. Eldjárn, G.H.; Ramsay, A.; Van der Hooft, J.J.J.; Duncan, K.R.; Soldatou, S.; Rousu, R.; Daly, R.; Wandy, J.; Rogers, S. Ranking microbial metabolomic and genomic links in the NPLinker framework using complementary scoring functions. *bioRxiv* **2020**. [CrossRef]
49. Männle, D.; McKinnie, S.M.K.; Mantri, S.S.; Steinke, K.; Lu, Z.; Moore, B.S.; Ziemert, N.; Kaysser, L. Comparative Genomics and Metabolomics in the Genus Nocardia. *mSystems* **2020**, *5*. [CrossRef]
50. Kautsar, S.A.; Blin, K.; Shaw, S.; Navarro-Muñoz, J.C.; Terlouw, B.R.; Van der Hooft, J.J.J.; Van Santen, J.A.; Tracanna, V.; Suarez Duran, H.G.; Pascal Andreu, V.; et al. MIBiG 2.0: A repository for biosynthetic gene clusters of known function. *Nucleic Acids Res.* **2020**, *48*, D454–D458. [CrossRef] [PubMed]
51. Schorn, M.A.; Verhoeven, S.; Ridder, L.; Huber, F.; Acharya, D.D.; Aksenov, A.A.; Aleti, G.; Amiri Moghaddam, J.; Aron, A.T.; Aziz, S.; et al. A community resource for paired genomic and metabolomic data mining. *Nat. Chem. Biol.* **2021**. [CrossRef]
52. Dejong, C.A.; Chen, G.M.; Li, H.; Johnston, C.W.; Edwards, M.R.; Rees, P.N.; Skinnider, M.A.; Webster, A.L.; Magarvey, N.A. Polyketide and nonribosomal peptide retro-biosynthesis and global gene cluster matching. *Nat. Chem. Biol.* **2016**, *12*, 1007–1014. [CrossRef] [PubMed]
53. Johnston, C.W.; Skinnider, M.A.; Wyatt, M.A.; Li, X.; Ranieri, M.R.; Yang, L.; Zechel, D.L.; Ma, B.; Magarvey, N.A. An automated Genomes-to-Natural Products platform (GNP) for the discovery of modular natural products. *Nat. Commun.* **2015**, *6*, 8421. [CrossRef] [PubMed]

54. Dührkop, K.; Nothias, L.F.; Fleischauer, M.; Reher, R.; Ludwig, M.; Hoffmann, M.A.; Petras, D.; Gerwick, W.H.; Rousu, J.; Dorrestein, P.C.; et al. Systematic classification of unknown metabolites using high-resolution fragmentation mass spectra. *Nat. Biotechnol.* **2020**. [CrossRef] [PubMed]
55. Tripathi, A.; Vázquez-Baeza, Y.; Gauglitz, J.M.; Wang, M.; Dührkop, K.; Nothias-Esposito, M.; Acharya, D.D.; Ernst, M.; Van der Hooft, J.J.J.; Zhu, Q.; et al. Chemically informed analyses of metabolomics mass spectrometry data with Qemistree. *Nat. Chem. Biol.* **2021**, *17*, 146–151. [CrossRef] [PubMed]
56. Reher, R.; Kim, H.W.; Zhang, C.; Mao, H.H.; Wang, M.; Nothias, L.F.; Caraballo-Rodriguez, A.M.; Glukhov, E.; Teke, B.; Leao, T.; et al. A Convolutional Neural Network-Based Approach for the Rapid Annotation of Molecularly Diverse Natural Products. *J. Am. Chem. Soc.* **2020**, *142*, 4114–4120. [CrossRef] [PubMed]
57. Danelius, E.; Halaby, S.; Van der Donk, W.A.; Gonen, T. MicroED in natural product and small molecule research. *Nat. Prod. Rep.* **2020**. [CrossRef]

marine drugs

Article

Comparative Metabologenomics Analysis of Polar Actinomycetes

Sylvia Soldatou [1,†], Grímur Hjörleifsson Eldjárn [2], Andrew Ramsay [2], Justin J. J. van der Hooft [3], Alison H. Hughes [1], Simon Rogers [2] and Katherine R. Duncan [1,*]

1 Strathclyde Institute of Pharmacy and Biomedical Sciences, University of Strathclyde, Glasgow G4 0RE, UK; s.soldatou@rgu.ac.uk (S.S.); a.hughes@strath.ac.uk (A.H.H.)
2 School of Computing Science, University of Glasgow, Glasgow G12 8RZ, UK; 2332462H@student.gla.ac.uk (G.H.E.); andrew.ramsay@glasgow.ac.uk (A.R.); Simon.Rogers@glasgow.ac.uk (S.R.)
3 Bioinformatics Group, Wageningen University, 6708 PB Wageningen, The Netherlands; justin.vanderhooft@wur.nl
* Correspondence: katherine.duncan@strath.ac.uk
† Current address: School of Pharmacy and Life Sciences, Robert Gordon University, Aberdeen AB10 7GJ, UK.

Abstract: Biosynthetic and chemical datasets are the two major pillars for microbial drug discovery in the *omics* era. Despite the advancement of analysis tools and platforms for multi-strain metabolomics and genomics, linking these information sources remains a considerable bottleneck in strain prioritisation and natural product discovery. In this study, molecular networking of the 100 metabolite extracts derived from applying the OSMAC approach to 25 Polar bacterial strains, showed growth media specificity and potential chemical novelty was suggested. Moreover, the metabolite extracts were screened for antibacterial activity and promising selective bioactivity against drug-persistent pathogens such as *Klebsiella pneumoniae* and *Acinetobacter baumannii* was observed. Genome sequencing data were combined with metabolomics experiments in the recently developed computational approach, NPLinker, which was used to link BGC and molecular features to prioritise strains for further investigation based on biosynthetic and chemical information. Herein, we putatively identified the known metabolites ectoine and chrloramphenicol which, through NPLinker, were linked to their associated BGCs. The metabologenomics approach followed in this study can potentially be applied to any large microbial datasets for accelerating the discovery of new (bioactive) specialised metabolites.

Keywords: Actinobacteria; marine; Polar; genomics; metabolomics; specialised metabolites

Citation: Soldatou, S.; Eldjárn, G.H.; Ramsay, A.; van der Hooft, J.J.J.; Hughes, A.H.; Rogers, S.; Duncan, K.R. Comparative Metabologenomics Analysis of Polar Actinomycetes. *Mar. Drugs* **2021**, *19*, 103. https://doi.org/10.3390/md19020103

Academic Editor: Max Crüsemann

Received: 21 January 2021
Accepted: 8 February 2021
Published: 10 February 2021

Publisher's Note: MDPI stays neutral with regard to jurisdictional claims in published maps and institutional affiliations.

1. Introduction

More than 80 years after the first reported case of sulphonamide-resistant bacterial strains [1], antibiotic resistance is now a global threat to human health, projected to cause 10 million deaths annually by 2050 [2,3]. Historically, microorganisms have been a source of over 22,000 biologically active metabolites, including antibiotics, isolated from terrestrial and marine strains [4]. In particular, the order Actinomycetales (actinomycetes) has been shown to produce structurally diverse specialised metabolites which exhibit a wide range of biological activities. Indeed, more than 7000 metabolites have been isolated from the genus *Streptomyces* and approximately 3000 metabolites from the "rare" (due to their lower isolation frequency) actinomycete genera [5]. Actinomycetes have an average genome size of over 5 Mb. However, this number varies greatly between genomes which can reach up to 12 Mb in some *Streptomyces* species [6]. Actinomycetes dedicate 0.8–3.0 Mb of their whole genome to specialised metabolite production, which has been shown to result in 20–50 Biosynthetic Gene Clusters (BGCs) per strain [7]. A recent study of 21 rare marine actinomycetes isolated from temperate and sub-tropic marine environments unveiled diverse and numerous BGCs, with *Actinomadura* spp. and *Nocardia* spp. containing 44 and 38 BGCs per strain, respectively. Interestingly, only three percent of the BGC families overlapped between the *Streptomyces* strains and the rare actinomycetes, suggesting an exciting resource for biosynthetic novelty [8]. Moreover, analysis of 119 genomes of the rare actinomycete genus *Salinispora* derived from various sub-tropic and tropic locations revealed 176 BGCs, of which only 24 were linked to their respective products [9], indicating a potential resource for novel metabolites.

Although actinomycetes from the (sub-)tropics have been extensively studied and shown to be a promising source of biological and chemical novelty, Actinobacteria isolated from Polar regions also show potential for affording new biologically active specialised metabolites. Actinobacteria accounted for 5% of the total microbial community present in Antarctic sediment samples as revealed by high-throughput 16S rRNA gene sequencing, with the *Salinibacterium* genus being amongst the most abundant [10]. In terms of isolating rare actinomycetes from Polar habitats, a study of ancient Antarctic and sub-Arctic sediment samples yielded 50 bacterial strains, of which 39 belonged to rare actinomycetes genera (*Microbacterium*, *Dietzia*, *Rhodococcus*, and *Pseudonocardia*) [11]. Regarding the chemical potential, molecular networking indicated rare actinomycetes from sub-Arctic and Antarctic sediments to be a rich source of metabolites [11,12]. Since 2001, a total of twenty-nine new metabolites have been isolated from Antarctic and sub-Arctic bacteria, with 13 being produced by marine actinomycetes [13]. For example, the rare actinomycete *Nocardia dassonvillei* BM-17 isolated from an Arctic sediment sample yielded a new phenazine derivative with significant antifungal and cytotoxic activity [14]. Two new α-pyrones were isolated from an Antarctic *Nocardiopsis* strain [15], whereas the seaweed-derived *Nocardiopsis* sp. 03N67 collected in the Arctic Ocean afforded a new diketopiperazine, cyclo-(L-Pro-L-Met), which showed promising anti-angiogenesis activity [16].

It is widely known that variations in cultivation parameters can induce the expression of so-called 'silent' BGCs, for which the biosynthetic enzymes have been identified but no natural product has been isolated from laboratory cultures [17]. Hence, changes in abiotic factors such as nutrient availability (carbon, nitrogen, trace-elements), temperature, salinity, and pH have been shown to influence the production of such 'cryptic' specialised metabolites. Moreover, the chemical profile of a microorganism can depend on the culture vessels, shaking conditions, and aeration, as well as on co-culturing techniques [18]. For example, when glucose was substituted for glycerol in the ISP2 growth medium, the liquid culture of *Streptomyces* sp. C34 isolated from the Atacama Desert, yielded ansamycin-type polyketides [19]. Furthermore, the marine-derived *Streptomyces* sp. CHQ-64 was found to produce new biologically active polyene-polyols and hybrid isoprenoid alkaloids when cultured under shaking, whereas static fermentation yielded only one new metabolite [20,21]. Therefore, the "One Strain Many Compounds" (OSMAC) approach [22] has been a successful addition in the microbial drug discovery pipeline

Mass spectrometry approaches are often used to compare multi-strain metabolomics. Molecular networking using the Global Natural Products Social Molecular Networking (GNPS) infrastructure [23] has been deemed a valuable tool in the discovery of new metabolites [24] as it provides rapid dereplication [25] and identification of unknown parent ions. Clarinoside, a new pentalogin from the plant *Mitracarpus scaber* Zucc [26], retimycin A, a non-ribosomal peptide from *Salinispora arenicola* [27], and deoxyphorbol ester derivatives from *Euphorbia dendroides* [28] are a few of the specialised metabolites discovered using MS-guided isolation based on the GNPS platform. Recently, further analysis tools have been implemented on the GNPS infrastructure, such as MS2LDA which provides fragmentation patterns of commonly co-occurring mass fragment peaks and/or neutral losses that often represent molecular substructures (Mass2Motifs) [29], and Network Annotation Propagation (NAP) [30] which improves in silico fragmentation of the input data. The MolNetEnhancer workflow was introduced to combine the outputs of the above-mentioned tools and add (putative) chemical class annotations to molecular families in the molecular network [31].

The sequencing of the first *Streptomyces* genome in 2002 [32] paved the way for the discovery of further microbial natural products based on genomic data. The continuous development of genome sequencing technology has led to a wealth of genomic data which has motivated the development of sophisticated mining tools that can augment the search and discovery of novel specialised metabolites [33,34]. Several of these [35] are publicly accessible, enabling thorough and targeted genome mining of complex bacterial genomes, including antiSMASH for the identification of secondary metabolites BGCs [36], ARTS for high-throughput screening of bacterial genomes in reference to antibiotic production [37], and BiG-SCAPE for clustering BGCs into Gene Cluster Families (GCFs) [38].

The linking of genome and metabolome mining outcomes to accelerate natural products discovery has shown great promise over the last decade, with several tools contributing to bridging the gap between BGCs and mass spectra [39]. Although the term "metabologenomics" was officially introduced in 2016 to describe correlations between BGCs and metabolites [40], research on this approach started earlier. A study of actinomycete strains in which their genomic data were linked with MS profiles, led to the identification of GCFs for the previously reported natural products desertomycins and oasamycins, for which the corresponding BGCs were unknown [41]. The authors were also able to isolate and characterise a new chlorinated metabolite, tambromycin, and correlate it with its BGC in 11 actinomycete strains using metabologenomics [40]. Another successful study used a combination of molecular networking and pattern-based genome mining approach from which arenicolide A was linked to an uncharacterised BGC (PKS28) and the new metabolite, retimycin A was identified, characterised and linked to the known NRPS40 pathway [27].

Herein, we introduce a novel unsupervised *-omics* integration method to link tandem mass spectrometry data to BGCs to accelerate the analysis of large microbial natural products datasets. NPlinker, a newly introduced software framework [42] was applied for the first time to bridge the large metabolomics and genomics datasets of marine Polar Actinobacteria. With the aid of the novel approach Rosetta, links between spectra and BGCs for chloramphenicol and ectoine were established. Molecular networking of the 100 metabolite extracts derived from applying the OSMAC approach, showed growth media specificity and potential chemical novelty was suggested. Moreover, the metabolite extracts were screened for antibacterial activity and promising selective bioactivity against drug-persistent pathogens such as *Klebsiella pneumoniae* and *Acinetobacter baumannii* was observed.

2. Results

2.1. Phylogenetic Analysis

Twenty-five strains, 14 Antarctic and 11 Arctic, were selected from a larger collection of Polar marine sediment bacteria mainly consisting of Actinobacteria [11], based on taxonomy, isolation location (depths ranging from 388 to 4730 m) and previously known metabolic profile of the strains. The selected strains belonged to seven rare actinomycete genera—*Pseudonocardia* (eight strains), *Micrococcus* (seven strains), *Rhodococcus* (three strains), *Microbacterium* (three strains), *Kocuria* (one strain), *Agrococcus* (one strain), *Dietzia* (one strain). This genus-level delineation was well supported with bootstrap values over 67% and all strains clade with their respective reference sequences. Additionally, one strain of the phylum Proteobacteria, belonging to the *Halomonas* genus, was included in the study (Figure 1, Table S1). In terms of core depth (Figure 1), the two *Agrococcus*, one *Kocuria* and the eight *Pseudonocardia* strains were only isolated from the deepest sediment cores at a depth greater than 4000 m, and the one *Halomonas* and the two *Microbacterium* strains were only isolated from core depths of 1000–4000 m, while no pattern was observed for the genera *Micrococcus* and *Rhodococcus*. Although these observations are interesting, larger strain numbers would be required to draw statistical conclusions.

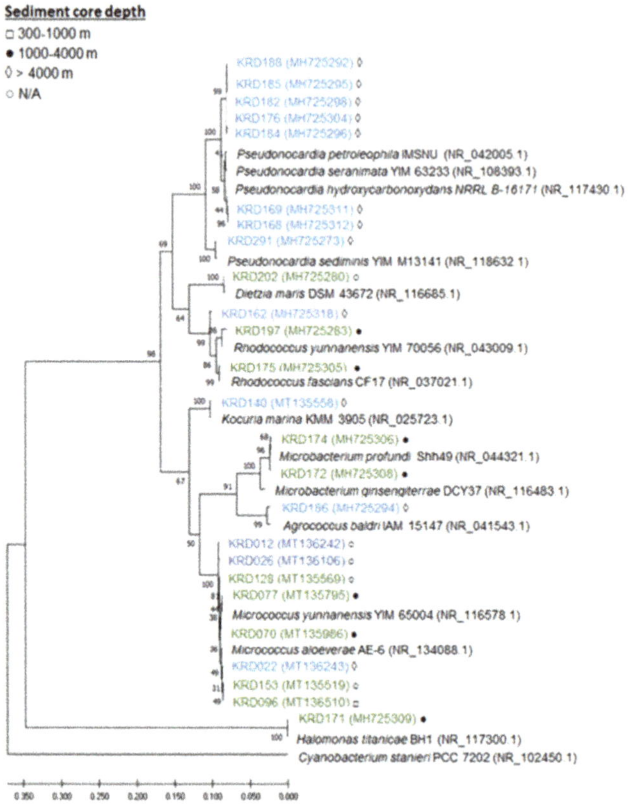

Figure 1. Maximum likelihood tree based on 16S rRNA gene sequences of 25 strains isolated from Antarctic (blue) and Arctic (green) sediment samples. Strain numbers are followed by a symbol indicating the depth at which the sediment samples were collected from: □ 300–1000 m, • 1000–4000 m, ◊ > 4000 m and ○ N/A (information missing). The accession number is shown in brackets following the strain name.

2.2. Genome Mining

Genome assembly was carried out using SPAdes and due to the large numbers of contigs obtained, MeDuSa was utilised for genome scaffolding, using reference strains with >95% similarity based on 16S rRNA sequencing data (Table S2). No reference strains with >95% sequence similarity could be identified for the *Pseudonocardia* strains; therefore, they were eliminated from genome mining to avoid possible discrepancies.

Genome mining of the seventeen Polar rare Actinobacteria and the Proteobacteria (*Pseudonocardia* strains excluded) revealed a total of 133 BGCs including NRPS, PKS, terpene and RiPP classes. Interestingly, 37% of the total BGCs showed no homology to any BGC within the MiBIG database and a further 30% suggested homology ranging from 2% to 63% to known antibiotics. The biosynthetic diversity per strain is shown in the Circos diagram (Figure 2). The width of the bands indicates the number of BGCs within each Natural Product (NP) class which, as expected, is positively correlated to genome size. The lowest number of BGCs was observed for small genomes such as the *Micrococcus* (2.4–2.7 Mbp) and *Agrococcus* (3.1 Mbp) both of which had five BGCs, whereas the three *Rhodococcus* strains (5.4–6.7 Mbp) revealed the largest number (17–22) of BGCs. Moreover, strains belonging to the same genus showed BGCs of the same NP class (Table S3). The ectoine pathway was observed in almost all genomes except the *Kocuria* (KRD140) and the *Microbacterium*

(KRD174) strains. A similar pattern was observed for the terpene BGC which was present in the genome of all Polar isolates except the *Halomonas* strain (KRD171) (Table S3). The most abundant NP class was NRPSs which were not evenly distributed among all strains, as the smaller genomes such as *Micrococcus* and *Microbacterium* did not show any NRPS BGCs, although at least one NRPS-like fragment was identified in their genomes. On the other hand, larger genomes such as the *Rhodococcus* strains revealed a high number of NRPS BGCs (up to 10). Identification of siderophores based on bioinformatic analysis can often be challenging as many siderophores are produced through NRPS pathways, thus antiSMASH identifies them as NRPS and not siderophores [8,43]. Indeed, antiSMASH identified two NRPS clusters in one *Halomonas* strain (KRD 171) and one *Rhodococcus* strain (KRD 197) that have 53% and 63% gene homology to the serobactin and heterobactin siderophore pathways, respectively. Only 10 BGCs belonging to the PKS family were observed, of these, five were identified as Type I PKS, one Type II PKS, three Type III PKS, and one heterocyst glycolipid synthase-like PKS (hgIE-KS).

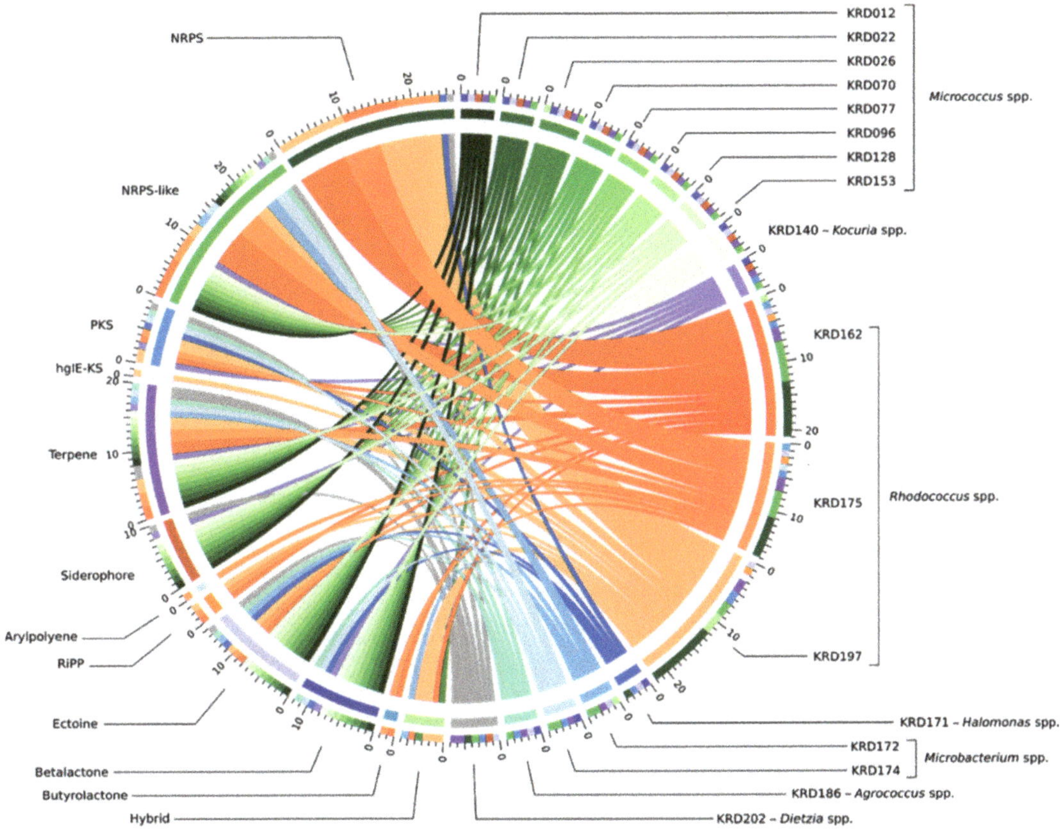

Figure 2. BGC diversity by NP class and strain taxonomy across 17 Polar strains. The band colour depicts taxonomy at the genus-level *Micrococcus* spp. (green), *Kocuria* sp. (purple), *Rhodococcus* spp. (orange), *Halomonas* sp. (dark blue), *Microbacterium* spp. (light blue), *Agrococcus* sp. (teal) and *Dietzia* sp. (grey). Each coloured band can be traced from the organism (right half of the circle) to the types of BGCs found in that genome (left half of the circle). The width of the band represents the number of BGCs of that NP class. The outer rings on the left of the diagram show the number of the BGC types found in each microbial genome. BGCs are colour coded based on the NP classification.

The BGCs of the 17 Polar strains were further analysed using BiG-SCAPE, which resulted in 80 GCFs, with 46% shown as singletons. As expected, there were BGCs present in strains belonging to the same genus, that clustered in the same GCF. For example, the ectoine BGCs present in the eight Micrococcus strains clustered in one GCF and the ectoine BGCs of the three *Rhodococcus* strains were represented as an additional GCF (green circles in Figure 3). The three *Rhodococcus* strains had a terpene BGC which showed low homology (6%) to SF2575 BGC from the soil-derived *Streptomyces* sp. SF2575 [44] (blue circle in Figure 3). Although the homology with the known biosynthetic pathway is low, the fact that it is shared by all three BGCs from the different *Rhodococcus* strains, implies that the strains may produce the same or similar metabolite(s) to the tetracycline antibiotic SF2575 [45]. Additionally, the three *Rhodococcus* strains (KRD12, KRD175, KRD197) showed an NRPS BGC that shows low homology (11%) to the chloramphenicol BGC from *Streptomyces venezuelae* ATCC 10712 [46]. Interestingly, only the gene clusters of KRD175 and KRD162 were grouped in the same family, whereas the corresponding BGC of KRD197 was shown as a singleton (red circles in Figure 3) even running BiG-SCAPE with a high cut off (0.7). Further investigation of the antiSMASH data showed that the predicted metabolites for the NRPS genes of interest could be cyclic lipopeptides, which often exhibit antibiotic properties [47].

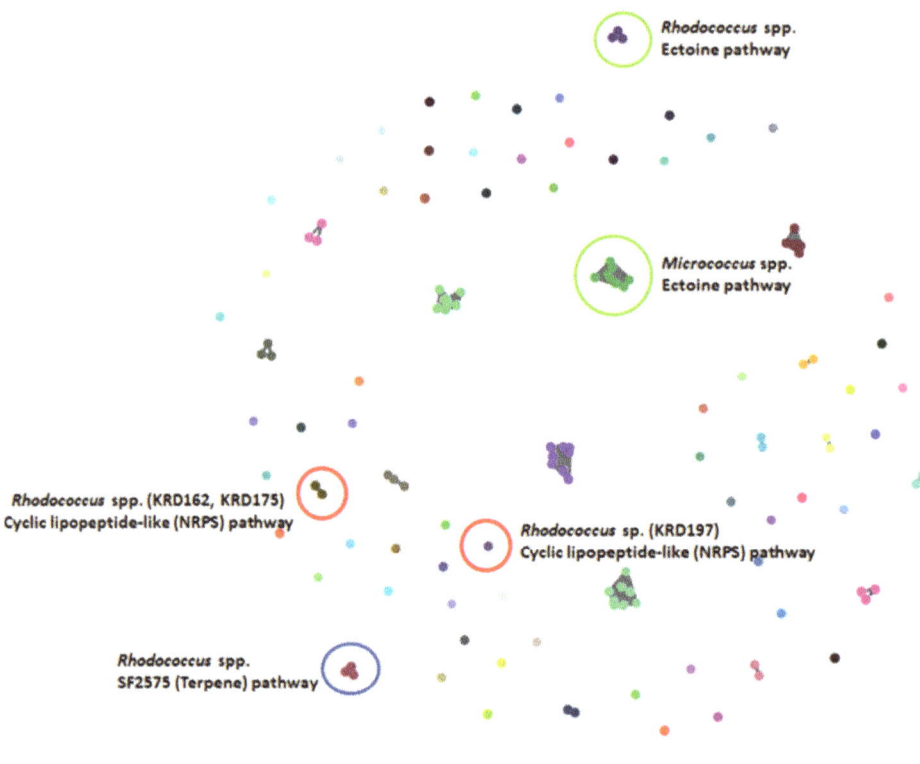

Figure 3. BiG-SCAPE analysis of 17 strains. The 133 BGCs; 53 NRPS/NRPS-like, 20 Terpene, 10 PKS, 3 RiPP and 47 others (including BGCs such as ectoine, siderophore, betalactone) were clustered in 80 GCFs. Examples of GCFs of interest are highlighted in coloured circles; red represents the *Rhodococcus* spp. NRPS BGC corresponding to a potentially new cyclic lipopeptide, green represents the ectoine pathway found in all strains (here highlighted for the *Micrococcus* and *Microbacterium* spp.) and blue the terpene BGC found in all three *Rhodococcus* strains with low homology to the known antibiotic SF2575.

2.3. Antibacterial Activity and Parent Ion Distribution

Culturing all strains in four growth media resulted in 100 metabolite extracts, of which 72% exhibited activity against six pathogenic bacteria (*Escherichia coli*, *Staphylococcus aureus*, *Klebsiella pneumoniae*, *Acinetobacter baumanii*, *Pseudomonas aeruginosa* and *Enterococcus faecalis*) known as the "ESKAPE" pathogens [48]. Specifically, 39% of the biologically active strains (28% of the total number) showed antibacterial activity against only one pathogen. The same percentage of active extracts inhibited the growth of one or more pathogens under only one cultivation condition. The inhibition zones ranged from 0.1 to 2.1 cm (Table S4). Most of the bacterial metabolite extracts were active against *S. aureus* with the *Pseudonocardia* strain KRD185 showing the largest inhibition zone (2.1 cm). Moreover, the 10-fold diluted TSB extract of strain KRD185 showed promising antibacterial activity against *K. pneumoniae* (0.9 cm) and *A. baumannii* (1.5 cm), whereas the A1M1 and 10-fold diluted TSB extracts of *Rhodococcus* strain KRD175 were selectively active against *K. pneumoniae* (Table S4). The occurrence of parent ions in relation to the bioactive extract is shown in Figure 4 where Hinton diagrams are illustrating the number of parent ions produced only by each strain (strain specific), as well as shared between two strains (Figure 4A). Strains belonging to the same genus shared the highest number of produced parent ions, which of course varies between the genera. For example, within the *Micrococcus* genus, strains KRD022 and KRD026 share the highest number of parent ions (649 in total), whereas strains KRD128 and KRD096 share only 287 parent ions. For the *Pseudonocardia* spp. isolates, there is a wide variation in the number of shared parent ions (163–632), where strain KRD176 shares 632 ions with KRD196 and only 163 with KRD291. Variations ranging from 104 to 649 shared parent ions also occurred between strains of different genera, as expected. The *Microbacterium* sp. strain KRD174 shared 104 and 123 parent ions with *Micrococcus* sp. KRD096 and *Pseudonocardia* sp. KRD291, respectively, representing the lowest number of shared ions. On the other hand, the *Rhodococcus* strain KRD175 showed the largest number of shared parent ions (649) with strain KRD022 of the *Micrococcus* genus. The sole *Kocuria* sp. isolate, KRD140, shared only 199 parent ions with *Pseudonocardia* strain KRD176, but shared more than 400 ions with three *Pseudonocardia* strains (KRD182, KRD185, KRD188). Amongst the *Pseudonocardia* strains, KRD182 showed the highest number of shared parent ions with *Micrococcus* spp. (356–607 parent ions), and *Rhodococcus* strains (465–612 parent ions). The Hinton diagram in Figure 4B demonstrates the number of parent ions produced by strains under each growth condition (white box), as well as the number of specific parent ions per strain grown under each growth condition (purple box) and the observed bioactivity (black outline). The 10-fold diluted TSB metabolite extract of KRD185 (*Pseudonocardia* sp.) had the highest bioactivity, with a zone of inhibition of 2.1 cm, and it produced the highest number of total (803) and unique (29) parent ions in that growth condition when compared to the rest of the studied isolates. Although the *Micrococcus* strain KRD022 produced the highest numbers of parent ions in ISP2 (819) and A1M1 (864) media, it did not exhibit any biological activity against the pathogenic bacteria. These two examples indicate that bioactivity is not necessarily related to the highest number of produced metabolites (parent ions).

2.4. Molecular Networking

A molecular network of all 100 microbial metabolite extracts (25 strains cultured in four media), in addition to the media and solvent blanks, consisted of 3107 parent ions (nodes). There were 721 nodes that were excluded from the data analysis as they corresponded to parent ions present in the media and solvent blanks. Of the total number of parent ions produced (i.e., not present in the blanks, 2386), 414 of these nodes were singletons indicating that their fragmentation pattern did not correlate with that of any other parent ion, suggesting chemical novelty within the dataset. After ions in the media controls were excluded, 23% (549) of ions were produced by strains grown in all four media. A further 65% (1551) of ions were produced in more than one medium (i.e., not media specific). Interestingly, the percentage of nodes which were media-specific was almost constant across ISP2 (8.3%), ISP3 (8.8%), and 10-fold diluted TSB (8.0%) media, whereas 6.3% of the produced ions were present in the metabolite extracts derived from A1M1 medium. The MolNetEnhancer workflow showed 38 (putative) chemical classes annotated in the molecular network (Figure 5B and Figure S2). Almost 71% of the produced ions did not match any chemical classification which implies chemical novelty and is in accordance with the low number of library hits generated by the GNPS molecular network. Fatty acyls, and benzene and substituted derivatives represented 4% and 5% of the produced ions, whereas prenol lipids covered 6% of the chemical classes identified in the network.

2.5. Computational Pattern Matching

A recently introduced software framework, NPLinker, was utilised to suggest links between spectra of interest and their corresponding GCFs and therefore BGCs [42]. Initially, analysis was carried out using the standardised strain correlation scoring method which yielded potential MF-GCF links based upon correlating strain presence and absence. This approach greatly narrowed the space of links requiring investigation. Further analysis of the suggested links based on biosynthetic knowledge allowed the BGCs to be identified that were likely to be most relevant to the metabolite of interest. Specifically, the GNPS infrastructure allows parent ion clustering into molecular families and comparison of observed spectra with GNPS embedded libraries. Simultaneously, BGCs were clustered into GCFs via BiG-SCAPE. The generated MFs and GCFs were then uploaded to NPLinker where potential MF-GCF links were ranked based on two scoring functions; standardised strain correlation scoring and the here introduced, novel approach named Rosetta scoring (Figure 6A).

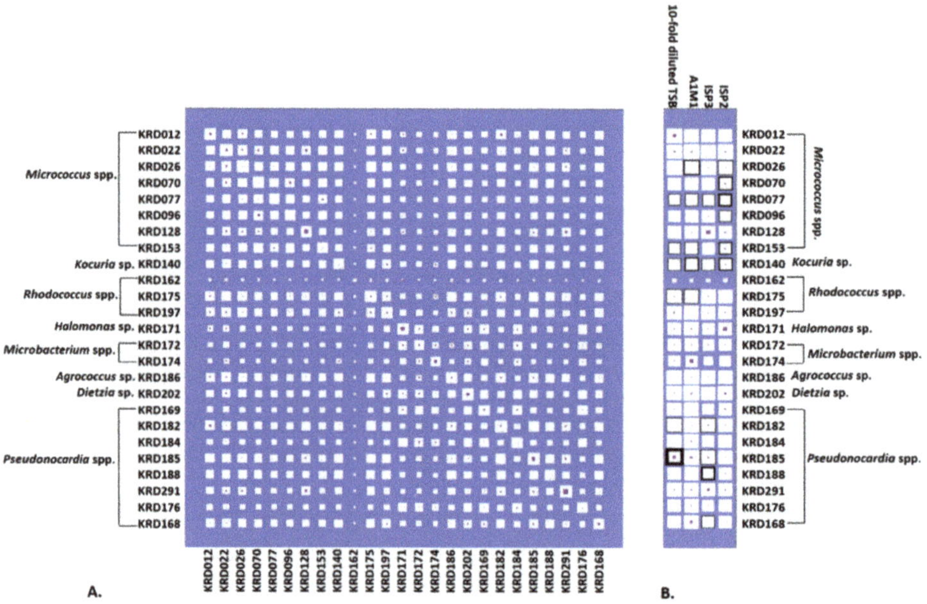

Figure 4. (A) Hinton diagram showing the number of parent ions (proportional to the size of white box) produced by each strain (max. 1041, min. 543 parent ions) and shared by each pair of strains (max. 670, min. 104 parent ions. Number of parent ions specific to that strain (or pair) are proportional to the size of the inner purple box. (B) Hinton diagram showing the number of parent ions by strain across each media (white box). Parent ions specific to only that strain-medium are also shown (purple box). The thickness of black box outline corresponds to the number of ESKAPE pathogens bioactivity was observed against (ranging from 1 to 6). For example, the bacterial metabolite extract for KRD185 in diluted TSB was found to be bioactive against all six pathogens, but no bioactivity was observed when the same strain was cultured in any of the other tested media.

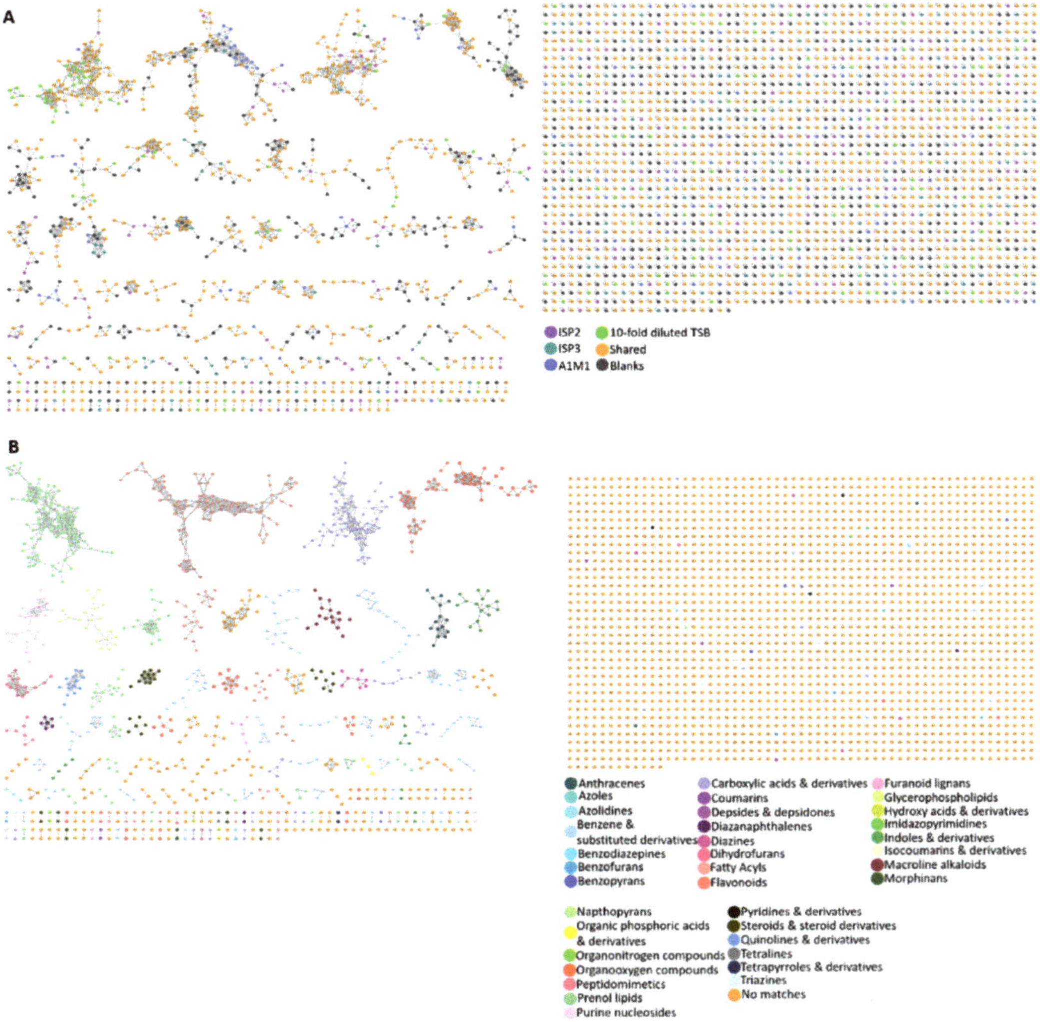

Figure 5. (**A**) Molecular network of 3107 parent ions produced by 25 strains cultured in four media and those found in media and solvent blanks. Nodes are colour coded based on media: ISP2, ISP3, A1M1 and 10-fold diluted TSB. Grey nodes represent media components, whereas orange nodes represent parent ions that are found in more than one different medium. (**B**) Nodes are colour coded based on 36 chemical class terms annotated using MolNetEnhancer workflow. Orange nodes represent parent ions that had no matches with any chemical class.

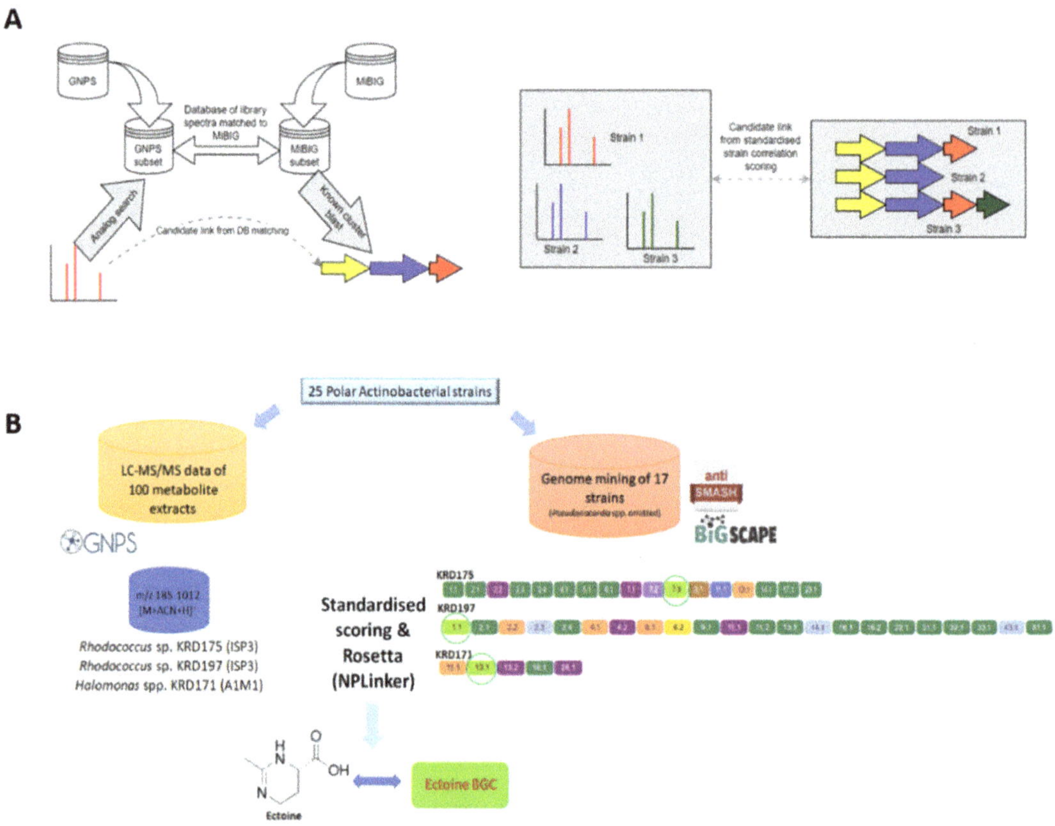

Figure 6. (**A**) Molecular families (MFs) are created through molecular networking using the GNPS infrastructure and parent ions of interest are identified through dereplication using GNPS embedded libraries and the Rosetta tool. Genome mining data (antiSMASH) of the Polar strains were clustered in GCFs using BiG-SCAPE. The GNPS (MFs) and BiG-SCAPE (GCFs) outputs are then analysed with NPLinker to rank potential MF-GCF links using two scoring functions (standardised strain correlation linking and Rosetta scoring). (**B**) The ectoine metabolite produced by two *Rhodococcus* spp. (KRD175 and KRD197) when cultured in ISP3 and one *Halomonas* sp. (KRD171) cultured in A1M1 was linked with its corresponding ectoine BGC via NPLinker.

2.5.1. Computational Pattern Matching Using the Standardised Strain Correlation Scoring Method

The parent ion (m/z 547.3815) produced by *Microbacterium* sp. KRD174 cultured in A1M1 showed spectral similarity to the GNPS spectrum CCMSLIB00000569369 suggesting it was an antimycin-related metabolite. Through NPLinker, it was shown that this metabolite could potentially be linked with the NRPS-like, betalactone, t3PKS and terpene BGCs (KRD174). Although the standardised strain correlation score for all links was high (2.7–4, with 4 being the maximum value observed in the dataset), when this information was combined with the fact that antimycins are produced by an NRPS/PKS hybrid [49], it was hypothesised that the betalactone and terpene BGCs were less likely to be involved in the biosynthesis of the metabolite of interest. Of course, further validation studies are required to confirm the responsible BGC. Similarly, another metabolite (m/z 521.3294) showed similarity with GNPS spectrum CCMSLIB00004710288 for conglobatin (MIBiG ID: BGC0001215), suggested that it could potentially be structurally related to the known macrolide conglobatin originally isolated from the antibiotic-producing *Streptomyces con-*

globatus [50]. The metabolite of interest was produced by two *Micrococcus* strains, KRR022 and KRD026 (diluted TSB medium), in addition to *Rhodococcus* sp. KRD175 (diluted TSB medium) and two *Pseudonocardia* strains KRD184 and KRD291 (ISP2 medium). Using the standardised strain correlation scoring method, the spectrum was potentially linked with 14 GCFs; two from *Micrococcus* sp. (KRD026) and 12 from *Rhodococcus* sp. (KRD175). However, the highest standardised strain correlation linking score (2.1) was observed for the hybrid BGC arylpolyene-NRPS (KRD026) as well as for the NRPS, NRPS-like, arylpolyene and butyrolactone BGCs (KRD175). Considering that conglobatin biosynthesis is governed by an NRPS/PKS BGC [51], the arylpolyene-NRPS BGCs are most likely to be involved in the biosynthesis, but further studies would be required to validate this. These examples demonstrate that using spectral library matches with the standardised scoring method included within NPLinker can narrow down possible MF-GCF links and thus enable a more focused downstream analysis.

2.5.2. Computational Pattern Matching Using Standardised Strain Correlation Scoring and the Rosetta Method

To further investigate the potential links between the genomics and metabolomics datasets of the Polar strains, an additional filter layer was added into NPLinker which allowed the use of the standardised strain correlation scoring method and the Rosetta hit list simultaneously. This approach led to linking spectrum ID 219769 (m/z 185.1012), putatively identified as ectoine ($[M + CAN + H]^+$ adduct), via Rosetta, with the ectoine BGC in two *Rhodococcus* sp. (KRD175, KRD197) and Halomonas sp. (KRD171) strains. Interestingly, when using only the standardised scoring the same spectrum was linked to 40 GCFs. However, applying the additional Rosetta scoring method narrowed it down to two GCFs (Figure 6B). Moreover, Rosetta identified that spectrum ID 111427 (m/z 380.2794) could be structurally related to the known antibiotic chloramphenicol, originally isolated from *Streptomyces venezuelae* [52]. The parent ion of interest was present in the metabolite extracts of *Rhodococcus* sp. KRD175 and *Micrococcus* sp. KRD128 and was linked with the NRPS BGC (KRD175) which showed homology to the chloramphenicol BGC. It is important to note that the Rosetta scoring approach is limited by the number of MiBIG BGCs for which experimental spectra are available. Due to the relatively low number of publicly available spectra of microbial metabolites [53], the combined filtering approach (standardised score and Rosetta) could only identify links for ectoine and chloramphenicol to their corresponding BGCs. It must be pointed out that the Rosetta hits were a result of matching single MS fragments to publicly available MS/MS datasets (Table S5), hence the aforementioned metabolites could be only putatively identified. However, this workflow clearly shows the promise of the implemented method for analysing large genomics and metabolomics datasets.

3. Discussion

Over the years, it has been shown that the Arctic and Antarctic marine environment host a vast variety of Actinobacteria with great potential for producing novel chemistry with a wide range of biological activities [11–13]. Bioprospecting for new specialised metabolites from Polar strains has greatly improved by the advancement of publicly available tools for untargeted metabolomics [23] and genome mining [54], which are continuously under development to meet the rapidly evolving field of microbial natural products discovery. One of the main challenges of genome mining is the quality of the genome assembly and annotation which can affect the outcome of the analysis [55,56]. A large number of contigs in the genome assembly can lead to BGCs, especially PKS-I and NRPS, to be broken across pieces and not being identified by available software and tools. A great example of such issue was demonstrated by Baltz who showed that draft genomes containing large NRPS/PKS-I genes were incorrectly assembled due to being largely fragmented which resulted in overestimation of such BGCs by antiSMASH 3.0 [57]. However, since then, new updated versions of antiSMASH have been released in which the location of the gene cluster close to the contig edge is flagged. Moreover, the need for closed genomes is of paramount importance for accurate and reliable genome mining. However, long-read technologies are often required to achieve this, which comes with greater expense and their own drawbacks such as high error frequencies and reliability [58]. A recent study of nine Actinobacterial species, including three *Pseudonocardia* strains used short-read (Illumina MiSeq) and long-read (Oxford Nanopore MinION) sequencing technologies to analyse BGC fragmentation. The authors found that the MinION-based genome assemblies increased the sensitivity related to BGC annotation and reduced the number of fragmented BGCs. [56]. In this present study we omitted the *Pseudonocardia* strains from the genomic analysis due to lack of reference strains for genome scaffolding. Genome mining of the 17 non-*Pseudonocardia* strains revealed a wide diversity of BGCs with most of them having low homology to known BGCs which suggests biosynthetic and chemical novelty. Terpene BGCs were present in almost every genome, which was not surprising as recent studies have revealed a wide distribution of terpene synthases in bacteria which has led to the development of a new hidden Markov model for terpene synthases identification in bacterial genomes [58,59]. As expected, the number and variety of BGCs increased for larger genome sizes such as the *Rhodococcus* strains. However, it was unexpected to notice that smaller genomes such as *Micrococcus*, *Halomonas* and *Kocuria* were lacking PKS and NRPS BGCs as actinomycetes are known to produce metabolites encoded by those pathways [60,61]. A similar observation was made by Schorn et al. when studying rare marine actinomycetes [8]. Although small genomes might not look as promising from a natural products discovery perspective, it does not necessarily mean that they are not worth further investigation. The sponge-associated *Micrococcus* sp. was reported to produce a new antibacterial xanthone named microluside A [62] and marine *Halomonas* strains have yielded new antibacterial and cytotoxic metabolites named loihichelins A−F and aminophenoxazinones, respectively [63,64].

To further explore and investigate the observed BGCs in our Polar strains, analysis showed the ectoine BGC present in all genomes; this is known to be ubiquitous as the metabolite aids survival under extreme osmotic stress [65]. Moreover, the terpene BGC with high homology (66%) to a known carotenoid BGC was present in all *Micrococcus* strains and clustered in the same GCF. Carotenoids are terpenoids produced by all photosynthetic organisms and some non-phototrophic organisms, and have several applications as food colorants, feed supplements, nutraceuticals, and pharmaceuticals [66]. Terpene BGCs with homology (>37%) to the isorenieratene BGC were observed in the *Rhodococcus* strains and were clustered in the same GCF. Actinobacteria, and particularly *Streptomyces* spp., often bear isorenieratene BGCs in their genome that are usually silent, and there have been only a few cases in which these BGCs have been activated [67,68]. Furthermore, the genomic data of the three strains belonging to the genus *Rhodococcus* suggest the presence of NRPS BGCs which could potentially encode for cyclic lipopeptides. Such metabolites are of great importance in drug discovery with the example of daptomycin, originally isolated from the soil-derived *Streptomyces roseosporus* [69], which has been approved by the FDA as an antibacterial agent against Gram positive pathogens [70].

For over 30% of the BGCs within our dataset, the most similar known cluster encoded for an antibiotic. Of this, almost half showed low homology (<10%) with known BGCs. This is an exciting finding suggesting that the rare actinomycete strains derived from Polar marine sediments can potentially be a fruitful source of novel chemistry. It is worth noting that extracting metabolites from culture broth in organic solvents was proven to be a more effective and reliable method to assess biological activity (disc diffusion assay) than an agar plug assay [71]. Although genome mining of the *Rhodococcus* spp. showed promising potential for producing metabolites, the bioassay data did not fully support this. As only strain KRD175 exhibited moderate but selective activity against *K. pneumoniae*. This could be because the BGCs encoding for antibiotics remained silent or the biologically active compounds were produced in low amounts that were not sufficient to inhibit the growth of the pathogens. Moreover, the bacterial metabolite extracts mostly inhibited the growth of *S. aureus*, whereas only a few showed inhibitory effects against *K. pneumoniae* and *A.*

baumannii, which are two of the most drug-persistent pathogenic bacteria [72,73]. To the best of our knowledge, there are only a few published reports on the inhibitory effects of microbial specialised metabolites on *A. baumannii* [74–76] but none on *K. pneumoniae*; and therefore, the Polar strains with such activity show promise to combat these pathogens.

Linking genomic and metabolomics datasets of actinomycete strains for specialised metabolite discovery has been introduced only recently [41]. However, there is increased interest in the scientific community to further explore this niche research field by generating automated methods for correlating these complex datasets and ranking promising MF-GCF links for further investigation. Targeted linking and automated approaches for accelerating drug discovery have been reviewed [39,53]. Recently, metabolomic and genomic data of 72 isolates belonging to the rare actinomycete genus *Planomonospora* were analysed using publicly available tools to link specialised metabolites to their corresponding BGCs [77]. The authors were able to manually pair siomycin congeners to a RiPP BGC and a new salinichelin-like metabolite to the known BGC encoding for erythrochelin. In the present study, the newly developed software, NPLinker, was used to link our experimental datasets and prioritise strains for further chemical and biosynthetic investigation. The filtering approaches that were implemented (standardised strain correlation score and Rosetta) established links for ectoine and chloramphenicol to their corresponding BGCs but were not yet sufficient to link the potentially new identified metabolites (antimycins-like and conglobatin-like compounds) to GCFs as publicly available spectra of microbial metabolites are almost non-existent and remain mostly hidden in supplemental figures in literature. Van Santen et al. [78], among others, discussed the need for data sharing within the scientific community which will allow the field of natural products to catch up with data-centric approaches used in other research fields and further flourish. It is worth pointing out that limiting number of Rosetta hits obtained within this metabolomics dataset is indicative of the potential novel chemistry of the Polar strains which is further supported by the large number of nodes that could not be annotated to specific chemical classes. However, our findings agree with a recent literature review which reported only 29 new metabolites isolated from Antarctic and Arctic bacteria, of which 13 have been discovered from marine actinomycetes [13]. A future direction for NPLinker could be the integration of bioassay data along with metabolomics and genomics datasets, as previously suggested by others [79], which will give the opportunity to users to explore possible MF-GCF links based on bioactivity and target the BGCs and therefore the metabolite(s) responsible for the biological effect.

4. Materials and Methods

4.1. Phylogenetic Analysis

Twenty-four rare actinomycete strains and a marine strain of the phylum *Proteobacteria* (Table S1) were previously isolated and taxonomically identified (through 16S rRNA gene sequencing) from the Antarctic and sub-Arctic sediment core collection from two separate studies in conjunction with the Scottish Association for Marine Sciences [11,12]. These strains were selected based on taxonomy and isolation location. Using the 16S rRNA gene sequences, a maximum likelihood (ML) phylogenetic tree was constructed (Kimura 2-parameter model, 1000 bootstraps) using Mega 7 (v 7.0.26) (https://www.megasoftware.net/ (accessed on 9 November 2020)) [80,81] with visualisation and annotation using FigTree (v 1.4.3) (http://tree.bio.ed.ac.uk/software/figtree (accessed on 9 November 2020)). The GenBank accession numbers for the 16S rRNA gene sequences are the following: MT135519 (KRD153), MT135569 (KRD128), MT135795 (KR077), MT135986 (KRD070), MT136106 (KRD026), MT136242 (KRD012), MT136243 (KRD022), MT136510 (KRD096). The remaining strains were deposited in GenBank as mentioned in [11].

4.2. Fermentation and Metabolite Extraction

All twenty-five strains were pre-cultured (5 mL, 28 °C, 160 rpm for 7 days) in ISP2 medium [82], ISP3 medium [82] A1M1 medium [27] and 10-fold diluted TSB medium

(BD™) prepared in distilled water. Instant ocean (18 g/L) was added in each of them. Each culture [ISP2/ISP3/A1M1/10-fold dil. TSB medium (50 mL) with activated HP-20 resin (Sigma) (2.5 g)] was inoculated (5% *v*/*v* pre-culture) and fermented (14 days, 28 °C, 160 rpm). The culture was then centrifuged (4000 rpm, 20 min), the supernatant removed, and the cell/resin pellet lyophilised until dry (Thermo Savant MicroModulyo, Thermo Fisher Scientific, Waltham, MA, USA). The lyophilised cell/resin pellet was extracted twice with ethyl acetate (Fisher Scientific, Loughborough, UK, reagent grade) (20 mL, 100 rpm, 25 °C). The extracts were combined, dried (under N_2), the weight recorded and stored (4 °C).

4.3. Bioactivity Disc Diffusion Assay

Cultures in TSB (BD™) were prepared for *Escherichia coli*, *Staphylococcus aureus*, *Klebsiella pneumoniae*, *Acinetobacter baumanii*, and *Pseudomonas aeruginosa*, whereas cultures in LB [peptone 10 g/L, yeast extract 5g/L, sodium chloride 5 g/L] (5 mL, 30 °C, 1200 rpm, 12 h) were prepared for *Enterococcus faecalis*. Nutrient agar (NA, 5 mL, ThermoFisher Scientific) was inoculated with 0.1 mg/mL of the pathogen and was poured onto NA Petri plates (10 mL). The ethyl acetate metabolite extracts were re-dissolved in ethyl acetate at a concentration of 5 mg/mL and 20 µL was added onto each sterile disc (5 mm). The plates were incubated overnight at 30 °C and the zones of inhibition were recorded (cm).

4.4. Bioactivity Agar Plug Assay

The 25 Polar strains were cultured in ISP2, ISP3, 10-fold diluted TSA and A1M1 media in 6-well plates (38 mm diameter/3 mL of media) until a uniform lawn was formed (25 °C, 7–14 days). Cultures in TSB (BD™) and LB [peptone 10 g/L, yeast extract 5g/L, NaCl 5 g/L] (5 mL, 30 °C, 1200 rpm, 12 h) were prepared for *Escherichia coli*, *Staphylococcus aureus*, *Klebsiella pneumoniae*, *Acinetobacter baumanii*, *Pseudomonas aeruginosa* and *Enterococcus faecalis*, respectively. NA (5 mL, Thermo Fisher Scientific) was inoculated with 0.1 mg/mL of the pathogen and poured onto NA (10 mL). Plugs (8 mm) from each bacterial lawn (grown for 14 days) were placed on the seeded pathogen plates and incubated overnight at 30 °C and the zones of inhibition were measured (cm).

4.5. Mass Spectral Data Acquisition

LC–MS/MS was performed using a Thermo Scientific Accela LC system coupled to a Thermo Finnigan LTQ Orbitrap mass spectrometer with an ESI source. Bacterial metabolite extracts and control media extracts (no bacteria) were prepared at 1 mg/mL in ACN and were injected onto an ACE 5 (Hichrom) C18 column (5 µm, 75 × 3.0 mm) using the following gradient: 1–5 min (5% ACN in H_2O), 5–25 min (5–100% ACN), 25–30 min (100% ACN). Mass data were collected in positive ion mode using ESI and mass range 150–1500 m/z (15,000 resolution). Data-dependent MS2 scans were obtained using collision-induced dissociation (CID) with an energy of 35 eV and activation time of 30,000 ms for the first, second, and third most intense peaks.

4.6. Mass Spectral Data Processing

Mass spectral data were processed using MZmine v2.38 freeware (http://mzmine.sourceforge.net/ (accessed on 9 November 2020)) for peak detection, deconvolution, deisotoping, filtering, alignment and gap filling to make multiple data files comparable. Throughout the data processing, the m/z tolerance used was 0.01, peaks were detected above 3.00E3 and the minimum time span and tR tolerance was 0.1 min. Mass detection was performed using a centroid mass detector with a noise level set at 2.00×10^3.

4.7. Molecular Networking

The MS/MS data were converted from raw to mzXML file format using Proteowizard MSConvert [83] and the data were uploaded to the GNPS server [23]. A molecular network was created with the feature-based molecular networking workflow on the GNPS website (http://gnps.ucsd.edu (accessed on 9 November 2020)). The data were filtered by removing all MS/MS fragment ions within +/−17 Da of the precursor m/z. MS/MS spectra were window filtered by choosing only the top 6 fragment ions in the +/−150 Da window throughout the spectrum. The precursor ion mass tolerance was set to 0.2 Da and a MS/MS fragment ion tolerance of 0.2 Da. A network was then created where edges were filtered to have a cosine score above 0.6 and at least 1 matched peak. Further, edges between two nodes were kept in the network if and only if each of the nodes appeared in each other's respective top 10 most similar nodes. Finally, the maximum size of a molecular family was set to 100, and the lowest scoring edges were removed from molecular families until the molecular family size was below this threshold. The spectra in the network were then searched against GNPS' spectral libraries. The library spectra were filtered in the same manner as the input data. All matches kept between network spectra and library spectra were required to have a score above 0.6 and at least 1 matched peak (https://gnps.ucsd.edu/ProteoSAFe/status.jsp?task=124de327f32f474291a5037f41ac991d (accessed on 9 November 2020)). For molecular network visualisation, Cytoscape version 3.6.1 was utilised [84] where each node corresponds to a consensus spectrum and each edge represents a modified cosine similarity score between nodes. The data used for the molecular networking analysis were deposited in the MassIVE Public GNPS database under access number MSV000086584.

4.8. MolNetEnhancer Workflow Description for Chemical Class Annotation of Molecular Networks

To enhance chemical structural information within the molecular network, information from in silico structure annotations from GNPS Library Search and Network Annotation Propagation (NAP) were incorporated into the network using the GNPS MolNetEnhancer workflow (https://ccms-ucsd.github.io/GNPSDocumentation/molnetenhancer/ (accessed on 9 November 2020)) on the GNPS website [31]. Chemical class annotations were performed using the ClassyFire chemical ontology [85]. (https://gnps.ucsd.edu/ProteoSAFe/status.jsp?task=adbadc0707e7449dbe4de1562ecd7bd3 (accessed on 9 November 2020)).

4.9. Genomic DNA Extraction

All 25 Polar strains were cultured in ISP2 medium (5 mL, 30 °C, 200 rpm for 3 days). High quality genomic DNA was isolated using an in-house protocol based on chemical cell lysis followed by phenol/chloroform extraction [86]. The *Pseudonocardia* sp. strains underwent cell lysis by vigorous vortexing (10 min) of the bacterial cultures with zirconium oxide beads (~0.5 g) (Sigma-Aldrich Ltd., Dorset, UK). The purity and concentration of the obtained genomic DNA was determined using a Nanodrop 2000 spectrophotometer (Thermo Fisher Scientific) followed by measurements on Qubit 2.0 Fluorometer (Invitrogen, Thermo Fisher Scientific, Waltham, MA, USA).

4.10. Genome Sequencing and Alignment

Whole-genome sequencing was carried out by Microbes NG (https://microbesng.com/ (accessed on 9 November 2020)) as follows: Genomic DNA libraries were prepared using Nextera XT Library Prep Kit (Illumina, San Diego, CA, USA) following the manufacturer's protocol with the following modifications: two nanograms of DNA instead of one were used as input, and PCR elongation time was increased to 1 min from 30 s. DNA quantification and library preparation were carried out on a Hamilton Microlab STAR automated liquid handling system. Pooled libraries were quantified using the Kapa Biosystems Library Quantification Kit for Illumina on a Roche light cycler 96 qPCR machine. Libraries were sequenced on the Illumina HiSeq using a 250 bp paired-end protocol. Reads were adapter trimmed using Trimmomatic 0.30 with a sliding window quality cut off of Q15 [87]. The closest available reference genome was identified using Kraken [88] the reads were mapped with BWA mem for assessing the quality of the data. De novo assembly of the reads was carried out utilising SPAdes [89]. MeDuSa [90] was utilised for genome scaffolding, using reference strains with >95% similarity based on 16S rRNA sequencing data. The

Pseudonocardia isolates were not analysed by MeDuSa as no reference strains were identified. The whole genome sequences for the polar strains have been deposited to GenBank with the following accession numbers: SAMN14679891-SAMN14679907 (Table S2).

4.11. Biosynthetic Gene Cluster Mining and Comparison

The identification of BGCs was carried out using antiSMASH 5 beta [91]. The variety and number of BGCs each Polar strain was visualised using the Circos diagram [92]. The detected BGCs were grouped into Gene Cluster Families (GCF) using BiG-SCAPE 1.0 beta (Navarro-Munoz et al. 2019), with the underlying assumption that similar BGCs, i.e., BGCs that belong to the same GCF, produce similar metabolites. BiG-SCAPE was run using Longest Common Subcluster alignment mode, and cluster analysis carried out at the default cutoff of 0.3.

4.12. Computational Pattern Matching

Computational prioritisation of links between BGCs and candidate products made use of two complementary approaches. Firstly, the standardised strain correlation score described in [42] was used to compute a score between each spectrum and each GCF. The original strain correlation score introduced in [41] is heavily influenced by the number of strains present in each spectrum or GCF making the ranking of links between spectra and a particular GCF problematic. The standardised score overcomes this limitation, permitting a more balanced ranking of spectra for each GCF independent of their size. Significance values for each link were computed as described in [42]. Secondly, a novel approach named Rosetta (code available here: https://github.com/sdrogers/nplinker/tree/master/prototype/rosetta_data_prep (accessed on 9 November 2020)) based upon a set of collated matches between the GNPS [23] library spectra and the MiBIG database of characterised BGCs allows for putative links between individual spectra and BGCs to be highlighted. The set consists of 2960 links, 2069 unique spectra, 249 unique MIBiG IDs. To establish this set of collated links, the structural annotations available for both databases were used. A pair of objects from the two datasets were matched if the first blocks of the InChIKeys of the molecules in the GNPS library spectra and MiBIG validated gene cluster products matched. Matching was restricted to the first block to avoid distinguishing between molecules based on chemical properties that would not show up in the MS/MS spectra (e.g., stereochemistry). With this set of collated links, observed spectra and BGCs were putatively matched as follows: spectral similarity between measured MS2 spectra and the relevant subset of the GNPS spectra was computed using the modified cosine score (equivalent to "Analog search" in the GNPS framework). Results from antiSMASH were parsed to extract the known cluster blast results and Rosetta links between spectra and BGCs were generated where the spectra showed similarity to the GNPS spectrum and the MiBIG entry was found in the known cluster blast record for the BGC. All analysis was performed with the NPLinker framework [42] in which potential can be reported using either one of these two scoring methods, or both simultaneously, with user-defined thresholds.

Supplementary Materials: The following are available online at https://www.mdpi.com/1660-3397/19/2/103/s1, Figure S1: Molecular network of 3107 parent ions produced by 25 Polar actinomycete strains. Nodes are colour coded based on genus: *Agrococcus*, *Dietzia*, *Halomonas*, *Kocuria*, *Microbacterium*, *Micrococcus*, *Pseudonocardia* and *Rhodococcus*. Grey nodes represent media components, whereas orange nodes represent parent ions that are produced by more than one different medium. Figure S2: Pie chart showing the distribution of parent ions (%) between the 36 chemical class terms shown in the legend as annotated by MolNetEnhancer. The percentage of parent ions with no chemical class match (70.5%) is not shown in the pie chart Each class has been colour coded to match the molecular network generated through MolNetEnhancer workflow analysis (Figure 5B). Table S1: Isolation and collection data of the 25 polar bacteria. Table S2: Genome quality of the Polar strains (*Pseudonocardia* strains were not analysed by MeDuSa as no reference strains were available). Table S3: Identified BGCs using antiSMASH 5 clusters after genome scaffolding using MeDuSa.

Table S4: Bioactive bacterial extracts organised by genus, strain name (KRD) and growth medium ISP3, A1M1, ISP2, and 10-fold dil. TSB. Antibiotic activity against the clinical pathogens *E. faecalis*, *S. aureus*, *K. pneumoniae*, *A. baumannii*, *P. aeruginosa* and *E. coli* is shown as zones of inhibition (cm) and colour coded by inhibition zone size. Table S5: Putatively identified metabolites using the Rosetta approach.

Author Contributions: Conceptualisation, K.R.D. and S.R.; methodology, S.S., G.H.E., S.R., and K.R.D.; formal analysis, S.S., G.H.E., S.R., and K.R.D.; investigation, S.S., G.H.E., A.H.H., S.R., and K.R.D.; writing—original draft preparation, S.S., G.H.E., S.R., and K.R.D.; writing—review and editing, S.S., G.H.E., A.R., J.J.J.v.d.H., A.H.H., S.R., and K.R.D.; supervision, K.R.D. and S.R.; project administration, K.R.D. and S.R. funding acquisition, K.R.D. and S.R. All authors have read and agreed to the published version of the manuscript.

Funding: This research was funded by Carnegie Trust Collaborative Research Grant (KRD, SR, SS). AR, KRD and SR were supported by the Biotechnology and Biological Sciences Research Council (BB/R022054/1). Additionally, genome sequencing was provided by MicrobesNG (http://www.microbesng.uk (accessed on 21 January 2021)) which was supported by the Biotechnology and Biological Sciences Research Council (BB/L024209/1).

Data Availability Statement: The code for Rosetta is available at https://github.com/sdrogers/nplinker/tree/master/prototype/rosetta_data_prep (accessed on 21 January 2021). The genomes have been deposited to GenBank with the following accession numbers: SAMN14679891-SAMN14679907 (Table S2). The GenBank accession numbers for the 16S rRNA gene sequences are the following: MT135519 (KRD153), MT135569 (KRD128), MT135795 (KR077), MT135986 (KRD070), MT136106 (KRD026), MT136242 (KRD012), MT136243 (KRD022), and MT136510 (KRD096) (Figure 1). The LC–MS data are available at the MassIVE dataset under access number MSV000086584.

Conflicts of Interest: The authors declare no conflict of interest.

References

1. Davies, J.; Davies, D. Origins and Evolution of Antibiotic Resistance. *Microbiol. Mol. Biol. Rev.* **2010**, *74*, 417–433. [CrossRef]
2. O' Neil, J. *Review on Antibiotic Resisitance. Antimicrobial Resistance: Tackling a Crisis for the Health and Wealth of Nations*; The Wellcome Trust and the UK Department of Health: London, UK, 2014.
3. O' Neill, J. *Tackling Drug-Resistant Infections Globally: Final Report and Recommendations*; The Wellcome Trust and the UK Department of Health: London, UK, 2016.
4. Jackson, S.A.; Crossman, L.; Almeida, E.L.; Margassery, L.M.; Kennedy, J.; Dobson, A.D.W. Diverse and Abundant Secondary Metabolism Biosynthetic Gene Clusters in the Genomes of Marine Sponge Derived *Streptomyces* spp. *Isolates. Mar. Drugs* **2018**, *16*, 67. [CrossRef]
5. Baltz, R.H. Renaissance in Antibacterial Discovery from Actinomycetes. *Curr. Opin. Pharmacol.* **2008**, *8*, 557–563. [CrossRef] [PubMed]
6. Lewin, G.R.; Carlos, C.; Chevrette, M.G.; Horn, H.A.; McDonald, B.R.; Stankey, R.J.; Fox, B.G.; Currie, C.R. Evolution and Ecology of Actinobacteria and Their Bioenergy Applications. *Annu. Rev. Microbiol.* **2016**, *70*, 235–254. [CrossRef] [PubMed]
7. Baltz, R.H. Gifted Microbes for Genome Mining and Natural Product Discovery. *J. Ind. Microbiol. Biotechnol.* **2017**, *44*, 573–588. [CrossRef] [PubMed]
8. Schorn, M.A.; Alanjary, M.M.; Aguinaldo, K.; Korobeynikov, A.; Podell, S.; Patin, N.; Lincecum, T.; Jensen, P.R.; Ziemert, N.; Moore, B.S. Sequencing Rare Marine Actinomycete Genomes Reveals High Density of Unique Natural Product Biosynthetic Gene Clusters. *Microbiology* **2016**, *162*, 2075–2086. [CrossRef] [PubMed]
9. Letzel, A.-C.; Natalie, M.-A.; Amos, G.C.; Millán-Aguiñaga, N.; Ginigini, J.; Abdelmohsen, U.R.; Gaudêncio, S.P.; Ziemert, N.; Moore, B.S.; Jensen, P.R. Genomic Insights into Specialized Metabolism in the Marine *Actinomycete salinispora*. *Environ. Microbiol.* **2017**, *19*, 3660–3673. [CrossRef] [PubMed]
10. Li, A.-Z.; Han, X.-B.; Zhang, M.-X.; Zhou, Y.; Chen, M.; Yao, Q.; Zhu, H.-H. Culture-Dependent and -Independent Analyses Reveal the Diversity, Structure, and Assembly Mechanism of Benthic Bacterial Community in the Ross Sea, Antarctica. *Front. Microbiol.* **2019**, *10*, 2523. [CrossRef]
11. Millán-Aguiñaga, N.; Soldatou, S.; Brozio, S.; Munnoch, J.T.; Howe, J.A.; Hoskisson, P.A.; Duncan, K.R. Awakening Ancient Polar Actinobacteria: Diversity, Evolution and Specialized Metabolite Potential. *Microbiology* **2019**, *165*, 1169–1180. [CrossRef] [PubMed]
12. Purves, K.; Macintyre, L.; Brennan, D.; Hreggviðsson, G.; Kuttner, E.; Ásgeirsdóttir, M.E.; Young, L.C.; Green, D.H.; Edrada-Ebel, R.; Duncan, K.R. Using Molecular Networking for Microbial Secondary Metabolite Bioprospecting. *Metabolites* **2016**, *6*, 2. [CrossRef]
13. Tian, Y.; Taglialatela-Scafati, O.; Zhao, F. Secondary Metabolites from Polar Organisms. *Mar. Drugs* **2017**, *15*, 28. [CrossRef]

14. Gao, X.; Lu, Y.; Xing, Y.; Ma, Y.; Lu, J.; Bao, W.; Wang, Y.; Xi, T. A Novel Anticancer and Antifungus Phenazine Derivative from a Marine Actinomycete BM-17. *Microbiol. Res.* **2012**, *167*, 616–622. [CrossRef] [PubMed]
15. Zhang, H.; Saurav, K.; Yu, Z.; Mándi, A.; Kurtán, T.; Li, J.; Tian, X.; Zhang, Q.; Zhang, W.; Zhang, C. α-Pyrones with Diverse Hydroxy Substitutions from Three Marine-Derived Nocardiopsis Strains. *J. Nat. Prod.* **2016**, *79*, 1610–1618. [CrossRef] [PubMed]
16. Shin, H.J.; Mondol, M.M.; Yu, T.K.; Lee, H.-S.; Lee, Y.-J.; Jung, H.J.; Kim, J.H.; Kwon, H.J. An Angiogenesis Inhibitor Isolated from a Marine-Derived Actinomycete, *Nocardiopsis sp.* 03N67. *Phytochem. Lett.* **2010**, *3*, 194–197. [CrossRef]
17. Hoskisson, P.A.; Seipke, R.F. Cryptic or Silent? The Known Unknowns, Unknown Knowns, and Unknown Unknowns of Secondary Metabolism. *mBio* **2020**, *11*, 02642–20. [CrossRef]
18. Romano, S.; Jackson, S.A.; Patry, S.; Dobson, A.D.W. Extending the "One Strain Many Compounds" (Osmac) Principle to Marine Microorganisms. *Mar. Drugs* **2018**, *16*, 244. [CrossRef]
19. Rateb, M.E.; Houssen, W.E.; Harrison, W.T.A.; Deng, H.; Okoro, C.K.; Asenjo, J.A.; Andrews, B.A.; Bull, A.T.; Goodfellow, M.; Ebel, R.; et al. Diverse Metabolic Profiles of aStreptomycesStrain Isolated from a Hyper-Arid Environment. *J. Nat. Prod.* **2011**, *74*, 1965–1971. [CrossRef] [PubMed]
20. Che, Q.; Li, J.; Li, D.; Gu, Q.; Zhu, T. Structure and Absolute Configuration of Drimentine I, an Alkaloid from *Streptomyces* sp. CHQ-64. *J. Antibiot.* **2016**, *69*, 467–469. [CrossRef]
21. Che, Q.; Zhu, T.; Qi, X.; Mándi, A.; Kurtán, T.; Mo, X.; Li, J.; Gu, Q.; Li, D. Hybrid Isoprenoids from a Reeds Rhizosphere Soil Derived Actinomycete *Streptomyces* sp. CHQ-64. *Org. Lett.* **2012**, *14*, 3438–3441. [CrossRef]
22. Bode, H.B.; Bethe, B.; Höfs, R.; Zeeck, A. Big Effects from Small Changes: Possible Ways to Explore Nature's Chemical Diversity. *ChemBioChem* **2002**, *3*, 619–627. [CrossRef]
23. Wang, M.; Carver, J.J.; Phelan, V.V.; Sanchez, L.M.; Garg, N.; Peng, Y.; Nguyen, D.D.; Watrous, J.; Kapono, C.A.; Luzzatto-Knaan, T.; et al. Sharing and Community Curation of Mass Spectrometry Data with Global Natural Products Social Molecular Networking. *Nat. Biotechnol.* **2016**, *34*, 828–837. [CrossRef]
24. Quinn, R.A.; Nothias, L.F.; Vining, O.; Meehan, M.; Esquenazi, E.; Dorrestein, P.C. Molecular Networking As a Drug Discovery, Drug Metabolism, and Precision Medicine Strategy. *Trends Pharmacol. Sci.* **2017**, *38*, 143–154. [CrossRef] [PubMed]
25. Yang, J.Y.; Sanchez, L.M.; Rath, C.M.; Liu, X.; Boudreau, P.D.; Bruns, N.; Glukhov, E.; Wodtke, A.; De Felicio, R.; Fenner, A.; et al. Molecular Networking as a Dereplication Strategy. *J. Nat. Prod.* **2013**, *76*, 1686–1699. [CrossRef]
26. Audoin, C.; Zampalégré, A.; Blanchet, N.; Giuliani, A.; Roulland, E.; Laprévote, O.; Genta-Jouve, G. MS/MS-Guided Isolation of Clarinoside, a New Anti-Inflammatory Pentalogin Derivative. *Molecules* **2018**, *23*, 1237. [CrossRef] [PubMed]
27. Duncan, K.R.; Crüsemann, M.; Lechner, A.; Sarkar, A.; Li, J.; Ziemert, N.; Wang, M.; Bandeira, N.; Moore, B.S.; Dorrestein, P.C.; et al. Molecular Networking and Pattern-Based Genome Mining Improves Discovery of Biosynthetic Gene Clusters and their Products from Salinispora Species. *Chem. Biol.* **2015**, *22*, 460–471. [CrossRef] [PubMed]
28. Nothias, L.-F.; Nothias-Esposito, M.; Da Silva, R.; Wang, M.; Protsyuk, I.; Zhang, Z.; Sarvepalli, A.; Leyssen, P.; Touboul, D.; Costa, J.; et al. Bioactivity-Based Molecular Networking for the Discovery of Drug Leads in Natural Product Bioassay-Guided Fractionation. *J. Nat. Prod.* **2018**, *81*, 758–767. [CrossRef]
29. Hooft, V.D.J.J.J.; Wandy, J.; Barrett, M.P.; Burgess, K.E.V.; Rogers, S. Topic Modeling for Untargeted Substructure Exploration in Metabolomics. *Proc. Natl. Acad. Sci.USA* **2016**, *113*, 13738–13743. [CrossRef]
30. Marchisio, M.A. In Silico Implementation of Synthetic Gene Networks BT-Synthetic Gene Networks: Methods and Protocols. *Methods Mol. Biol.* **2012**, *813*, 3–21.
31. Ernst, M.; Bin Kang, K.; Caraballo-Rodríguez, A.M.; Nothias, L.-F.; Wandy, J.; Chen, C.; Wang, M.; Rogers, S.; Medema, M.H.; Dorrestein, P.C.; et al. MolNetEnhancer: Enhanced Molecular Networks by Integrating Metabolome Mining and Annotation Tools. *Metabolites* **2019**, *9*, 144. [CrossRef]
32. Bentley, S.D.; Chater, K.F.; Cerdeño-Tárraga, A.-M.; Challis, G.L.; Thomson, N.R.; James, K.D.; Harris, D.E.; Quail, M.; Kieser, H.M.; Harper, D.P.; et al. Complete Genome Sequence of the Model Actinomycete Streptomyces Coelicolor A3(2). *Nat. Cell Biol.* **2002**, *417*, 141–147. [CrossRef]
33. Machado, H.; Tuttle, R.N.; Jensen, P.R. Omics-Based Natural Product Discovery and the Lexicon of Genome Mining. *Curr. Opin. Microbiol.* **2017**, *39*, 136–142. [CrossRef] [PubMed]
34. Ziemert, N.; Alanjary, M.; Weber, T. The Evolution of Genome Mining in Microbes—A Review. *Nat. Prod. Rep.* **2016**, *33*, 988–1005. [CrossRef] [PubMed]
35. Medema, M.H.; Fischbach, M.A. Computational Approaches to Natural Product Discovery. *Nat. Chem. Biol.* **2015**, *11*, 639–648. [CrossRef] [PubMed]
36. Blin, K.; Medema, M.H.; Kottmann, R.; Lee, S.Y.; Weber, T. The AntiSMASH Database, a Comprehensive Database of MI-Crobial Secondary Metabolite Biosynthetic Gene Clusters. *Nucleic Acids Res.* **2017**, *45*, D555–D559. [CrossRef] [PubMed]
37. Alanjary, M.; Kronmiller, B.; Adamek, M.; Blin, K.; Weber, T.; Huson, D.H.; Philmus, B.; Ziemert, N. The Antibiotic Resistant Target Seeker (ARTS), An Exploration Engine for Antibiotic Cluster Prioritization and Novel Drug Target Discovery. *Nucleic Acids Res.* **2017**, *45*, W42–W48. [CrossRef]
38. Navarro-Muñoz, J.C.; Selem-Mojica, N.; Mullowney, M.W.; Kautsar, S.A.; Tryon, J.H.; Parkinson, E.I.; Santos, E.L.C.D.L.; Yeong, M.; Cruz-Morales, P.; Abubucker, S.; et al. A Computational Framework to Explore Large-Scale Biosynthetic Diversity. *Nat. Chem. Biol.* **2020**, *16*, 60–68. [CrossRef]

39. Soldatou, S.; Eldjarn, G.H.; Huerta-Uribe, A.; Rogers, S.; Duncan, K.R. Linking Biosynthetic and Chemical Space to Accelerate Microbial Secondary Metabolite Discovery. *FEMS Microbiol. Lett.* **2019**, *366*, 142. [CrossRef]
40. Goering, A.W.; McClure, R.A.; Doroghazi, J.R.; Albright, J.C.; Haverland, N.A.; Zhang, Y.; Ju, K.S.; Thomson, R.J.; Metcalf, W.W.; Kelleher, N.L. Metabologenomics: Correlation of Microbial Gene Clusters with Metabolites Drives Discovery of a Non-Ribosomal Peptide with an Unusual Amino Acid Monomer. *ACS Cent. Sci.* **2016**, *2*, 99–108. [CrossRef]
41. Doroghazi, J.R.; Albright, J.C.; Goering, A.W.; Ju, K.S.; Haines, R.R.; Tchalukov, K.A.; Labeda, D.P.; Kelleher, N.L.; Metcalf, W.W. Aroadmap for Natural Product Discovery Based on Large-Scale Genomics and Metabolomics. *Nat. Chem. Biol.* **2014**, *10*, 963–968. [CrossRef]
42. Eldjárn, G.H.; Ramsay, A.; van der Hooft, J.J.J.; Duncan, K.R.; Soldatou, S.; Rousu, J.; Daly, R.; Wandy, J.; Rogers, S. Ranking Microbial Metabolomic and Genomic Links in the NPLinker Framework Using Complementary Scoring Functions. *bioRxiv* **2020**. [CrossRef]
43. Fenical, W.; Jensen, P.R. Developing a New Resource for Drug Discovery: Marine Actinomycete Bacteria. *Nat. Chem. Biol.* **2006**, *2*, 666–673. [CrossRef] [PubMed]
44. Pickens, L.B.; Kim, W.; Wang, P.; Zhou, H.; Watanabe, K.; Gomi, S.; Tang, Y. Biochemical Analysis of the Biosynthetic Pathway of an Anticancer Tetracycline SF2575. *J. Am. Chem. Soc.* **2009**, *131*, 17677–17689. [CrossRef] [PubMed]
45. Hatsu, M.; Sasaki, T.; Watabe, H.-O.; Miyadoh, S.; Nagasawa, M.; Shomura, T.; Sezaki, M.; Inouye, S.; Kondo, S. A New Tetracycline Antibiotic with Antitumor Activity. I. Taxonomy and Fermentation of the Producing Strain, Isolation and Characterization of SF2575. *J. Antibiot.* **1992**, *45*, 320–324. [CrossRef] [PubMed]
46. Fernández-Martínez, L.T.; Borsetto, C.; Gomez-Escribano, J.P.; Bibb, M.J.; Al-Bassam, M.M.; Chandra, G.; Bibb, M. New Insights into Chloramphenicol Biosynthesis in Streptomyces venezuelae ATCC 10712. *Antimicrob. Agents Chemother.* **2014**, *58*, 7441–7450. [CrossRef]
47. Kleijn, L.H.J.; Martin, N.I. The Cyclic Lipopeptide Antibiotics. In *Antibacterials. Topics in Medicinal Chemistry*; Fisher, J.F., Mobashery, S., Miller, M.J., Eds.; Springer International Publishing: Cham, Switzerland, 2018; pp. 27–53. ISBN 978-3-319-70839-3.
48. Rice, L.B. Federal Funding for the Study of Antimicrobial Resistance in Nosocomial Pathogens: No ESKAPE. *J. Infect. Dis.* **2008**, *197*, 1079–1081. [CrossRef] [PubMed]
49. Yan, Y.; Zhang, L.; Ito, T.; Qu, X.; Asakawa, Y.; Awakawa, T.; Abe, I.; Liu, W. Biosynthetic Pathway for High Structural Diversity of a Common Dilactone Core in Antimycin Production. *Org. Lett.* **2012**, *14*, 4142–4145. [CrossRef]
50. Westley, J.W.; Liu, C.-M.; Evans, R.H.; Blount, J.F. Conglobatin, a Novel Macrolide Dilactone from *Streptomyces conglobatus* ATCC 31005. *J. Antibiot.* **1979**, *32*, 874–877. [CrossRef]
51. Zhou, Y.; Murphy, A.C.; Samborskyy, M.; Prediger, P.; Dias, L.C.; Leadlay, P.F. Iterative Mechanism of Macrodiolide Formation in the Anticancer Compound Conglobatin. *Chem. Biol.* **2015**, *22*, 745–754. [CrossRef] [PubMed]
52. Rebstock, M.C.; Crooks, H.M.; Controulis, J.; Bartz, Q.R. Chloramphenicol (Chloromycetin).1IV.1aChemical Studies. *J. Am. Chem. Soc.* **1949**, *71*, 2458–2462. [CrossRef]
53. Van Der Hooft, J.J.J.; Mohimani, H.; Bauermeister, A.; Dorrestein, P.C.; Duncan, K.R.; Medema, M.H. Linking Genomics and Metabolomics to Chart Specialized Metabolic Diversity. *Chem. Soc. Rev.* **2020**, *49*, 3297–3314. [CrossRef]
54. Medema, M.H.; Blin, K.; Cimermancic, P.; De Jager, V.; Zakrzewski, P.; Fischbach, M.A.; Weber, T.; Takano, E.; Breitling, R. antiSMASH: Rapid Identification, Annotation and Analysis of Secondary Metabolite Biosynthesis Gene Clusters in Bacterial and Fungal GE-Nome Sequences. *Nucleic Acids Res.* **2011**, *39*, W339–W346. [CrossRef]
55. Klassen, J.L.; Currie, C.R. Gene Fragmentation in Bacterial Draft Genomes: Extent, Consequences and Mitigation. *BMC Genom.* **2012**, *13*, 14. [CrossRef] [PubMed]
56. Goldstein, S.; Beka, L.; Graf, J.; Klassen, J.L. Evaluation of Strategies for the Assembly of Diverse Bacterial Genomes Using Minion Long-Read Sequencing. *BMC Genom.* **2019**, *20*, 23. [CrossRef] [PubMed]
57. Baltz, R.H. Molecular Beacons to Identify Gifted Microbes for Genome Mining. *J. Antibiot.* **2017**, *70*, 639–646. [CrossRef] [PubMed]
58. Smits, T.H.M. The Importance of Genome Sequence Quality to Microbial Comparative Genomics. *BMC Genom.* **2019**, *20*, 1–4. [CrossRef]
59. Yamada, Y.; Kuzuyama, T.; Komatsu, M.; Shin-ya, K.; Omura, S.; Cane, D.E.; Ikeda, H. Terpene Synthases Are Widely Dis-Tributed in Bacteria. *Proc. Natl. Acad. Sci. USA* **2015**, *112*, 857–862. [CrossRef]
60. Blodgett, J.A.V.; Oh, D.-C.; Cao, S.; Currie, C.R.; Kolter, R.; Clardy, J. Common Biosynthetic Origins for Polycyclic Tetramate Macrolactams from Phylogenetically Diverse Bacteria. *Proc. Natl. Acad. Sci. USA* **2010**, *107*, 11692–11697. [CrossRef]
61. Li, S.; Li, Y.; Lu, C.; Zhang, J.; Zhu, J.; Wang, H.; Shen, Y. Activating a Cryptic Ansamycin Biosynthetic Gene Cluster To Produce Three New Naphthalenic Octaketide Ansamycins with n-Pentyl and n-Butyl Side Chains. *Org. Lett.* **2015**, *17*, 3706–3709. [CrossRef]
62. Eltamany, E.E.; Abdelmohsen, U.R.; Ibrahim, A.K.; Hassanean, H.A.; Hentschel, U.; Ahmed, S.A. New Antibacterial Xan-Thone from the Marine Sponge-Derived *Micrococcus sp.* EG45. *Bioorg. Med. Chem. Lett.* **2014**, *24*, 4939–4942. [CrossRef]
63. Homann, V.V.; Sandy, M.; Tincu, J.A.; Templeton, A.S.; Tebo, B.M.; Butler, A. Loihichelins A−F, a Suite of Amphiphilic Siderophores Produced by the Marine *Bacterium Halomonas* LOB-5. *J. Nat. Prod.* **2009**, *72*, 884–888. [CrossRef]
64. Bitzer, J.; Grosse, T.; Wang, L.; Lang, S.; Beil, W.; Zeeck, A. New Aminophenoxazinones from a Marine *Halomonas sp.*: Fermentation, Structure Elucidation, and Biological Activity. *J. Antibiot.* **2006**, *59*, 86–92. [CrossRef] [PubMed]

65. Czech, L.; Hermann, L.; Stöveken, N.; Richter, A.A.; Höppner, A.; Smits, S.H.J.; Heider, J.; Bremer, E. Role of the Extremolytes Ectoine and Hydroxyectoine as Stress Protectants and Nutrients: Genetics, Phylogenomics, Biochemistry, and Structural Analysis. *Genes* **2018**, *9*, 177. [CrossRef] [PubMed]
66. Schweiggert, R.; Carle, R. Carotenoid Deposition in Plant And Animal Foods and Its Impact on Bioavailability. *Crit. Rev. Food Sci. Nutr.* **2015**, *57*. [CrossRef] [PubMed]
67. Iftime, D.; Kulik, A.; Härtner, T.; Rohrer, S.; Niedermeyer, T.H.J.; Stegmann, E.; Weber, T.; Wohlleben, W. Identification and Activation of Novel Biosynthetic Gene Clusters by Genome Mining in the Kirromycin Producer *Streptomyces collinus* Tü 365. *J. Ind. Microbiol. Biotechnol.* **2016**, *43*, 277–291. [CrossRef]
68. Myronovskyi, M.; Tokovenko, B.; Brötz, E.; Rückert, C.; Kalinowski, J.; Luzhetskyy, A. Genome Rearrangements of Streptomyces Albus J1074 Lead to the Carotenoid Gene Cluster Activation. *Appl. Microbiol. Biotechnol.* **2014**, *98*, 795–806. [CrossRef]
69. Debono, M.; Barnhart, M.; Carrell, C.B.; Hoffmann, J.A.; Occolowitz, J.L.; Abbott, B.J.; Fukuda, D.S.; Hamill, R.L.; Biemann, K.; Herlihy, W.C. A21978C, A Complex of New Acidic Peptide Antibiotics. Isolation, Chemistry, and Mass Spectral Structure Elucidation. *J. Antibiot.* **1987**, *40*, 761–777. [CrossRef]
70. Kosmidis, C.; Levine, D.P. Daptomycin: Pharmacology and Clinical Use. *Expert Opin. Pharmacother.* **2010**, *11*, 615–625. [CrossRef]
71. Balouiri, M.; Sadiki, M.; Ibnsouda, S.K. Methods for in Vitro Evaluating Antimicrobial Activity: A Review. *J. Pharm. Anal.* **2016**, *6*, 71–79. [CrossRef]
72. Paczosa, M.K.; Mecsas, J. *Klebsiella pneumoniae*: Going on the Offense with a Strong Defense. *Microbiol. Mol. Biol. Rev.* **2016**, *80*, 629–661. [CrossRef]
73. Chapartegui-González, I.; Lázaro-Díez, M.; Bravo, Z.; Navas, J.; Icardo, J.M.; Ramos-Vivas, J. Acinetobacter Baumannii Maintains Its Virulence after Long-Time Starvation. *PLoS ONE* **2018**, *13*, e0201961. [CrossRef]
74. Liaw, C.-C.; Chen, P.-C.; Shih, C.-J.; Tseng, S.-P.; Lai, Y.-M.; Hsu, C.-H.; Dorrestein, P.C.; Yang, Y. Vitroprocines, New Antibiotics against Acinetobacter Baumannii, Discovered from Marine Vibrio SP. QWI-06 Using Mass-Spectrometry-Based Metabolomics Approach. *Sci. Rep.* **2015**, *5*, 12856. [CrossRef]
75. Vila-Farres, X.; Chu, J.; Ternei, M.A.; Lemetre, C.; Park, S.; Perlin, D.S.; Brady, S.F. An Optimized Synthetic-Bioinformatic Natural Product Antibiotic Sterilizes Multidrug-Resistant Acinetobacter baumannii-Infected Wounds. *mSphere* **2018**, *3*, e00528-17. [CrossRef]
76. Wu, W.-S.; Cheng, W.-C.; Cheng, T.-J.R.; Wong, C.-H. Affinity-Based Screen for Inhibitors of Bacterial Transglycosylase. *J. Am. Chem. Soc.* **2018**, *140*, 2752–2755. [CrossRef]
77. Zdouc, M.M.; Iorio, M.; Maffioli, S.I.; Crüsemann, M.; Donadio, S.; Sosio, M. Planomonospora: A Metabolomics Perspective on an Underexplored Actinobacteria Genus. *J. Nat. Prod.* **2021**. [CrossRef] [PubMed]
78. Van Santen, J.A.; Kautsar, S.A.; Medema, M.H.; Linington, R.G. Microbial Natural Product Databases: Moving Forward in the Multiomics Era. *Nat. Prod. Rep.* **2021**, *38*, 264–278. [CrossRef] [PubMed]
79. Kurita, K.L.; Glassey, E.; Linington, R.G. Integration of High-Content Screening and Untargeted Metabolomics for ComPre-hensive Functional Annotation of Natural Product Libraries. *Proc. Natl. Acad. Sci. USA* **2015**, *112*, 11999–12004. [CrossRef]
80. Kimura, M. A Simple Method for Estimating Evolutionary Rates of Base Substitutions through Comparative Studies of Nucle-Otide Sequences. *J. Mol. Evol.* **1980**, *16*, 111–120. [CrossRef] [PubMed]
81. Kumar, S.; Stecher, G.; Tamura, K. MEGA7: Molecular Evolutionary Genetics Analysis Version 7.0 for Bigger Datasets. *Mol. Biol. Evol.* **2016**, *33*, 1870–1874. [CrossRef]
82. Shirling, E.B.; Gottlieb, D. Methods for Characterization of Streptomyces Species. *Int. J. Syst. Bacteriol.* **1966**, *16*, 313–340. [CrossRef]
83. Adusumilli, R.; Mallick, P. Data Conversion with Proteo Wizard msConvert. In *Proteomics*; Springer: Berlin/Heidelberg, Germany, 2017; pp. 339–368.
84. Cline, M.S.; Smoot, M.; Cerami, E.; Kuchinsky, A.; Landys, N.; Workman, C.; Christmas, R.; Avila-Campilo, I.; Creech, M.; Gross, B.; et al. Integration of Biological Networks and Gene Expression Data Using Cytoscape. *Nat. Protoc.* **2007**, *2*, 2366–2382. [CrossRef]
85. Djoumbou Feunang, Y.; Eisner, R.; Knox, C.; Chepelev, L.; Hastings, J.; Owen, G.; Fahy, E.; Steinbeck, C.; Subramanian, S.; Bolton, E.; et al. Classyfire: Automated Chemical Classification with a Comprehensive, Computable Taxonomy. *J. Cheminform.* **2016**, *8*, 61. [CrossRef]
86. Sambrook, J.; Maniatis, T.; Fritsch, E.F. *Molecular Cloning: A Laboratory Manual*, 2nd ed.; Cold Spring Harbor Laboratory Press: New York, NY, USA, 1989.
87. Bolger, A.M.; Lohse, M.; Usadel, B. Trimmomatic: A Flexible Trimmer for Illumina Sequence Data. *Bioinformatics* **2014**, *30*, 2114–2120. [CrossRef]
88. Wood, E.; Salzberg, D.E.; Kraken, S.L. Ultrafast Metagenomic Sequence Classification Using Exact Alignments. *Genome Biol.* **2014**, *15*, R46. [CrossRef] [PubMed]
89. Bankevich, A.; Nurk, S.; Antipov, D.; Gurevich, A.A.; Dvorkin, M.; Kulikov, A.S.; Lesin, V.M.; Nikolenko, S.I.; Pham, S.; Prjibelski, A.D.; et al. SPAdes: A New Genome Assembly Algorithm and Its Applications to Single-Cell Sequencing. *J. Comput. Biol.* **2012**, *19*, 455–477. [CrossRef] [PubMed]
90. Bosi, E.; Donati, B.; Galardini, M.; Brunetti, S.; Sagot, M.-F.; Lió, P.; Crescenzi, P.; Fani, R.; Fondi, M. MeDuSa: A Multi-Draft Based Scaffolder. *Bioinformatics* **2015**, *31*, 2443–2451. [CrossRef]

91. Blin, K.; Shaw, S.; Steinke, K.; Villebro, R.; Ziemert, N.; Lee, S.Y.; Medema, M.H.; Weber, T. antiSMASH 5.0: Updates to the Secondary Metabolite Genome Mining Pipeline. *Nucleic Acids Res.* **2019**, *47*, W81–W87. [CrossRef] [PubMed]
92. Krzywinski, M.; Schein, J.; Birol, I.; Connors, J.; Gascoyne, R.; Horsman, D.; Jones, S.J.; Marra, M.A. Circos: An Information Aesthetic for Comparative Genomics. *Genome Res.* **2009**, *19*, 1639–1645. [CrossRef] [PubMed]

marine drugs

MDPI

Article

Mining Indonesian Microbial Biodiversity for Novel Natural Compounds by a Combined Genome Mining and Molecular Networking Approach

Ira Handayani [1,2,†], Hamada Saad [3,4,†], Shanti Ratnakomala [5], Puspita Lisdiyanti [2], Wien Kusharyoto [2], Janina Krause [1], Andreas Kulik [1], Wolfgang Wohlleben [1], Saefuddin Aziz [3], Harald Gross [3], Athina Gavriilidou [6], Nadine Ziemert [6,7] and Yvonne Mast [1,7,8,9,*]

1 Department of Microbiology/Biotechnology, Interfaculty Institute of Microbiology and Infection Medicine, Tübingen (IMIT), Cluster of Excellence 'Controlling Microbes to Fight Infections', University of Tübingen, Auf der Morgenstelle 28, 72076 Tübingen, Germany; irahndyn@gmail.com (I.H.); Janina.Krause-d1j@rub.de (J.K.); andreas.kulik@uni-tuebingen.de (A.K.); wolfgang.wohlleben@biotech.uni-tuebingen.de (W.W.)
2 Research Center for Biotechnology, Indonesian Institute of Sciences (LIPI), Jl. Raya Jakarta-Bogor KM.46, Cibinong, West Java 16911, Indonesia; puspita.lisdiyanti@bioteknologi.lipi.go.id (P.L.); wien.kyoto@gmail.com (W.K.)
3 Department of Pharmaceutical Biology, Institute of Pharmaceutical Sciences, University of Tübingen, Auf der Morgenstelle 8, 72076 Tübingen, Germany; Hamada.saad@pharm.uni-tuebingen.de (H.S.); azizgene@gmail.com (S.A.); harald.gross@uni-tuebingen.de (H.G.)
4 Department of Phytochemistry and Plant Systematics, Division of Pharmaceutical Industries, National Research Centre, Dokki, Cairo 12622, Egypt
5 Research Center for Biology, Indonesian Institute of Sciences (LIPI), Jl. Raya Jakarta-Bogor KM.46, Cibinong, West Java 16911, Indonesia; shanti_ratna01@yahoo.com
6 Applied Natural Products Genome Mining, Interfaculty Institute of Microbiology and Infection Medicine Tübingen (IMIT), Cluster of Excellence 'Controlling Microbes to Fight Infections', University of Tübingen, Auf der Morgenstelle 28, 72076 Tübingen, Germany; athina.gavriilidou@uni-tuebingen.de (A.G.); nadine.ziemert@uni-tuebingen.de (N.Z.)
7 German Center for Infection Research (DZIF), Partner Site Tübingen, 72076 Tübingen, Germany
8 Department of Bioresources for Bioeconomy and Health Research, Leibniz Institute DSMZ-German Collection of Microorganisms and Cell Cultures, Inhoffenstraße 7B, 38124 Braunschweig, Germany
9 Department of Microbiology, Technical University of Braunschweig, 38124 Braunschweig, Germany
* Correspondence: yvonne.mast@dsmz.de; Tel.: +49-531-2616-358
† Ira Handayani and Hamada Saad contributed equally to this work.

Citation: Handayani, I.; Saad, H.; Ratnakomala, S.; Lisdiyanti, P.; Kusharyoto, W.; Krause, J.; Kulik, A.; Wohlleben, W.; Aziz, S.; Gross, H.; et al. Mining Indonesian Microbial Biodiversity for Novel Natural Compounds by a Combined Genome Mining and Molecular Networking Approach. *Mar. Drugs* **2021**, *19*, 316. https://doi.org/10.3390/md19060316

Academic Editors: Ipek Kurtboke, Orazio Taglialatela-Scafati and Max Crüsemann

Received: 29 April 2021
Accepted: 25 May 2021
Published: 28 May 2021

Publisher's Note: MDPI stays neutral with regard to jurisdictional claims in published maps and institutional affiliations.

Abstract: Indonesia is one of the most biodiverse countries in the world and a promising resource for novel natural compound producers. Actinomycetes produce about two thirds of all clinically used antibiotics. Thus, exploiting Indonesia's microbial diversity for actinomycetes may lead to the discovery of novel antibiotics. A total of 422 actinomycete strains were isolated from three different unique areas in Indonesia and tested for their antimicrobial activity. Nine potent bioactive strains were prioritized for further drug screening approaches. The nine strains were cultivated in different solid and liquid media, and a combination of genome mining analysis and mass spectrometry (MS)-based molecular networking was employed to identify potential novel compounds. By correlating secondary metabolite gene cluster data with MS-based molecular networking results, we identified several gene cluster-encoded biosynthetic products from the nine strains, including naphthyridinomycin, amicetin, echinomycin, tirandamycin, antimycin, and desferrioxamine B. Moreover, 16 putative ion clusters and numerous gene clusters were detected that could not be associated with any known compound, indicating that the strains can produce novel secondary metabolites. Our results demonstrate that sampling of actinomycetes from unique and biodiversity-rich habitats, such as Indonesia, along with a combination of gene cluster networking and molecular networking approaches, accelerates natural product identification.

Keywords: Indonesia; biodiversity; novel antibiotics; drug screening; bioactivity; gene cluster networking; GNPS

1. Introduction

It is now 80 years ago that Selman Waksman and Boyd Woodruff discovered actinomycin from *Actinomyces (Streptomyces) antibioticus*, which was the first antibiotic that was isolated from an actinomycete [1]. Since then, actinomycetes have been widely used as sources for drug discovery and development [2]. Most antibiotics and other useful natural products applied in human medicine, veterinary, and agriculture are derived from these filamentous bacteria [3,4]. Within the family of Actinomycetales, *Streptomyces* is the most prominent genus in respect to the production of bioactive secondary metabolites since it is the origin of more than 50% of all clinically useful antibiotics [5]. Successfully, the intensive screening campaigns of soil-derived streptomycetes yielded many currently recognized drugs, such as the antibacterial substance streptomycin, the antifungal metabolite nystatin, and the anticancer compound doxorubicin during the golden era of antibiotics [6,7]. However, in the last few decades, discovering and developing new drugs from these soil microorganisms has declined immensely, while the need for new drugs to overcome multidrug resistance has become greater than ever [8]. Nowadays, one of the major problems in antibiotic screening programs, in particular with streptomycetes, is the high rediscovery rate of already-known antibacterial compounds through the classical bioactivity-guided paradigms [3].

Sampling actinomycetes from conventional environments such as soils often leads to the rediscovery of known species producing already-known antibiotics [9]. Thus, gaining access to unusual unique habitats with the pursuit to isolate new strains as sources of novel bioactive compounds represents a current barrier in drug discovery research [9]. In recent years, the bioprospection of underexplored niches such as extreme or marine environments has become an efficient approach to find novel *Streptomyces* species that might produce novel compounds [10,11]. *S. asenjonii* strain KNN 42.f, isolated from a desert soil sample, is one example of a novel *Streptomyces* species from an extreme habitat, which produces the three new bioactive compounds asenjonamides A–C [12]. Another example displays the marine *S. zhaozhouensis* CA-185989 that produces three new bioactive polycyclic tetramic acid macrolactams [13]. *Micromonospora* sp. as turbinimicin producer represents a further example of prolific marine bacteria that can deliver new antifungal compounds [14]. These are only a few examples demonstrating that unusual or aquatic territories can be promising avenues as new natural products reservoirs.

Indonesia is the world's largest archipelagic country, spanning into three time zones, covering more than 17,000 islands, with 88,495,000 hectares of tropical forest, 86,700 square kilometers of coral reefs, and 24,300 square kilometers of mangrove areas [15,16]. It has the second-highest level of terrestrial biodiversity globally after Brazil [17], while being ranked as first if marine diversity is taken into account [16,17]. With the given species-rich flora and fauna besides endemic and ecologically adapted species, mega biodiversity of microbial species is gratifyingly represented across various unique habitats [18–20], such as acidic hot springs [21], peatland forests [22], the Thousand Islands reef complex [23], Enggano Island [24], fish species [25], and leaves of traditional medicinal plants [26]. Thus, since unique Indonesian niches are expected to deliver untapped potential actinomycetal strains that may produce novel bioactive secondary metabolites, different locations were targeted for the sampling of actinomycetes in this study.

The latest analyses of genome sequence data from actinomycetes revealed a remarkable discrepancy between the genetic potential of the secondary metabolism, known to be encoded by biosynthetic gene clusters (BGCs), and the actual natural compound production capacity of such isolates, upon their growth under standard laboratory conditions. This is attributed to the fact that numerous BGCs are not expressed under conventional lab parameters and occur as so-called "silent" or "cryptic" BGCs [27]. The activation of these silent clusters allows one to unlock the chemical diversity of the tested organisms and enables the discovery of new molecules for medical and biotechnological purposes [28]. Thus, several efforts, e.g., involving genetic and cultivation methods, are employed to activate the expression of silent gene clusters [29]. One cultivation-based approach to exploit the metabolic capacity of the natural compound producers is the "one strain many compounds (OSMAC)" strategy [3,28,30]. Such a strategy simply relies on the variation of media compositions as a basis to test for different natural compound production profiles since global changes in the specialized metabolic pathways can occur under variable cultivation conditions [31]. The OSMAC concept represents a well-established model that was suggested nearly two decades ago; however, it still leads to the discovery of new chemotypes, such as the novel aromatic polyketide lugdunomycin from *Streptomyces* sp. QL37 [32] or an eudesmane sesquiterpenoid and a new homolog of the Virginiae Butanolides (VB-E) from from *Lentzea violacea* strain AS 08 [33]. Along the lines of the OSMAC concept, an elicitor screening approach has recently been suggested, which intends to mimic natural trigger molecules that can induce the biosynthesis of formerly unknown metabolites. This format has been conducted in a high-throughput approach and was coupled with MALDI-MS analysis. In the case of *S. ghanaensis*, this strategy led to the discovery of the antibiotically active depsipeptide cinnapetide [34].

Besides the variable trials to elicit the BGCs via pleiotropic approaches, a mass spectrometry dereplication step is frequently included in the current screening programs to address the formerly stated challenge of the high rediscovery rate prior to the tedious screening, isolation, and purification processes [35–37]. The utility of such a platform is to pinpoint known compounds in the initial phase of the discovery pipeline and leverage the process of finding new drugs. Integrated genomic and metabolomic mining methods have proven as an efficient dereplication strategy for compound identification in recent years [38–41]. While genome mining involves the identification of putative BGCs based on the genome sequences of the natural compound producers [42,43] using in silico bioinformatics tools such as antiSMASH [44], metabolome mining encompasses sorting out the chemical compounds in extracts of natural compound producers via their mass fragmentation patterns. Counting on the fact that metabolites with a similar chemical architecture tend to generate similar mass fragmentation patterns in mass spectrometry (MS) analysis, the implementation of the computational platform Global Natural Product Social (GNPS) to group the structurally related entities, often derive from a common biosynthetic origin, as a connected set of a molecular family cluster is an overgrowing necessity [45]. Such a platform iteratively proves its effectiveness to arrange seamlessly large numbers of samples enabling dereplication and tentative structural identification and/or classification [46]. The combinatorial employment of both computational tools side by side empowers the rapid identification of new substances, which can be highlighted by discovering the antibacterial substance thiomarinol from *Pseudoalteromonas luteoviolacea* [38] and microviridin 1777, a chymotrypsin inhibitor from *M. aeruginosa* EAWAG 127a [47].

Taken all together with the promises that highly biodiverse habitats can offer in synergy with an effective and practical mining technique, this study aimed to characterize the secondary metabolomes of selected actinomycetes isolated from three different locations within Indonesia. A collection of 422 actinomycetes from Lombok, Bali, and Enggano Islands were sampled and preliminary filtered with different bioactivity tests, where nine actinomycetes with the most bioactive potential were nominated for a hybrid genome mining and molecular networking approach in order to assess their biosynthetic capacity for the production of novel natural compounds.

2. Results and Discussion

2.1. Isolation and Characterization of Indonesian Actinomycetes

To isolate actinomycetes, soil samples were collected from two specific habitats (terrestrial and marine) in three different geographic areas of Indonesia using standard isolation protocols [48–52]. Enggano Island was chosen as a sampling location for terrestrial habitats since it is a pristine island with many endemic species and high biodiversity [53,54], whereas Bali and Lombok Island were selected as sampling sites for marine habitats resulting in 422 strains in total (Table 1). Among all sampling locations, the Enggano Island soil samples contributed to the highest number of actinomycetes isolates (56.2%), followed by sediment samples from Lombok (37.2%) and Bali island (6.6%).

Table 1. Indonesian strains, isolation method, source of isolation (compare Figure 1), and most closely related species (%) based on 16S rRNA gene sequence phylogenetic analysis with EzTaxon.

Strain (*Streptomyces* sp.)	Isolation Method	Source of Isolation	Most Closely Related Species Based on 16S rDNA Analysis
SHP 22-7	phenol	Soil under a ketapang tree (*Terminalia catappa*) from Desa Meok (B1), Enggano Island	*Streptomyces rochei* NBRC 12908^T (99.59%)
SHP 20-4	phenol	Soil under a kina tree (*Cinchona* sp.), Desa Banjarsari (B2), Enggano Island	*Streptomyces hydrogenans* NBRC 12908^T (99.68%)
SHP 2-1	phenol	Soil under a hiyeb tree (*Artocarpus elastica*) near Bak Blau water spring, Desa Meok (B3), Enggano Island	*Streptomyces griseoluteus* NBRC 13375^T (98.96%)
DHE 17-7	dry heat	Soil under a ficus tree (*Ficus* sp.), Desa Boboyo (B4), Enggano Island	*Streptomyces lannensis* TA4-8^T (99.78%)
DHE 12-3	dry heat	Soil under a cempedak tree (*Artocarpus integer*), Desa Boboyo (B4), Enggano Island	*Streptomyces coerulescens* ISP 51446^T (98.87%)
DHE 7-1	dry heat	Soil under a terok tree (*Artocarpus elastica*), desa Boboyo (B4), Enggano Island	*Streptomyces adustus* WH-9^T (99.59%)
DHE 6-7	dry heat	Soil under forest snake fruit tree (*Salacca* sp.), Desa Malakoni (B5), Enggano Island	*Streptomyces parvulus* NBRC 13193^T (98.55%)
DHE 5-1	dry heat	Soil under a banana tree (*Musa* sp.), Desa Banjar sari (B2), Enggano Island	*Streptomyces parvulus* NBRC 13193^T (99.79%)
BSE 7-9	NBRC medium 802	Mangrove sediment near plant rhizosphere, Kuta (C1), Bali Island	*Streptomyces bellus* ISP 5185^T (99.06%)
BSE 7F	NBRC medium 802	Mangrove sediment near plant rhizosphere, Kuta (C1), Bali Island	*Streptomyces matensis* NBRC 12889^T (99.72%)
I3	humic acid-vitamin + chlorine 1%	Mangrove sediment from Pantai Tanjung Kelor, Sekotong (D2), West Lombok Island	*Streptomyces longispororuber* NBRC 13488^T (99.23%)
I4	humic acid-vitamin + chlorine 1%	Mangrove sediment from Pantai Tanjung Kelor, Sekotong (D2), West Lombok Island	*Streptomyces griseoincarnatus* LMG 19316^T (99.89%)
I5	humic acid-vitamin + chlorine 1%	Mangrove sediment from Pantai Tanjung Kelor, Sekotong (D2), West Lombok Island	*Streptomyces viridodiasticus* NBRC13106^T (99.31%)
I6	humic acid-vitamin + chlorine 1%	Mangrove sediment from Pantai Tanjung Kelor, Sekotong (D2), West Lombok Island	*Streptomyces spongiicola* HNM0071^T (99.78%)
I8	humic acid-vitamin	Sea sands from Pantai Koeta (D3), Lombok Island	*Streptomyces smyrnaeus* SM3501^T (98.44%)
I9	humic acid-vitamin	Sea sands from Pantai Koeta (D3), Lombok Island	*Streptomyces gancidicus* NBRC 15412^T (98.82%)

Within the frame of a preliminary bioactivity screening, all 422 isolates were evaluated for their antimicrobial activities in agar plug diffusion bioassays against selected Gram-positive (*Bacillus subtilis, Micrococcus luteus,* and *Staphylococcus carnosus*) and Gram-negative bacteria (*Escherichia coli* and *Pseudomonas fluorescens*). The 16 most potent isolates were selected based on their antimicrobial activity against the tested organisms, indicated by the largest inhibition zones around the agar plug. All 16 isolates showed bioactivity against the Gram-positive test organism *B. subtilis* (Figure 2A), and nine exerted further activity against Gram-negative test strains (Figure 2B), while only four strains (BSE 7–9, BSE 7F, I3, and I6) displayed potency against both (Figure 2).

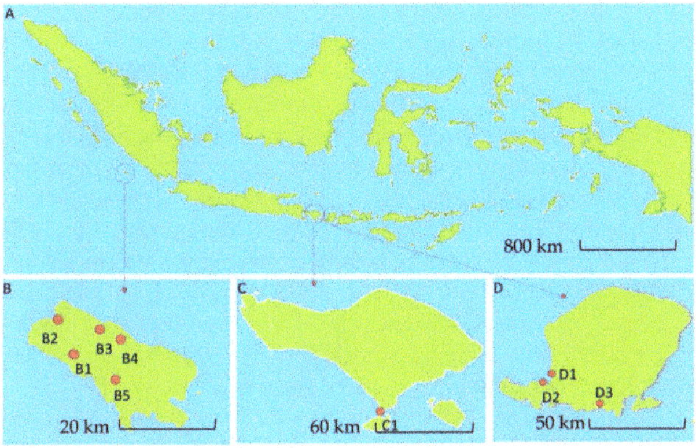

Figure 1. Map of Indonesia showing three geographical regions (**A**). Sampling site location in Enggano Island (**B**), Bali Island (**C**), and Lombok Island (**D**). Red dot shows the sampling locations at Enggano Island, B1: Desa Meok; B2: Desa Banjar Sari; B3: Bak Blau Waterspring, Desa Meok; B4: Desa Boboyo; B5: Desa Malakoni; at Bali Island C1 for Kuta; and Lombok Island D1: Pantai Cemara, Lembar; D2: Pantai Tanjung Kelor, Sekotong; D3: Pantai Koeta.

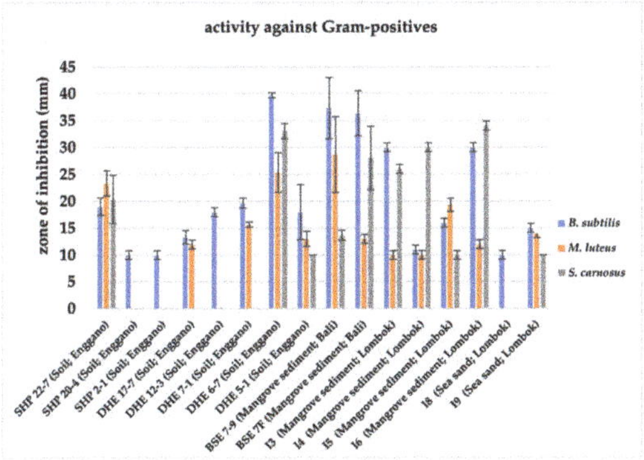

(**A**)

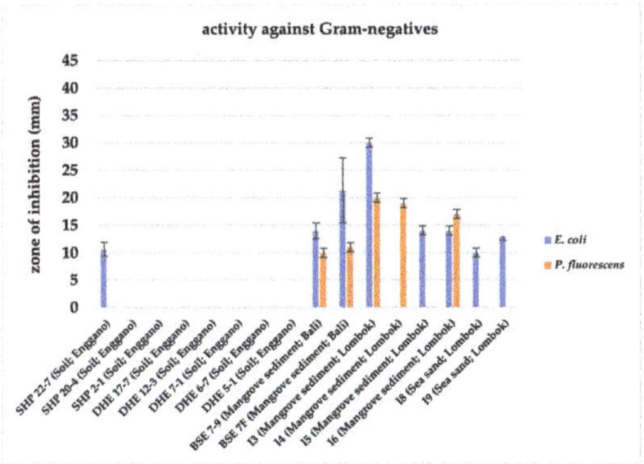

(**B**)

Figure 2. Antimicrobial bioassays with 16 Indonesian actinomycetes strain samples against Gram-positive (**A**) and Gram-negative test strains (**B**). Inhibition zone diameters of agar plug test assays are given in mm. Agar plugs were used after ten days of growth of the respective actinomycetes strains. Data shown are as the result of three independent biological replicates.

To investigate the phylogenetic relationship of the 16 bioactive actinomycetal isolates, 16S rRNA gene sequence analyses were performed. For this purpose, the genomic DNA was isolated from each and was used as a template in a PCR approach with 16S rRNA gene-specific primers. The resulting 16S rRNA gene amplifications were sequenced, and the 16S rRNA gene sequences were compared using the EzTaxon database (www.ezbiocloud.net/, accessed on 28 May 2018) to determine the phylotype of the strains [55]. EzTaxon analysis revealed that all isolates belong to the genus *Streptomyces* with similarity values amongst the various predicted related species ranging from 98.44–99.89% (Table 1).

Subsequently, nine strains were prioritized based on their bioactivity profile and taxonomic position. Strains SHP 22-7, BSE 7-9, BSE 7F, I3, I4, I5, and I6 were selected since they showed antibacterial activity against Gram-positive and Gram-negative bacteria (Figure 2A,B). DHE 17-7 and DHE 7-1 were selected as they exerted bioactivity against at least two different Gram-positive test strains. DHE 6-7 and DHE 5-1, which showed bioactivity against all Gram-positive test strains, were not chosen for further analysis because both strains showed a close phylogenetic relationship to *Streptomyces parvulus* (Table 1), which is a known producer of the polypeptide antibiotic actinomycin D [56]. In an initial attempt with HPLC-MS analysis of the methanolic extracts of culture samples from DHE 6-7 and DHE 5-1, actinomycin D was detected as a product (Figure S1), ruling out both strains from further investigations.

2.2. Phylogenomic Analysis of Nine Prioritized Indonesian Streptomyces Strains

To obtain a better understanding of the phylogenetic relationship about the prioritized nine *Streptomyces* strains, a phylogenetic analysis based on their full-length genomes sequences was performed. For this purpose and the genome mining studies mentioned below, the genomic DNA was isolated from each sample and sequenced by using the Pacific Biosciences RS II (PacBioRSII) platform [57–59]. The resultant genome sequences ranged in sizes between 7.05 Mbp (*Streptomyces* sp. I6) and 8.36 Mbp (DHE 17-7) and GC contents between 72.08% (DHE 7-1) and 72.47% (*Streptomyces* sp. I6) (Table S1), which share comparable values reported for *Streptomyces* species (genome sizes of 6-12 Mb [60] and GC contents of 72–73% [61,62]).

In order to run a whole-genome phylogenetic analysis, the genome sequences were submitted to the Type (Strain) Genome Server (TYGS) (https://tygs.dsmz.de, accessed on 13 December 2019) [63], which allows a phylogenetic analysis based on full-length genome sequences and compares genomic data with the database genomes. The resulting phylogenetic information is more authentic than those obtained from 16S rDNA- or multi-locus sequence analysis (MLSA)-based classifications, which only use small sequence fragments as a basis for sequence comparisons [63]. The TYGS analysis provides information on the similarity of a strain to its nearest related type strain, derived from the digital DNA-DNA hybridization (dDDH) values calculated by the genome-to-genome distance calculator (GGDC) 2.1 (http://ggdc.dsmz.de, accessed on 13 December 2019) [64]. TYGS phylogenomic analysis revealed that all nine isolates belong to the genus *Streptomyces*. The dDDH values between the nine Indonesian strains and their closest relatives ranged between 31.4% (*Streptomyces* sp. I4) and 51.5% (*Streptomyces* sp. I6) (using GGDC distance formula *d4*) (Table 2), which is below the threshold of 70% used for species delineation [65,66], proposing a novel collection of *Streptomyces* species.

Table 2. Data from pairwise comparisons between genome sequences from nine Indonesian strains and their closest related strains based on dDDH analysis. "Query strain" refers to analyzed strain, and "subject strain" refers to most closely related Indonesian strain sample. Degree of relatedness is given as dDDH distance formula *d4* as previously described by Meyer-Kolthoff et al. [66].

Query Strain	Subject Strain	dDDH (d_4, in %)
I3	I4	99.6
BSE 7-9	BSE 7F	95.7
DHE 17-7	SHP 22-7	86.7
I4	I5	82.6
I3	I5	82.5
BSE 7F	I5	78.4
BSE 7-9	I5	78.4
BSE 7-9	I4	77.2
BSE 7F	I4	77.2
BSE 7F	I3	77
BSE 7-9	I3	77
I6	*Streptomyces spongiicola* HNM0071	51.5
SHP 22-7	*Streptomyces luteus* TRM 45540	43.6
DHE 17-7	*Streptomyces luteus* TRM 45540	40.3
DHE 7-1	*Streptomyces bungoensis* DSM 41781	32.3
I3	*Streptomyces capillispiralis* DSM 41695	31.5
BSE 7-9	*Streptomyces capillispiralis* DSM 41695	31.5
I5	*Streptomyces capillispiralis* DSM 41695	31.5
I4	*Streptomyces capillispiralis* DSM 41695	31.4
BSE 7F	*Streptomyces capillispiralis* DSM 41695	31.4

According to the TYGS phylogenomic tree, the terrestrial Enggano Island strains SHP 22-7 and DHE 17-7 belong to the same clade (clade A) (Figure 3) and most likely resemble the same type of species with a dDDH value of 86.7% (Table 2). Both bacteria are found to be closely related to *S. luteus* TRM 45540, isolated from a soil sample from China [67]. All mangrove isolates originating from sediments of Lombok Island (*Streptomyces* sp. I3, I4, and I5) and Bali Island (BSE 7F, and BSE 7-9) were allied in clade B, suggesting a correlative connection (Figure 3). Additionally, the dDDH analysis showed that BSE 7F is closely related to BSE 7-9 with a value of 95.7% and thus most likely represent the same subspecies (Table 2), while *Streptomyces* sp. I3 and I4 probably represent the same species having a dDDH score of almost 100% (Table 2). The nearest related type strain of all five mangrove strains is *S. capillispiralis* DSM 41695 isolated from a Sweden soil sample [68].

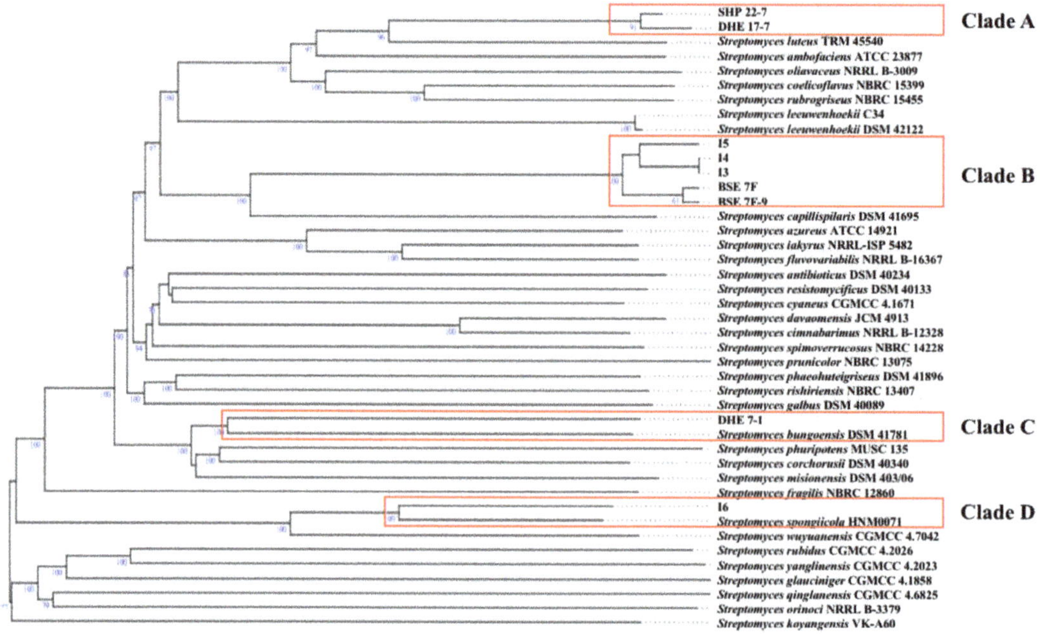

Figure 3. Whole-genome sequence tree generated with the TYGS web server for nine Indonesian *Streptomyces* isolates (highlighted by red boxes) and closely related type strains. Tree inferred with FastME from GBDP distances was determined from genome sequences. The branch lengths are scaled in terms of GBDP distance formula d_5. The numbers above branches indicate GBDP pseudobootstrap support values > 60% from 100 replications, with an average branch support of 84.4%. The tree was rooted at the midpoint.

By contrast, the soil sample DHE 7-1 and mangrove *Streptomyces* sp. I6 were found to group separately in distinct clades (clade C and D, respectively) (Figure 3). The soil *S. bungoensis* DSM 41781 collected in Japan [69] shares a dDDH value of 32.3% as the closest related strain to DHE 7-1 (Table 2), while the nearest related neighbor of *Streptomyces* sp. I6 is *S. spongiicola* HNM0071, isolated from a marine sponge collected from China [70] with a dDDH value of 51.5% (Table 2). Additional information on the specific polyphasic characteristics of the representative type strains from each clade can be found in the Supplementary Material. Altogether, 16S rRNA gene-based phylogenetic and phylogenomic studies revealed that all nine prioritized isolates belong to the genus *Streptomyces* and, based on dDDH analysis, represent novel species (Figure 3).

2.3. Genetic Potential for Secondary Metabolite Biosynthesis of Nine Indonesian *Streptomyces* Strains

To infer the genetic potential of the strains for the biosynthesis of secondary metabolites, the genomes were analyzed bioinformatically using the web tool antiSMASH version 5.0 (https://antismash.secondarymetabolites.org, accessed on 13 November 2019) [44]. The antiSMASH analysis yielded a sum of 206 potential BGCs for the nine isolates (Table 3) with the lowest BGC count of 17 for strain *Streptomyces* sp. I3 and the highest number of 30 BGCs for strain DHE 17-7 (Table 3). On average, this makes 23 BGCs per strain, which is lower than the average value of 40 BGCs reported for *Streptomyces* genomes [71]. However, the lower BGC count is most likely a result of the underlying PacBio genome sequences, which generally yield less contigs than other sequencing technologies, resulting in less interrupted BGCs and thus less BGC counts in antiSMASH analyses. The genome of DHE 17-7 exhibited a slight correlation between genome size (8.4 Mbp) and the observable number of BGCs

(30 BGCs) (Table 3 and Table S1). Several of the identified BGCs from the nine Indonesian isolates showed a high similarity (>60%) to already-known BGCs (Figure 4), e.g., all strains harbored BGCs encoding compounds that are commonly produced by streptomycetes, such as desferrioxamine, which is a vital siderophore for the growth and development [72], hopene, as a substance of the cytoplasmic membrane modulating membrane fluidity and stability [73], and a spore pigment for protection against UV radiation [74]. This result is consistent with previous observations, where these BGCs have been reported for most analyzed *Streptomyces* genomes [71]. Ectoine and geosmin BGCs were found in all Indonesian isolates except for *Streptomyces* sp. I6 (Figure 4). Moreover, albaflavenone BGCs were uncovered in all strains, excluding *Streptomyces* sp. I6 and DHE 7-1. Interestingly, in the genomes of the mangrove-derived isolates BSE 7F, BSE 7-9, I3, I4, and I5, two ectoine BGC were identified, suggesting that the additional ectoine BGCs may play a role in the adaptation of these organisms to the osmotic stress of such high-salinity environments.

Table 3. List of Indonesian actinomycetes strains with number and type of BGCs as predicted by antiSMASH analysis.

Strain	Total BGCs	PKS	NRPS	Hybrid BGC	Terpene	RiPP	Siderophore	Others
DHE 17-7	30	6	7	-	6	3	3	5
DHE 7-1	27	6	6	3	5	-	3	4
SHP 22-7	25	5	6	1	4	1	2	6
I4	19	3	2	-	4	4	2	5
I3	17	4	2	1	4	2	2	3
I5	19	3	2	1	4	4	2	3
BSE 7F	23	3	1	4	5	4	2	4
BSE 7-9	22	4	2	3	4	1	2	6
I6	24	3	6	1	2	1	2	9

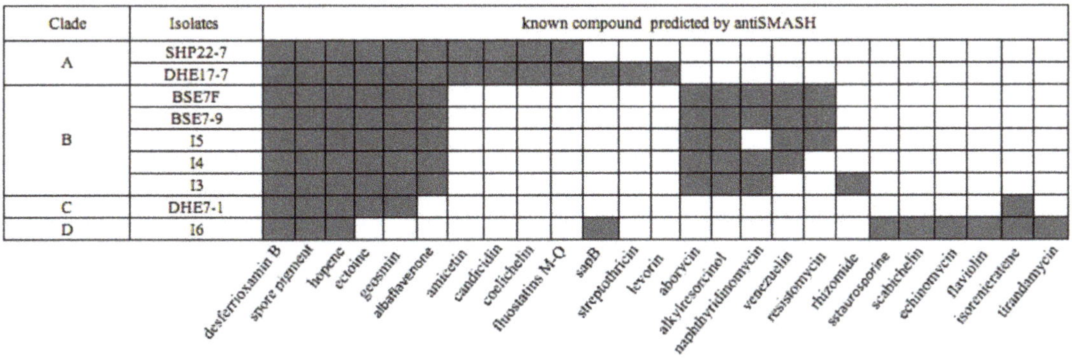

Figure 4. Presence (grey color) and absence (white color) of BGCs in nine Indonesian strains as predicted by antiSMASH analysis with similarity above 60%.

Aborycin and alkylresorcinol gene clusters were discovered in the five mangrove *Streptomyces* strains, whereas amicetin, candicidin, coelichelin, and fluostatin M-Q BGCs were only detected for the soil-based isolates SHP 22-7 and DHE 17-7. Candicidin, as an example of a fungizide [75], is most likely produced by terrestrial streptomycetes in order to defend themselves against local fungal competitors. Coelichelin is a further spotted siderophore which might be necessary for the soil-living streptomycetes to sequester poorly soluble environmental Fe^{3+} [76], which is quite scarce and highly contested by other microorganisms in soils. The discovery of the same BGC composition in strains derived from the same habitat, such as soil or mangroves, is probably attributed to the fact that each biosynthetic product has its specific biochemical relevance in the respective environment. Of the nine strains, only *Streptomyces* sp. I6 harbored a staurosporine, scabichelin, echinomycin, flaviolin, and tirandamycin BGC. Likewise, DHE 7-1 together with *Streptomyces* sp. I6 were the only representatives comprising an isorenieratene BGC among the nine strains (Figure 4). Both strains, I6 and DHE 7-1, were found to be phylogenetically distant from the other strains (Figure 3), outlining that phylogenetically related isolates tend to have similar biosynthetic elements known as BGCs shaped by the environmental conditions. A similar finding has already been made by Meij et al., who reported that ecological conditions play an important role in controlling the formation of secondary metabolites in actinomycetes [77].

To glean a more detailed picture about the BGC distribution amongst the strains, the genome sequences from the nine strains have been analyzed using the BiG-SCAPE software (https://bigscape-corason.secondarymetabolites.org/, accessed on 13 November 2019) [78]. BiG-SCAPE allows fast computation and visual exploration of BGC similarities by grouping BGCs into gene cluster families (GCF) based on their sequences and Pfam protein families similarities [79]. Comparing all shared BGCs within the nine Indonesian strains with BiG-SCAPE allows visualization of the more common BGCs (large nodes) and the less frequent ones (doubletons, (singletons are not shown) (Figure 5). With this approach, we visualized the occurrence of eight GCFs with a similarity of less than 60% similarity to known BGCs as predicted by antiSMASH. Ectoine-butyrolactone-NRPS-T1PKS GCF, which has similarities with polyoxypeptin (48%) or aurantimycin A (51%), was distributed among strains I3, I4, I5 and BSE 7F (Figure 5, Tables S6, S7, S9 and S10). A type III polyketide (T3PKS) GCF was shared amongst the strains DHE 17-7, SHP 22-7, and DHE 7-1, which showed 7–8% BGC similarity to the herboxidiene BGC (Figure 5, Tables S4, S5 and S11). In the strains *Streptomyces* sp. I3 and I4 of clade B, we found the others-type I polyketide (otherks-T1PKS), which showed 48–55% BGC similarity to the nataxazole BGC, and an aminoglycoside/aminocyclitol (amglyccycl) BGC type, which led to 2% similarity to the BGC of cetoniacytone A (Figure 5, Tables S6 and S7). We identified two unique GCFs in the strains BSE 7F and BSE 7-9 of clade B, namely a transAT-PKS GCF, which showed 54–58% similarity to the weishanmycin and phenazine BGC types, and did not show any similarity to any BGC in the antiSMASH database (Figure 5, Tables S9 and S10). Moreover, we detected two GCFs of an indole, which showed 23–33% BGC similarity to the 5-isoprenylindole-3-carboxylate β-D-glycosyl ester BGC and other BGC type, which do not belong to any BGCs in the antiSMASH database for the phylogenetically related species of SHP 22-7 and DHE 17-7 of clade A (Figure 5, Tables S4 and S5). Altogether, the Big-SCAPE analysis revealed eight unique GCFs, which could not be associated with known BGCs and may have the potential to encode for new substances. Furthermore, the obtained data disclosed that phylogenetically related strains derived from a similar environmental habitat tend to share similar BGC composition profiles. Inferred from this observation, one can conclude that it is worth it to make an effort to sample actinomycetes from unique environmental habitats, since this may lead to the isolation of phylogenetically unique species, which have a higher potential of producing novel natural compounds, as also previously described by Hug et al. [9].

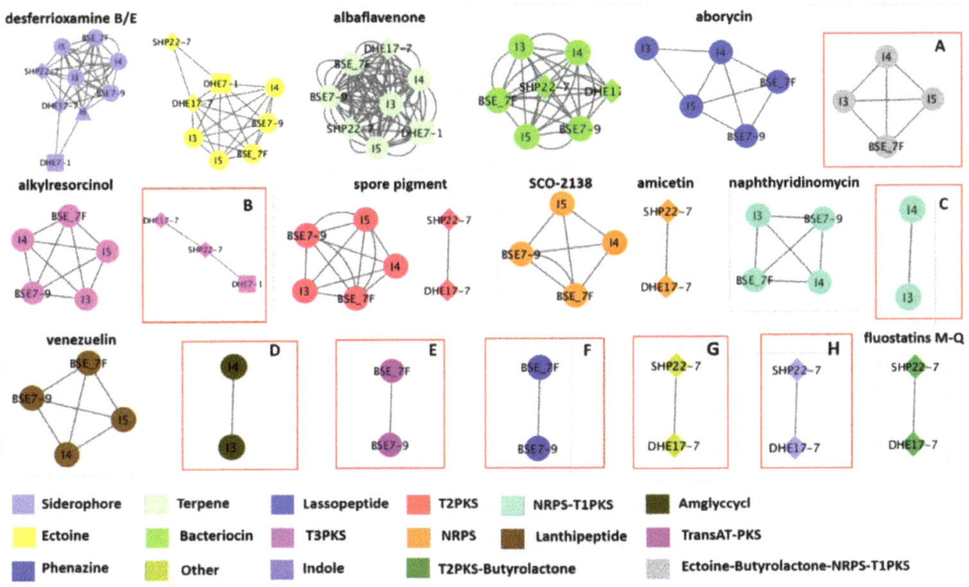

Figure 5. Similarity network of the predicted biosynthetic gene clusters (BGCs) of the nine Indonesian *Streptomyces* strains. Shared similar BGCs are indicated by a connected line. Each node represents a specific BGC type (labeled with different colors). The shape node represents the same species, i.e., clade A (SHP 22-7 and DHE 17-7) indicated with diamond, clade B (I4, I5, BSE 7F, and BSE 7-9) shown with ellipse, clade C (DHE 7-1) with a cube, and clade D (I6) indicated with a triangle. BGCs with similarities less than 60% are highlighted by red boxes: (**A**) Ectoine-butyrolactone-NRPS-T1PKS; (**B**) T3PKS; (**C**) Otherks-T1PKS, (**D**) Amglyccyc; (**E**) TransAT-PKS; (**F**) Phenazine; (**G**) Other; and (**H**) Indole.

2.4. Optimal Cultivation Conditions for Compound Production of Nine Indonesian Streptomyces Strains

In order to infer the biosynthetic capacity of the prioritized nine isolates in a bioactivity context, various media following the OSMAC strategy were screened to define the optimal production conditions [30,31]. For this purpose, SHP 22-7, DHE 17-7, DHE 7-1, BSE 7-9, BSE 7F, I3, I4, I5, and I6 were each grown in twelve different liquid cultivation media (SGG, YM, OM, R5, MS, TSG, NL19, NL300, NL330, NL500, NL550, and NL800 (Table S2)), and culture samples were harvested at different time points (48, 72, 96, and 168 h). Cell cultures were extracted with ethyl acetate, concentrated in vacuo, and then re-dissolved in methanol. Methanolic extracts were tested in bioassays against a selected panel of pathogenic strains *B. subtilis, M. luteus, S. carnosus, E. coli,* and *P. fluorescens*. Samples with the largest inhibition zones in bioassay tests were defined as the ones grown under optimal cultivation conditions. For each Indonesian *Streptomyces* strain, the optimal production conditions have been defined for cultivation in liquid media (Table S3). In addition, it is hypothesized that filamentous actinomycetes as soil organisms grow and develop better on solid nutrient substrates and that a well-grown healthy culture produces more diverse secondary metabolites [80]. Thus, to extend the probability of finding new substances by exploring the biosynthetic potential of the nine strains for secondary metabolite production, we recruited an antibiotic extraction also from solid media. For this purpose, each isolate was spread on agar plates consisting of the respective abovementioned media and incubated for 7–10 days at 28 °C until spores formed. Grown agar samples were squeezed out and concentrated. The aqueous phase of the solid medium extract was used for bioassays and further chemical analysis.

For *Streptomyces* sp. I3 and I4, the same cultivation parameters were found to be optimal. Both strains showed a promising potency upon their growth in liquid NL550 medium for 72 h on solid MS medium (Table S3). Such similar production behavior might be ascribed to their most possible likelihood to represent the same species as suggested above. Furthermore, we found that most of the nine isolates (*Streptomyces* sp. I3, I4, I5, and I6) produced best on solid MS medium (Table S3). In general, MS is a suitable medium for streptomycetes regarding spore isolation [81]. This would support the hypothesis that strains produce better, when they show healthy growth and development.

2.5. Identification of Natural Compounds from Nine Indonesian Actinomycetes

To putatively identify the specialized bioactive substances which are produced by the nine isolates under the various conditions, the culture extract samples were submitted to high-resolution mass spectrometry (HRMS) coupled with the GNPS platform. For this purpose, the obtained extracts from the optimal medium in liquid and solid were firstly fractionated by solid-phase extraction (SPE) and then qualitatively profiled against their main crudes and media controls using HPLC. Subsequently, the prioritized profiles and/or SPE fractions that mainly cover the whole metabolomes with fewer media components were chosen for further metabolomics mass identification through HRMS/MS. The acquired tandem-MS mass spectra from the positive mode were recruited to build a feature-based molecular network, while the negative ionization was consulted, if needed, during the annotation step to further validate the feature identities [45,82]. The dereplication of the known compounds, chemical analogues, and potential novel chemical structures was carried out either by matching their MS/MS spectra against the literature if available, GNPS spectral libraries [45] and/or assisted by manual in silico annotation via Sirius+CSI: FingerID 4.0.1 integrated with Antibase and Pubchem databases [83,84] (see Material and Methods).

Among the numerous identified secondary metabolites from the nine isolates, antimycins cluster were swiftly retrieved through the identical similarity of their MS/MS spectra to the publicly shared ones of GNPS libraries (Figures S2–S6). Tracking down such features in liquid BSE 7F fractions, particularly the one eluted with 100% MeOH in negative mode, expanded this set with further known members (Figures S5 and S6). In alignment with the formerly described positional and stereogenic isomers of the antimycin family entities, the extracted ion chromatograms (EICs) unambiguously displayed such an isomeric behavior under both modes (Figures S2, S4 and S5) [85–87]. In a similar fashion to antimycins, a different cluster comprising ferrioxamines was deciphered with the aid of GNPS spectral libraries. Ferroxamine D1, 656.2830 Da in size as $C_{27}H_{48}N_6O_9$ [88,89], was displayed as the primary ion linked with an additional unknown analogue, 627.3303 Da as $C_{26}H_{51}FeN_8O_6$ (Figures S7–S9). Despite the fact of observing these two features under only solid cultivation parameters across different isolates (*Streptomyces* sp. I3, I4, I6, BSE 7F, DHE 17-7, and SHP 22-7) with variable concentrations, two extra unknown amphiphilic trihydroxamate-containing siderophores were also grouped (Figures S7 and S10). Interestingly, BSE 7-9 was the sole producer of such amphiphilic entities under exclusive liquid conditions. Moreover, two additional unknown ferrioxamines were retrieved as unique features singly produced by the DHE 17-7 isolate (Figure S11).

Analogously, staurosporine, with two further congeners, was dereplicated from the I6 sample assisted by shared spectral repositories (Figure S12). Manual annotation of a pair of singletons, 1137.45 as $[M+H]^+$ and 560.22 as $[M + 2H]^{2+}$ from the I6 extract, uniquely grown under solid conditions, could decipher echinoserine and depsiechinoserine, respectively (Figures S13–S15) [90,91]. Although the two features were supposed to group together considering their skeletons, the MS/MS spectra of their triggered singly and doubly pseudomolecular ions were different enough not to serve such a purpose resulting in scattered self-looped nodes (Figures S13 and S14). Furthermore, traces of the structurally related echinomycin [92] were also observed within *Streptomyces* sp. I6 extracts, expanding in this way the molecular compound family (Figure S15). Likewise, a tirandamycins cluster was disclosed in *Streptomyces* sp. I6 extracts upon liquid cultivation depicting the known tirandamycin A in connectivity with further related chemotypes (Figure S16). In parallel, the observed UV absorbance of the annotated mass ion at m/z 418.18 as tirandamycin A was in alignment with its reported characteristic value [93,94], additionally confirming the identity of the dereplicated feature (Figure S17). Notably, the anticipated molecular formula of the grouped ions of the tirandamycin cluster, besides their degrees of unsaturation, was also reflected by their observed UV absorbances, which differed from the characteristic known one (Figure S17).

An additional constellation of ions mainly derived from isolates BSE 7-9 and I5 was uncovered through manual annotation as naphthyridinomycins cluster (Figure S18). The in silico annotation considering the molecular formula prediction and their MS^2 spectra deconvoluted naphthyridinomycin-A, aclidinomycin A, and bioxalomycin-β2 besides several unknown related products (Figures S19–S22) [95–97]. Similarly, the manual interrogation of an exclusive group of ions derived from DHE 17-7 led to the putative dereplication of ECO-501, a PKS product so far only reported from *Amycolatopsis orientalis* ATCC 43491 [98] (Figures S23–S26). Interestingly, the putative annotation of such a feature was in complete alignment regarding the observed UV absorbance and the formerly reported MS/MS spectra (Figures S27–S29). Moreover, amicetin and cytosaminomycins as structurally related entities were uncovered from SHP 22-7 samples as a big group of ions (Figures S27–S29), encompassing a wide scope of structural modifications as expected according to previous reports in addition to a putatively new set of congeners (Figure S30) [99–101].

The compound naphthyridinomycin was detected in several culture extract samples from strains of mangrove origin, such as *Streptomyces* sp. I3, I4, I5, BSE 7F, and BSE 7-9 (Figure 6, Table 4), while amicetin was detected as a biosynthetic product from the isolates SHP 22-7 and DHE 17-7 obtained from soil samples of Enggano Island (Figure 6, Table 4). Furthermore, we observed that *Streptomyces* sp. I6 produces echinomycin (Figure 6, Table 4), a substance also reported as the biosynthetic product from the closely related type strain *Streptomyces spongiicola* HNM0071, which was originally derived from a marine sponge [102]. These results underline our assumption that phylogenetically related strains are likely to produce similar compounds as a response to their natural-habitat environmental conditions. Specifically, the isolates *Streptomyces* sp. I3 and I4 have been found to most likely represent the same species derived from a similar habitat as indicated by the dDDH value of almost 100% and the high overall similarities of BGC composition and secondary metabolite production profile of both strains (see above). In this context, it should be mentioned that current antibiotic research often addresses the problem of dereplication of known compounds during drug-screening approaches [103–105]. However, what should also be taken into account is the fact that there is also an issue of dereplication of producer strains as observed in the current study. Thus, it is worth it to put effort into phylogenetic profiling at the beginning of the screening strategy in order to sort out known producer strains.

Interestingly, the ferrioxamine molecular family was only detected for samples of strains grown on solid media (Tables 4 and 5). In addition to the abovementioned metabolites, the solid media uniquely delivered a putative new molecular family consisting of likely three peptides with *m/z* 598.2834 $[M + 2H]^{2+}$, 662.8048 $[M + 2H]^{2+}$, and 727.3259 $[M + 2H]^{2+}$, for which no known substance could be associated. These compounds were detected in samples of strains I3, I5, and BSE 7F (Figure S31, Table 5), highlighting that cultivation conditions have a substantial effect on the chemical profiles. A further example of rendering the impact of the adopted cultivation method was represented with an additional cluster of unknown features from SHP 22-7 isolate, designated compound group I, which were exclusively produced under nonliquid fermentation (Figure S32).

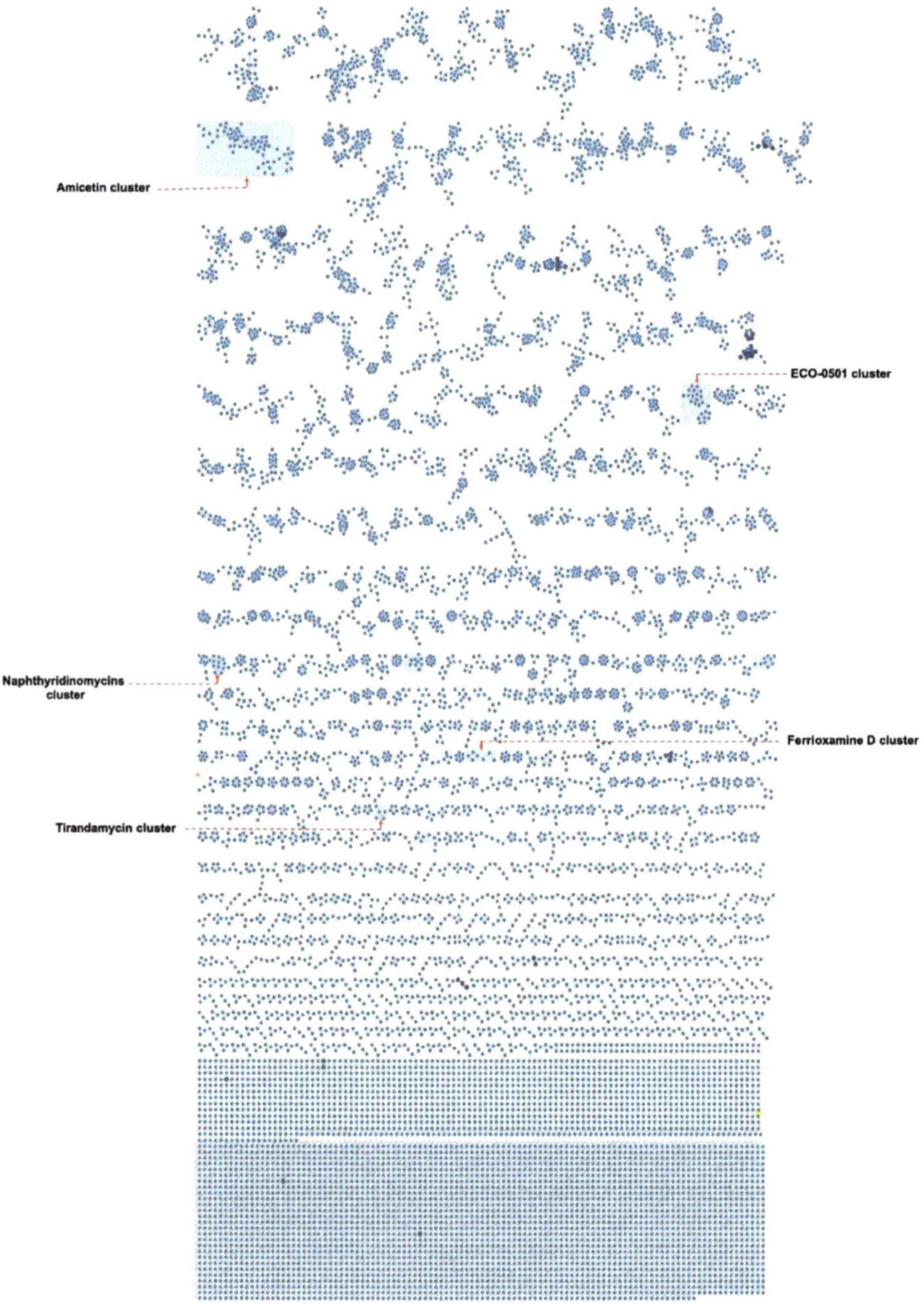

Figure 6. Molecular networking of extract and fraction samples from nine Indonesian *Streptomyces* strains. Molecular families containing a known substance are highlighted by blue boxes.

Table 4. Correlation between known compounds and BGC distribution in the nine Indonesian strains. A checkmark (√) indicates identified BGC in the studied strain, a question mark (?) indicates that BGC is not identified in the studied strain, and a minus sign (-) indicates the compound is not present in the medium.

Ion Cluster Name (Ion Formula)	*m/z* Measured	Adduct	Main Producer and Media Type		BGC Identified
			Solid	Liquid	
Ferrioxamine D1 ($C_{27}H_{48}N_6O_9$)	656.2830	$[M - 2H + Fe]^+$	SHP 22-7; I3; I4; I6	-	√
Naphthyridinomycin A ($C_{21}H_{28}N_3O_6$)	418.1980	$[M + H]^+$	I3; I4; I5	BSE 7F; BSE 7-9; I5	√
Amicetin ($C_{29}H_{43}N_6O_9$)	619.3100	$[M + H]^+$	-	SHP 22-7; DHE 17-7	√
Antimycin A2 ($C_{27}H_{39}N_2O_9$)	535.2659	$[M + H]^+$	-	BSE 7F	√
ECO-0501 ($C_{46}H_{69}N_4O_{10}$)	837.5022	$[M + H]^+$	-	DHE 17-7	?
Echinoserine ($C_{51}H_{69}N_{12}O_{14}S_2$)	1137.4504	$[M + H]^+$	I6	-	√
Echinomycin ($C_{51}H_{65}N_{12}O_{12}S_2$)	1101.4279	$[M + H]^+$	I6	-	√
Tirandamycin A ($C_{18}H_{25}O_6$)	337.1650	$[M + H]^+$	I6	-	√
Staurosporine ($C_{28}H_{27}N_4O_3$)	467.2070	$[M + H]^+$	I6		√

Table 5. Overview of analogs and putative new compounds identified for the nine Indonesian *Streptomyces* strains. A minus sign (-) indicates that the compound is not present in the medium.

Ion Cluster Description	*m/z* Measured	Adduct	Main Producer and Media Type	
			Solid	Liquid
Ferrioxamine analogs	627.3303	$[M - 2H + Fe]^+$	I3; I4; I6; DHE 17-7	-
	788.3753	$[M - 2H + Fe]^+$	BSE 7-9	-
	840.4060	$[M - 2H + Fe]^+$	-	BSE 7-9
	640.2520	$[M - 2H + Fe]^+$	-	DHE 17-7
	654.2685	$[M - 2H + Fe]^+$	DHE 17-7	-
Putative new peptides	598.2834	$[M + 2H]^{2+}$	I3, I5, BSE 7F	-
	662.8048	$[M + 2H]^{2+}$	I3, I5, BSE 7F	-
	727.3259	$[M + 2H]^{2+}$	I3, I5, BSE 7F	-
Putative new compound group I	821.3349	$[M + H]^+$	SHP 22-7	-
	734.3031	$[M + H]^+$	SHP 22-7	-
	679.2430	$[M + H]^+$	SHP 22-7	-
	647.2710	$[M + H]^+$	SHP 22-7	-
Putative new compound group II	435.2774	$[M + 2H]^{2+}$	-	DHE 17-7
	442.2857	$[M + 2H]^{2+}$	-	DHE 17-7
	449.2934	$[M + 2H]^{2+}$	-	DHE 17-7
	474.2833	$[M + 2H]^{2+}$	-	DHE 17-7

Within the same context, strain DHE 17-7 also offered several putative new compounds (compound group II) which were detected when grown in a liquid medium and presented themselves only as a set of doubly charged entities (Figure S33) (Table 5). Thus, in regard to drug-discovery efforts, strain DHE17-7 is the most promising strain to be investigated further. The potent biosynthetic capacity is also reflected by the genetically encoded biosynthetic potential since DHE17-7 has a total of 30 BGCs, which is the largest BGC set compared to the other Indonesian strains (Table 3). In summary, 16 potential novel compounds (Table 5) have been identified as biosynthetic products from the Indonesian strains, which could not be associated with any known compound and thus demonstrate the value of new strains for drug-discovery research.

Furthermore, we observed a correlation between growth conditions and compound production. It is known that sources of complex nitrogen such as soybean meal and corn steep liquor can increase ferrioxamine production in streptomycetes [106,107]. Interestingly, ferrioxamine B/D and its analogs has been mainly identified for strains grown on solid media, such as MS agar (*Streptomyces* sp. I3, I4, I6) and NL300 agar (SHP 22-7) (Tables 4 and S3), which contain soy flour and cotton seed powder, respectively (Table S2). We could detect ferrioxamines only in samples obtained from strains grown on solid medium. This might be because in liquid media iron (Fe^{3+}) is more evenly distributed compared to solid media. Thus, cells grown on solid media might be faced with local iron depletion conditions, which lead to induction of ferrioxamine biosynthesis [76]. In addition to ferrioxamine and its analogs, several known and unknown compounds were only discovered in samples from strains grown on solid medium, i.e., the three known compound echinomycin, staurosporine, and tirandamycin for *Streptomyces* sp. I6, and three putative new peptides for *Streptomyces* sp. I3; I5; BSE 7F, as well as the putative new compound group I for *S.* sp. SHP 22-7 (Tables 4 and 5). Apart from that, we also found some unknown and known compounds in strains grown in liquid media only, such as amicetin (SHP 22-7 and DHE 17-7), antimycin and its analogs (BSE 7F), ECO-0501 (DHE 17-7), or the putative new compound group II for strains *Streptomyces* sp. DHE 17-7 (Tables 4 and 5). This indicates that cultivation conditions significantly affect the formation of substances. Therefore, both the liquid and solid cultivation approach are feasible for increasing the probability of discovering new compounds.

2.6. Identification of Potential BGCs Responsible for Compound Production in the Nine Indonesian Streptomyces Strains

To identify the BGCs responsible for compound production in the nine Indonesian *Streptomyces* strains, we aimed to link the compound production profile and BGC composition by correlating the BGCs data with the MS-based molecular networking results. As described above, strains SHP 22-7, I3, I4, and I6 produce desferrioxamine B/D when grown on solid media (Table 4). We observed that the corresponding BGCs associated with desferrioxamine B/D biosynthesis were present in all of the four strains. Furthermore, we were able to assign the BGC responsible for the biosynthesis of naphthyridinomycin in the strains BSE 7F, BSE 7-9, I3, I4, and I5 (Table 4). Additional BGCs could be assigned to the compound formations of amicetin in SHP 22-7 and DHE 17-7, antimycin in BSE 7F, echinomycin, staurosporine, and tirandamycin A in I6 (Table 4). Furthermore, we could not identify the BGC encoding the biosynthesis of ECO-0501 in strain DHE 17-7 based on the antiSMASH output. A potential candidate gene cluster could be cluster region 24, which is a predicted type I PKS BGC that shows some similarity (<55%) to BGCs encoding structurally related macrolactam natural products, such as vicenistatin, sceliphrolactam, and streptovaricin (Figure S34).

In addition to the metabolites mentioned earlier, we also discovered a group of new peptides, which were detected in samples of strains *Streptomyces* sp. I3, I5, and BSE 7F grown on solid media (Table 5). Notably, for all three strains a bacteriocin BGC could be detected (Tables S6, S8 and S9), which showed 42–57% similarity to the informatipeptin BGC. Alternatively, all three strains also share a combined NRPS/ectoine/butyrolactone/other/T1PKS gene cluster (Tables S6, S8 and S9), and it is also conceivable that the peptide group might be encoded from this region. A similar cluster was found on regions 21 and 22 for the phylogenetically related strain BSE 7-9, for which, however, no respective compound was detected (Table S10). Moreover, we found the putative new compound group IIwith masses ranging from 435–474 Da, produced by strain DHE 17-7 when grown in liquid medium (Table 5). Five BGCs are present in DHE 17-7 (region 10, 16, 17, 22, and 28), which do not show any similarity to known BGCs in the antiSMASH database and nine BGCs (region 3, 4, 6, 11, 13, 19, 24, 25, and 26) have similarities of less than 50%. Thus, the so far unknown metabolites might be encoded by some of the unique BGCs from DHE 17-7 (Table S4). The same applies for the putative new compound group I detected in strain SHP 22-7. Its genome comprises 13 BGCs with similarities of less than 50% and therefore represents all putative candidates. Similar observations have been made in comparable studies, where it has been shown that BGCs encoding ectoine, desferrioxamine, spore pigment, and bacteriocin production are very abundant in actinobacterial natural compound producers; however, each strain still possesses numerous BGCs that code for potential yet unknown substances [108–110]. That Indonesian habitats can serve as a promising reservoir for antibiotic active substances has already been highlighted in several previous screening studies [111–115]. Especially Indonesian actinomycetes have been reported as producer strains of new secondary metabolites, as for example shown for the Indonesian *Streptomyces* sp. strains ICBB8230, ICBB8309, and ICBB8415, which produced new angucyclinones [116,117], *Streptomyces* sp. ICBB8198, producing new phenazine derivatives [118], and *Streptomyces* sp. ICBB9297, which produced new elaiophylin macrolides [119]. Furthermore, Indonesian non-*Streptomyces* strains, as for example *Micrococcus* sp. ICBB8177 and *Amycolatopsis* sp. ICBB8242, have also been reported to produce novel compounds, as for example the limazepines or succinylated apoptolidins, respectively [120,121]. Thus, Indonesian habitats can indeed be considered a promising source for new bioactive natural products.

Altogether, the combined GNPS and cluster networking approach disclosed several potentially novel compounds from the Indonesian strains *Streptomyces* sp. I3, I4, I5, I6, BSE 7F, BSE 7-9, and DHE 17-7—some of which could be assigned to potential encoding BGCs, and some are expected to be encoded by unique BGCs. The new Indonesian isolates thus represent a valuable resource for further drug research and development approaches. We conclude that the combined phylogenomic, GNPS, and cluster-networking approach is an efficient strategy to prioritize phylogenetically unique producer strains and focus on potentially novel compounds encoded by special BGCs.

3. Materials and Methods

3.1. Sample Collection and Treatment

Soil samples were collected from Enggano Island (5°22′57.0792″ S, 102°13′28.2792″ E), Indonesia, in December 2015 (Figure 1B). Marine samples were collected from marine sediments from Bali Island (8°43′5.5″ S, 115°10′7.8″ E), Indonesia, in May 2014 (Figure 1C), and Lombok Island West Nusa Tenggara (8°24′17.133″ S, 116°15′57.228″ E), Indonesia, in May 2017 (Figure 1D). Soil and sediment samples were taken aseptically from 10 cm depth of soil samples and the center of sediment in mangrove and tidal area. Soil and sediment samples were transferred into sterile 50 mL conical tubes and placed on ice and then stored at 4 °C until further treatment.

3.2. Isolation of Actinomycetes

Isolation and enumeration of actinomycetes were done using a serial dilution of Humic Acid-Vitamin (HV) medium [48] and/or NBRC No. 802 Medium [49] by using the direct method [50], the dry heat method [51], and the phenol method [51]. In the direct method, an air-dried soil sample or marine sediment was ground in a mortar and heated in a hot-air oven at 110 °C for 30 min. One gram of the heated samples was transferred to 10 mL of sterile water and mixed for 2 min, then diluted with sterile water to 10^{-1}, 10^{-2}, and 10^{-3} times. In total, 200 µL of each dilution was inoculated on isolation medium agar of HV [48] or NBRC No. 802 Medium [49] with or without the addition of 1% NaCl. The inoculated plates were incubated for 2–4 weeks at 28 °C. The colonies showing the *Streptomyces* morphological characteristics were selected and streaked on fresh plates of the modified *Streptomyces* International Project 2 (ISP2 ≙ YM) agar [52]. The cultures were resuspended in sterile 0.9% (w/v) saline supplemented with 15% (v/v) glycerol and stored at −80 °C. This dry-heat method [51] was used to isolate heat-tolerant actinomycetes spores. In the dry-heat method, the soil or sediment samples were incubated at 100 °C for 40 min and then cooled to 28 °C in a desiccator. The samples were distributed on HV medium agar plates with a spatula tip and incubated at 28 °C for 2–3 weeks. The phenol method was used to select for spores, which survive in the presence of phenol. In total, 1 mL of 10^{-1} dilution of one gram of oven-dried soil or marine sample was transferred to 9 mL of sterile 5 mM-phosphate buffer (pH 7.0) containing phenol at a final concentration of 1.5%. The sample was then heated and diluted in serial dilution (10^{-1}, 10^{-2}, 10^{-3}). Next, 100 or 200 µL of each dilution was spread over the surface of HV medium agar plates and incubated for 2–4 weeks at 28 °C.

3.3. Antimicrobial Bioassays

The preliminary screening of actinomycetal strains for antimicrobial activity was performed using the agar plug diffusion method (see Supplementary for test plate preparation). Gram-positive (*B. subtilis* ATCC6051, *M. luteus*, and *S. carnosus* TM300) and Gram-negative bacteria (*E. coli* K12 W3110 and *P. fluorescens*) were chosen as test organisms. The isolates were spread evenly over the agar plate surface of soya flour mannitol medium (MS) (mannitol 20 g, soy flour (full fat) 20 g, agar 16 g in 1 L of distilled water) [80] and incubated for 10 days at 28 °C. Agar discs of the 10 days inoculum were cut aseptically with a cork borer (9 mm diameter) and placed on the bioassay test plate. Bioassays to determine optimal cultivation conditions in the liquid culture were examined using a disc diffusion assay against the test Gram-positive (*B. subtilis* ATCC6051, *M. luteus*, and *S. carnosus* TM300) and Gram-negative bacteria (*E. coli* K12 W3110 and *P. fluorescens*). In total, 10 µL methanolic extract obtained from liquid cultures of the actinomycetal strains was pipetted on a filter disc (6 mm) and then placed on the respective test plates. In addition, 5 µL kanamycin (50 µg/mL) was used as positive control and 10 µl methanol as a negative control.

The bioassay plates were incubated overnight at 37 °C for *B. subtilis*, *E. coli*, and *S. carnosus* and at 28 °C for *M. luteus* and *P. fluorescens* to allow for the test organisms' growth. The antimicrobial activity of the isolates was assessed by measuring the diameter of the inhibition zone (mm) around the agar plug or the discs. All bioassay tests were carried out as three independent biological replicates.

3.4. Isolation of Genomic DNA and 16S rDNA Phylogenetic Analysis

For isolation of genomic DNA, the producer strains were grown for two days in 50 mL of R5 medium at 30 °C [81]. The genomic DNA was extracted and purified with the Nucleospin® Tissue kit from Macherey-Nagel (catalog number 740952.50) following the standard protocol from the manufacturer. The DNA was applied as a PCR template for 16S rRNA gene amplification using polymerase chain reaction (PCR). Primers used for PCR were 27Fbac (5′-AGAGTTTGATCMTGGCTCAG-3′) and 1492Runi (5′-TACGGTTACCTTAC GACTT-3′). The PCR amplicons were subcloned into the cloning vector pDrive (Qiagen) using basic DNA manipulation procedures as previously described by Sambrook et al. [122]. The respective 16S rDNA fragments were sequenced at MWG Eurofins (Ebersberg, Germany) with primers 27Fbac. The 16S rDNA sequence data were analyzed using the EzTaxon database (https://www.ezbiocloud.net, accessed on 28 May 2018).

3.5. Phylogenomic and Genome Mining Analysis

For phylogenomic and genome mining studies, full-genome sequence data have been obtained as reported previously [57–59]. Genomic DNA was isolated to construct a 10–20 kb paired-end library for sequencing by Macrogen (Seoul, South Korea) with the Pacific

Biosciences RS II technology (Pacbio). The genome was assembled using Hierarchical Genome Assembly (HGAP) V.3. and annotated with Prokka version 1.12b and the NCBI Prokaryotic Genome Annotation Pipeline (PGAP). The phylogenomic analysis of the nine selected strains was carried out with the Type (Strain) Genome Server (TYGS), a free bioinformatics tool (https://tygs.dsmz.de/, accessed on 13 December 2019) for whole-genome-based taxonomic analysis [63]. The identification of potential biosynthesis gene clusters (BGCs) was accomplished by analyzing the genome sequences with antiSMASH version 5.0 [44]. The antiSMASH results were further analyzed using the BiG-SCAPE platform [78] to cluster the predicted BGCs into gene cluster families (GCFs) based on their sequences and Pfam protein family similarities [79]. BiG-SCAPE was conducted on global mode with default parameters [78], with the exception of the raw distance cutoff and the "–mix"parameter. Raw distance cutoff was set to 0.4 to ensure that even clusters with a pairwise distance higher than 0.3 (the default) were included in the output. The resulting network of BiG-SCAPE was visualized with Cytoscape version 3.7.2 [82].

3.6. Cultivation Conditions for Optimal Compound Production of Nine Indonesian Strains

To determine optimal cultivation conditions in liquid culture, the nine Indonesian actinomycetes strains, SHP 22-7, DHE 17-7, DHE 7-1, BSE 7-9, BSE 7F, I3, I4, I5, and I6, were each cultivated in 50 mL inoculum medium (NL410) in 500-mL Erlenmeyer flasks (with steel springs) in an orbital shaker (180 rpm) at 28 °C. After 48 h, 10 mL of preculture was inoculated into 100 mL of twelve different production medium (SGG, YM, OM, R5, MS, TSG, NL19, NL300, NL330, NL500, NL550, and NL800 (Table S2) and cultivated for 48–168 h. Cell culture samples were harvested at different time points (48, 72, 96, and 168 h). In addition, 5 mL of each cell culture sample was extracted with the same volume of ethyl acetate (EtOAc) for 30 min at room temperature. The EtOAc was dried in a rotary evaporator and suspended in a total volume of 0.75 mL methanol. The methanolic extracts were used for bioassay experiments. The culture extract samples, which yielded the largest zone of inhibition in the bioassays against the test organisms, were used for further compound identification analysis. To determine optimal cultivation conditions on solid culture, the nine Indonesian strains were each spread on 100 mL agar plates consisting of the respective abovementioned cultivation media and then incubated for 7–10 days at 28 °C until spore formation was visible on agar plates. The overgrown agar was then used for bioassay experiments and further compound identification analysis.

3.7. Sample Preparation for Chemical Identification

For chemical identification in the liquid sample, the nine Indonesian isolates were each cultivated in 50 mL of NL410 medium. After 48 h, 10 mL of the preculture was inoculated into 100 mL of optimal production medium. The 100 mL whole broth of each cell culture was extracted as described above. Then, the extracts were used for further experiment. For chemical identification from samples grown on solid medium, overgrown agar was cut into pieces and transferred to 50 mL Falcon tubes. The Falcon tubes were centrifuged at 13,000 rpm for 30 min at room temperature. The aqueous phase was concentrated to 1/5 of the original volume in the Genevac Centrifugal Evaporator EZ-2 Elite (SP Scientific). The concentrated aqueous phase was used for further chemical profiling.

The culture extract samples obtained from liquid medium extraction and the aqueous phase of the solid medium extraction were separated by solid-phase extraction (SPE) columns. The columns were washed twice with 2 mL methanol and 2 mL distilled water for activating the columns. The samples were prepared by adding 100% methanol to the culture extract samples and the aqueous phase until the samples were dissolved completely. The methanolic samples were applied onto the activated columns with a flow rate of 2 mL/min. The column was washed twice with distilled water. The column was eluted consecutively with 2 mL of 100% methanol, 50% methanol, and distilled water. Samples from the elution column were defined as fractions. The column was eluted with 100% methanol as the 100% fraction, with 50% methanol as the 50% fraction, and distilled water as the distilled water fraction. The fractions were dried in the Genevac EZ-2 Elite (SP Scientific) and then dissolved with 0.5 mL methanol. The crude extracts and all fractions were analyzed with HPLC and high-resolution mass spectrometry (HRMS).

3.8. HPLC-HRMS/MS Analysis

The HRMS analysis was carried out on MaXis 4G instrument (Bruker Daltonics, Bremen, Germany) coupled to an Ultimate 3000 HPLC (Thermo Fisher Scientific, Bremen, Germany). HPLC-method was applied as follows: the spectrometer using a gradient (solvent A: 0.1% formic acid (FA) in H_2O, and solvent B: 0.06% formic acid in acetonitrile), a gradient of 10–100% B in 45 min, 100% B for an additional 10 min, using a flow rate of 0.3 mL/min; 5 μL injection volume and UV detector (UV/VIS) wavelength monitoring at 210, 254, 280, and 360 nm. The separation was carried out on a Nucleoshell 2.7 μm 150 × 2 mm column (Macherey-Nagel, Düren, Germany), and the range for MS acquisition was *m/z* 100–1800. A capillary voltage of 4500 V, nebulizer gas pressure (nitrogen) of 2 (1.6) bar, ion source temperature of 200 °C, the dry gas flow of 9 (7) l/min source temperature, and spectral rates of 3 Hz for MS1 and 10 Hz for MS^2 were used. For acquiring MS/MS fragmentation, the ten most intense ions per MS1 were selected for subsequent collision-induced dissociation (CID) with stepped CID energy applied. The employed parameters for tandem MS were applied as previously detailed by Garg et al. in 2015 [123]. Sodium formate was used as an internal calibrant and Hexakis (2,2-difluoroethoxy) phosphazene (Apollo Scientific Ltd., Stockport, UK) as the lock mass. Data processing was performed using Bruker Daltonics Data Analysis 4.1(Bremen, Germany).

3.9. MS/MS Molecular Networking

Mass-spectral data were analyzed using Compass Data Analysis 4.4 (Bruker Daltonik, Bremen, Germany), whereas MetaboScape 3.0 (Bruker Daltonik, Bremen, Germany) was consulted for molecular features selection. Raw data files were imported into MetaboScape 3.0 for the entire data treatment and preprocessing in which T-ReX 3D (time-aligned region complete extraction) algorithm is integrated for retention time alignment with an automatic detection to decompose fragments, isotopes, and adducts intrinsic to the same compound into one single feature. All the harvested ions were categorized as a bucket table with their corresponding retention times, measured *m/z*, molecular weights, detected ions, and their intensity within the sample. The Bucket table was prepared with an intensity threshold (1e3) for the positive measurements with a minimum peak length 3, possessing a mass range of 150–1800 Da. For detailed parameters employed for the MetaboScape analysis, see Table S13. The features list of the preprocessed retention time range was exported from MetaboScape as a single MGF file, which was in turn uploaded to the GNPS online platform where a feature-based molecular network (FBMN) was created. The precursor ion mass tolerance was set to 0.03 Da and a MS/MS fragment ion tolerance of 0.03 Da. A network was then created where edges were filtered to have a cosine score above 0.70 and more than 5 matched peaks. Further, edges between two nodes were kept in the network if and only if each of the nodes appeared in each other's respective top 10 most similar nodes. Finally, the maximum size of a molecular family was set to 100, and the lowest-scoring edges were removed from molecular families until the molecular family size was below this threshold. Cytoscape 3.5.1 was used for molecular network visualization.

4. Conclusions

In this study, we report on the isolation of 422 actinomycetes strains from three different unique areas in Indonesia. A combined genomics and metabolomics approach was applied to nine of the most potent antibiotic producer strains, which allowed us to uncover 16 so far unknown compounds. When cultivating the strains in various liquid and solid media, we found that culture conditions significantly affected the ability to produce specific compounds. Thus, the combination of both cultivation methods, solid and liquid cultivation, is a suitable approach to tap the full biosynthetic potential of actinomycetes.

By phylogeny-associated genome mining studies, we found that phylogenetically related species tend to have a similar BGC composition. Additional metabolomics data suggested that the ability of the strains to produce certain compounds may be influenced by the environmental conditions, where the producer strains have been derived from.

Overall, the described methodology represents an efficient strategy for drug discovery and the reported unknown compounds may serve as a basis for further drug development.

Supplementary Materials: The following are available online at https://www.mdpi.com/article/10.3390/md19060316/s1, Figure S1. Actinomycin D production in DHE 6-7 (a) and DHE 5-1 (b). Peaks in HPLC representing actinomycin are marked with red colour. Mass spectra of actinomycin D detected in DHE 6-7 (c); Figure S2. Positive extracted ion chromatograms (EICs), ions cluster and predicted molecular formula of antimycins; Figure S3. GNPS spectral libraries hits of antimycins; Figure S4. Positive MS2 spectra of the detected antimycins from isolate BSE7F; Figure S5. Negative EICs and predicted molecular formulae of antimycins; Figure S6. Negative MS2 spectra of the detected antimycins from isolate BSE7F; Figure S7. Ions cluster of ferrioxamines and GNPS spectral libraries hit of ferrioxamine D1; Figure S8. Positive EICs and molecular formula prediction of ferrioxamine D1; Figure S9. Positive EICs, molecular formula prediction and MS2 of an unknown ferrioxamine; Figure S10. Positive EICs and MS1 of unknown amphiphilic ferrioxamines; Figure S11. Positive EICs and MS2 of DHE 17-7 ferrioxamines; Figure S12. Ions cluster of staurosporines and GNPS spectral libraries hit of staurosporine; Figure S13. Ions clusters of echinoserine; Figure S14. Ion singleton of depsiechinoserine, positive EICs and MS2 of depsiechinoserine; Figure S15. Positive EICs and MS1 of echinomycin; Figure S16. Ions cluster, Positive EICs and MS1 of tirandamycin A in addition to its congeners; Figure S17. UV absorbance, and MS2 of tirandamycin A in addition to its congeners; Figure S18. Ion cluster of naphthyridinomycins and their predicted molecular formula (MF); Figure S19. Positive EICs and MS2 of naphthyridinomycin and their related entities from isolate BSE7-9; Figure S20. Positive EICs and MS1 of naphthyridinomycin from isolates BSE7-9 and I5; Figure S21. Positive EICs and MS1 of aclidinomycin A from isolates BSE7-9 and I5; Figure S22. Positive EICs and MS1 of bioxalomycin-β2 from isolates BSE7-9 and I5; Figure S23. Ions cluster of ECO-0501 and its related congeners from isolate DHE 17-7; Figure S24. UV absorbance, MS2 of ECO-0501 and its related congeners from isolate DHE 17-7; Figure S25. Comparative positive MS2 of ECO-0501 from isolate DHE 17-7 and its reported version from Amycolatopsis orientalis; Figure S26. Negative MS2 of ECO-0501 from isolate DHE 17-7 and its proposed fragmentation scheme; Figure S27. Ions cluster of amicetins and its related congeners from isolate SHP 22-7; Figure 28. Comparative positive MS2 of amicetin and streptocytosin A; Figure S29. Comparative negative MS2 of amicetin and streptocytosin A; Figure S30. Comparative positive MS2 of some unknown members of amicetin molecular family; Figure S31. Comparative positive MS2 of some unknowns of likely peptides; Figure S32. Comparative positive MS2 of some unknowns from isolate SHP 22-7; Figure S33. Comparative positive MS2 of some unknowns from isolate DHE 17-7; Figure S34. Cluster similarity between the DHE 17-7 gene region 24 (query sequence) and the streptovaricin, sceliphrolactam and vicenistatin cluster; Table S1. Genome characteristics from nine Indonesian actinomycetes strain isolates; Table S2. media tested for antibiotic production in agar and liquid culture. All data refer to 1 l H2Odeion. For solid media 16 g/l agar is added, except for R5 medium 18 g/l agar is added; Table S3. List of optimal culture conditions (media, time point) and bioactivity profile of nine Indonesian strain isolates; Table S4. List of predicted BGCs of strain DHE 17-7 derived from antiSMASH analysis. The minus sign (-) indicates the BGC did not have any similarity with any BGCs in the antiSMASH database; Table S5. List of predicted BGCs of strain SHP22-7 derived from antiSMASH analysis. The minus sign (-) indicates the BGC did not have any similarity with any BGCs in the antiSMASH database; Table S6. List of predicted BGCs of strain I3 derived from antiSMASH analysis. The minus sign (-) indicates the BGC did not have any similarity with any BGCs in the antiSMASH database; Table S7. List of predicted BGCs of strain I4 derived from antiSMASH analysis. The minus sign (-) indicates the BGC did not have any similarity with any BGCs in the antiSMASH database; Table S8. List of predicted BGCs of strain I5 derived from antiSMASH analysis. The minus sign (-) indicates the BGC did not have any similarity with any BGCs in the antiSMASH database; Table S9. List of predicted BGCs of strain BSE 7F derived from antiSMASH analysis. The minus sign (-) indicates the BGC did not have any similarity with any BGCs in the antiSMASH database; Table S10. List of predicted BGCs of strain BSE 7-9 derived from antiSMASH analysis. The minus sign (-) indicates the BGC did not have any similarity with any BGCs in the antiSMASH database; Table S11. List of predicted BGCs of strain DHE 7-1 derived from antiSMASH analysis. The minus sign (-) indicates the BGC did not have any similarity with any BGCs in the antiSMASH database; Table S12. List of predicted BGCs of strain I6 derived from antiSMASH analysis. The minus sign (-) indicates the BGC did not have any similarity with any BGCs in the antiSMASH database; Table S13. Parameters used in MetaboScape analysis;

Author Contributions: S.R. and S.A. isolated strains and performed preliminary bioassays; I.H. carried out phylogenetic analysis and antibiotic bioassays; I.H. and J.K. performed extraction of culture broths; A.K. and H.S. carried out HPLC-MS analysis, H.S. performed GNPS studies; I.H. and Y.M. performed genome-sequence-based bioinformatic analysis, A.G. performed BiG-SCAPE analysis; Y.M. and H.G. conceived the research. Y.M., W.W., H.G., P.L., W.K., and N.Z. supervised the work. I.H. wrote the original draft of paper, which was revised by Y.M., W.W., H.G., P.L., W.K., and N.Z. and approved by all authors. All authors have read and agreed to the published version of the manuscript.

Funding: We gratefully acknowledge the funding received from the BMBF German–Indonesian cooperation project NAbaUnAk (16GW0124K) and the German Center for Infection Research (DZIF) (TTU 09.811). I.H. is grateful for the RISET-Pro scholarship program from the Indonesian Ministry for Research and Technology (World Bank Loan No. 8245-ID). A.G. is grateful for the support of the Deutsche Forschungsgemeinschaft (DFG; Project ID # 398967434-TRR 261). S.A. is grateful for his Ph.D. scholarships (grant PKZ 91613866), generously provided by the German Academic Exchange Service (DAAD).

Institutional Review Board Statement: Not applicable.

Informed Consent Statement: Not applicable.

Data Availability Statement: The complete genomes sequence data were deposited at the National Center for Biotechnology (NCBI) information data base, https://www.ncbi.nlm.nih.gov/genome (29 December 2020 for all, except SHP 22-7 (7 September 2018) and BSE 7F (4 May 2018)) with the accession numbers QEQV00000000 for BSE 7F, QXMM00000000 for SHP 22-7, SAMN15691494 for DHE 7-1, SAMN15691533 for I3, SAMN15691540 for I4, SAMN15691656 for I5, SAMN15691724 for BSE 7-9, SAMN15692265 for DHE 17-7, and RHDP00000000 for I6. GNPS job data: https://gnps.ucsd.edu/ProteoSAFe/status.jsp?task=429506a1cc2c4a679b421cc455c0249b (accessed on 12 March 2021).

Acknowledgments: We thank R. Ort-Winklbauer for technical assistance and Dorothee Wistuba for support in HRMS experiments, and the Ministry of Research and Technology, Republic of Indonesia for the RISET-Pro Scholarship support of I.H. (World Bank Loan No. 8245-ID).

Conflicts of Interest: The authors declare no conflict of interest. The funders had no role in the design of the study; in the collection, analyses, or interpretation of data; in the writing of the manuscript, or in the decision to publish the results.

References

1. Waksman, S.A.; Woodruff, H.B. The Soil as a Source of Microorganisms Antagonistic to Disease-Producing Bacteria. *J. Bacteriol.* **1940**, *40*, 581–600. [CrossRef]
2. Kresge, N.; Simoni, R.D.; Hill, R.L. Selman Waksman: The Father of Antibiotics. *J. Biol. Chem.* **2004**, *279*, e7–e8. [CrossRef]
3. van Bergeijk, D.A.; Terlouw, B.R.; Medema, M.H.; van Wezel, G.P. Ecology and genomics of Actinobacteria: New concepts for natural product discovery. *Nat. Rev. Microbiol.* **2020**, *18*, 1–13. [CrossRef]
4. Newman, D.J.; Cragg, G.M. Natural Products as Sources of New Drugs over the Nearly Four Decades from 01/1981 to 09/2019. *J. Nat. Prod.* **2020**, *83*, 770–803. [CrossRef] [PubMed]
5. van der Heul, H.U.; Bilyk, B.L.; McDowall, K.J.; Seipke, R.F.; van Wezel, G.P. Regulation of antibiotic production in Actinobacteria: New perspectives from the post-genomic era. *Nat. Prod. Rep.* **2018**, *35*, 575–604. [CrossRef] [PubMed]
6. Baltz, R. Antibiotic discovery from actinomycetes: Will a renaissance follow the decline and fall? *SIM News* **2005**, *55*, 186–196.
7. Bérdy, J. Bioactive Microbial Metabolites. *J. Antibiot.* **2005**, *58*, 1–26. [CrossRef]
8. Baltz, R.H. Natural product drug discovery in the genomic era: Realities, conjectures, misconceptions, and opportunities. *J. Ind. Microbiol. Biotechnol.* **2019**, *46*, 281–299. [CrossRef]
9. Hug, J.J.; Bader, C.D.; Remškar, M.; Cirnski, K.; Müller, R. Concepts and methods to access novel antibiotics from actinomycetes. *Antibiotics* **2018**, *7*, 44. [CrossRef]
10. Sivalingam, P.; Hong, K.; Pote, J.; Prabakar, K. Extreme Environment *Streptomyces*: Potential Sources for New Antibacterial and Anticancer Drug Leads? *Int. J. Microbiol.* **2019**, *2019*, 5283948. [CrossRef]

11. Manivasagan, P.; Venkatesan, J.; Sivakumar, K. Pharmaceutically active secondary metabolites of marine. *Microbiol. Res.* **2014**, *169*, 262–278. [CrossRef]
12. Abdelkader, M.S.A.; Philippon, T.; Asenjo, J.A.; Bull, A.T.; Goodfellow, M.; Ebel, R.; Jaspars, M.; Rateb, M.E. Asenjonamides A-C, antibacterial metabolites isolated from *Streptomyces asenjonii* strain KNN 42.f from an extreme-hyper arid Atacama Desert soil. *J. Antibiot.* **2018**, *71*, 425–431. [CrossRef]
13. Lacret, R.; Oves-Costales, D.; Gómez, C.; Díaz, C.; De La Cruz, M.; Pérez-Victoria, I.; Vicente, F.; Genilloud, O.; Reyes, F. New ikarugamycin derivatives with antifungal and antibacterial properties from *Streptomyces Zhaozhouensis*. *Mar. Drugs* **2015**, *13*, 128–140. [CrossRef]
14. Zhang, F.; Zhao, M.; Braun, D.R.; Ericksen, S.S.; Piotrowski, J.S.; Nelson, J.; Peng, J.; Ananiev, G.E.; Chanana, S.; Barns, K.; et al. A marine microbiome antifungal targets urgent-threat drug-resistant fungi. *Science* **2020**, *370*, 974–978. [CrossRef] [PubMed]
15. Singh, S.B.; Pelaez, F. Biodiversity, chemical diversity and drug discovery. *Prog. Drug Res.* **2008**, *65*, 141, 143–174. [CrossRef] [PubMed]
16. Huffard, C.L.; Erdmann, M.V.; Gunawan, T. *Geographic Priorities for Marine Biodiversity Conservation in Indonesia*; Ministry of Marine Affairs and Fisheries and Marine Protected Areas Governance Program: Jakarta, Indonesia, 2012; ISBN 978-602-98450-6-8. Available online: https://www.coraltriangleinitiative.org/sites/default/files/resources/8_Geographic%20Priorities%20for%20Marine%20Biodiversity%20Conservation%20in%20Indonesia.pdf (accessed on 28 May 2021).
17. Convention on Biological Diversity Biodiversity Facts: Status and trends of biodiversity, including benefits from biodiversity and ecosystem services. Available online: https://www.cbd.int/countries/profile/?country=id (accessed on 20 January 2021).
18. von Rintelen, K.; Arida, E.; Häuser, C. A review of biodiversity-related issues and challenges in megadiverse Indonesia and other Southeast Asian countries. *Res. Ideas Outcomes* **2017**, *3*, e20860. [CrossRef]
19. De Bruyn, M.; Stelbrink, B.; Morley, R.J.; Hall, R.; Carvalho, G.R.; Cannon, C.H.; Van Den Bergh, G.; Meijaard, E.; Metcalfe, I.; Boitani, L.; et al. Borneo and Indochina are major evolutionary hotspots for Southeast Asian biodiversity. *Syst. Biol.* **2014**, *63*, 879–901. [CrossRef]
20. Lohman, D.J.; de Bruyn, M.; Page, T.; von Rintelen, K.; Hall, R.; Ng, P.K.L.; Shih, H.-T.; Carvalho, G.R.; von Rintelen, T. Biogeography of the Indo-Australian Archipelago. *Annu. Rev. Ecol. Evol. Syst.* **2011**, *42*, 205–226. [CrossRef]
21. Aditiawati, P.; Yohandini, H.; Madayanti, F. Akhmaloka Microbial diversity of acidic hot spring (kawah hujan B) in geothermal field of kamojang area, west java-indonesia. *Open Microbiol. J.* **2009**, *3*, 58–66. [CrossRef]
22. Liu, B.; Talukder, M.J.H.; Terhonen, E.; Lampela, M.; Vasander, H.; Sun, H.; Asiegbu, F. The microbial diversity and structure in peatland forest in Indonesia. *Soil Use Manag.* **2020**, *36*, 123–138. [CrossRef]
23. De Voogd, N.J.; Cleary, D.F.R.; Pol, A.R.M.; Gomes, N.C.M. Bacterial community composition and predicted functional ecology of sponges, sediment and seawater from the thousand islands reef complex, West Java, Indonesia. *FEMS Microbiol. Ecol.* **2015**, *91*, 1–12. [CrossRef]
24. Kanti, A.; Sumerta, I.N. Diversity of Xylose Assimilating Yeast From the Island of Enggano, Sumatera, Indonesia [Keragaman Khamir Pengguna Xilose Yang Diisolasi Dari Pulau Enggano, Sumatera, Indonesia]. *Ber. Biol.* **2016**, *15*. [CrossRef]
25. Hennersdorf, P.; Kleinertz, S.; Theisen, S.; Abdul-Aziz, M.A.; Mrotzek, G.; Palm, H.W.; Saluz, H.P. Microbial diversity and parasitic load in tropical fish of different environmental conditions. *PLoS ONE* **2016**, *11*, e0151594. [CrossRef]
26. Zam, S.I.; Agustien, A.; Djamaan, A.; Mustafa, I. The Diversity of Endophytic Bacteria from the Traditional Medicinal Plants Leaves that Have Anti-phytopathogens Activity. *J. Trop. Life Sci.* **2019**, *9*, 53–63. [CrossRef]
27. Baltz, R.H. Gifted microbes for genome mining and natural product discovery. *J. Ind. Microbiol. Biotechnol.* **2017**, *44*, 573–588. [CrossRef] [PubMed]
28. Romano, S.; Jackson, S.A.; Patry, S.; Dobson, A.D.W. Extending the "one strain many compounds" (OSMAC) principle to marine microorganisms. *Mar. Drugs* **2018**, *16*, 244. [CrossRef] [PubMed]
29. Krause, J.; Handayani, I.; Blin, K.; Kulik, A.; Mast, Y. Disclosing the Potential of the SARP-Type Regulator PapR2 for the Activation of Antibiotic Gene Clusters in Streptomycetes. *Front. Microbiol.* **2020**, *11*, 225. [CrossRef]
30. Bode, H.B.; Bethe, B.; Höfs, R.; Zeeck, A. Big effects from small changes: Possible ways to explore nature's chemical diversity. *ChemBioChem* **2002**, *3*, 619–627. [CrossRef]
31. Pan, R.; Bai, X.; Chen, J.; Zhang, H.; Wang, H.; Aon, J.C. Exploring Structural Diversity of Microbe Secondary Metabolites Using OSMAC Strategy: A Literature Review. *Front. Microbiol.* **2019**, *10*, 1–20. [CrossRef]
32. Wu, C.; van der Heul, H.U.; Melnik, A.V.; Lübben, J.; Dorrestein, P.C.; Minnaard, A.J.; Choi, Y.H.; van Wezel, G.P. Lugdunomycin, an Angucycline-Derived Molecule with Unprecedented Chemical Architecture. *Angew. Chem. Int. Ed.* **2019**, *58*, 2809–2814. [CrossRef]
33. Hussain, A.; Rather, M.A.; Dar, M.S.; Aga, M.A.; Ahmad, N.; Manzoor, A.; Qayum, A.; Shah, A.; Mushtaq, S.; Ahmad, Z.; et al. Novel bioactive molecules from *Lentzea violacea* strain AS 08 using one strain-many compounds (OSMAC) approach. *Bioorganic Med. Chem. Lett.* **2017**, *27*, 2579–2582. [CrossRef]
34. Zhang, C.; Seyedsayamdost, M.R. Discovery of a Cryptic Depsipeptide from *Streptomyces ghanaensis* via MALDI-MS-Guided High-Throughput Elicitor Screening. *Angew. Chem. Int. Ed.* **2020**, *59*, 23005–23009. [CrossRef] [PubMed]
35. Genilloud, O. Current challenges in the discovery of novel antibacterials from microbial natural products. *Recent Pat. Antiinfect. Drug Discov.* **2012**, *7*, 189–204. [CrossRef] [PubMed]
36. Beutler, J.A. Natural Products as a Foundation for Drug Discovery. *Curr. Protoc. Pharmacol.* **2009**, *46*, 9.11.1–9.11.21. [CrossRef]

37. Wohlleben, W.; Mast, Y.; Stegmann, E.; Ziemert, N. Antibiotic drug discovery. *Microb. Biotechnol.* **2016**, *9*, 541–548. [CrossRef] [PubMed]
38. Maansson, M.; Vynne, N.G.; Klitgaard, A.; Nybo, J.L.; Melchiorsen, J.; Nguyen, D.D.; Sanchez, L.M.; Ziemert, N.; Dorrestein, P.C.; Andersen, M.R.; et al. An Integrated Metabolomic and Genomic Mining Workflow To Uncover the Biosynthetic Potential of Bacteria. *mSystems* **2016**, *1*, e00028-15. [CrossRef]
39. Ong, J.F.M.; Goh, H.C.; Lim, S.C.; Pang, L.M.; Chin, J.S.F.; Tan, K.S.; Liang, Z.-X.; Yang, L.; Glukhov, E.; Gerwick, W.H.; et al. Integrated Genomic and Metabolomic Approach to the Discovery of Potential Anti-Quorum Sensing Natural Products from Microbes Associated with Marine Samples from Singapore. *Mar. Drugs* **2019**, *17*, 72. [CrossRef]
40. Tiam, S.K.; Gugger, M.; Demay, J.; Le Manach, S.; Duval, C.; Bernard, C.; Marie, B. Insights into the diversity of secondary metabolites of Planktothrix using a biphasic approach combining global genomics and metabolomics. *Toxins* **2019**, *11*, 498. [CrossRef]
41. Amiri Moghaddam, J.; Crüsemann, M.; Alanjary, M.; Harms, H.; Dávila-Céspedes, A.; Blom, J.; Poehlein, A.; Ziemert, N.; König, G.M.; Schäberle, T.F. Analysis of the Genome and Metabolome of Marine Myxobacteria Reveals High Potential for Biosynthesis of Novel Specialized Metabolites. *Sci. Rep.* **2018**, *8*, 16600. [CrossRef]
42. Albarano, L.; Esposito, R.; Ruocco, N.; Costantini, M. Genome mining as new challenge in natural products discovery. *Mar. Drugs* **2020**, *18*, 199. [CrossRef]
43. Ward, A.C.; Allenby, N.E.E. Genome mining for the search and discovery of bioactive compounds: The *Streptomyces* paradigm. *FEMS Microbiol. Lett.* **2018**, *365*, fny240. [CrossRef]
44. Blin, K.; Shaw, S.; Steinke, K.; Villebro, R.; Ziemert, N.; Lee, Y.; Medema, M.H.; Weber, T. antiSMASH 5.0: Updates to the secondary metabolite genome mining pipeline. *Nucleic Acid. Res.* **2019**, *47*, 81–87. [CrossRef] [PubMed]
45. Wang, M.; Carver, J.J.; Phelan, V.V.; Sanchez, L.M.; Garg, N.; Peng, Y.; Nguyen, D.D.; Watrous, J.; Kapono, C.A.; Luzzatto-Knaan, T.; et al. Sharing and community curation of mass spectrometry data with Global Natural Products Social Molecular Networking. *Nat. Biotechnol.* **2016**, *34*, 828–837. [CrossRef] [PubMed]
46. Yang, J.Y.; Sanchez, L.M.; Rath, C.M.; Liu, X.; Boudreau, P.D.; Bruns, N.; Glukhov, E.; Wodtke, A.; De Felicio, R.; Fenner, A.; et al. Molecular Networking as a Dereplication Strategy. *J. Nat. Prod.* **2013**, *76*, 1686–1699. [CrossRef]
47. Sieber, S.; Grendelmeier, S.M.; Harris, L.A.; Mitchell, D.A.; Gademann, K. Microviridin 1777: A Toxic Chymotrypsin Inhibitor Discovered by a Metabologenomic Approach. *J. Nat. Prod.* **2020**, *83*, 438–446. [CrossRef] [PubMed]
48. Hayakawa, M.; Nonomura, H. Efficacy of artificial humic acid as a selective nutrient in HV agar used for the isolation of soil actinomycetes. *J. Ferment. Technol.* **1987**, *65*, 609–616. [CrossRef]
49. Hamada, M.; Lino, T.; Tamura, T.; Iwami, T.; Harayama, S.; Suzuki, K.I. *Serinibacter salmoneus* gen. nov., sp. nov., an actinobacterium isolated from the intestinal tract of a fish, and emended descriptions of the families Beutenbergiaceae and Bogoriellaceae. *Int. J. Syst. Evol. Microbiol.* **2009**, *59*, 2809–2814. [CrossRef]
50. Hamada, M.; Shibata, C.; Nurkanto, A.; Ratnakomala, S.; Lisdiyanti, P.; Tamura, T.; Suzuki, K.I. *Serinibacter tropicus* sp. nov., an actinobacterium isolated from the rhizosphere of a mangrove, and emended description of the genus Serinibacter. *Int. J. Syst. Evol. Microbiol.* **2015**, *65*, 1151–1154. [CrossRef]
51. Hayakawa, M.; Sadakata, T.; Kajiura, T.; Nonomura, H. New methods for the highly selective isolation of Micromonospora and Microbispora from soil. *J. Ferment. Bioeng.* **1991**, *72*, 320–326. [CrossRef]
52. Shirling, E.B.; Gottlieb, D. Methods for characterization of *Streptomyces* species. *Int. J. Syst. Bacteriol.* **1966**, *16*, 313–340. [CrossRef]
53. Grismer, L.L.; Riyanto, A.; Iskandar, D.T.; Mcguire, J.A. A new species of *Hemiphyllodactylus Bleeker*, 1860 (Squamata: Gekkonidae) from Pulau Enggano, southwestern Sumatra, Indonesia. *Zootaxa* **2014**, *3821*, 485–495. [CrossRef] [PubMed]
54. Jakl, S. New cetoniine beetle from Enggano and Simeuleu Islands west of Sumatra (Coleoptera: Scarabaeidae: Cetoniinae). *Stud. Rep. Dist. Museum Prague-East Taxon. Ser.* **2008**, *4*, 103–110.
55. Yoon, S.H.; Ha, S.M.; Kwon, S.; Lim, J.; Kim, Y.; Seo, H.; Chun, J. Introducing EzBioCloud: A taxonomically united database of 16S rRNA gene sequences and whole-genome assemblies. *Int. J. Syst. Evol. Microbiol.* **2017**, *67*, 1613–1617. [CrossRef] [PubMed]
56. Shetty, P.R.; Buddana, S.K.; Tatipamula, V.B.; Naga, Y.V.V.; Ahmad, J. Production of polypeptide antibiotic from *Streptomyces parvulus* and its antibacterial activity. *Braz. J. Microbiol.* **2014**, *45*, 303–312. [CrossRef]
57. Handayani, I.; Ratnakomala, S.; Lisdiyanti, P.; Fahrurrozi; Kusharyoto, W.; Alanjary, M.; Ort-Winklbauer, R.; Kulik, A.; Wohlleben, W.; Mast, Y. Complete Genome Sequence of *Streptomyces* sp. Strain SHP22-7, a New Species Isolated from Mangrove of Enggano Island, Indonesia. *Microbiol. Resour. Announc.* **2018**, *7*, e01317-18. [CrossRef]
58. Handayani, I.; Ratnakomala, S.; Lisdiyanti, P.; Fahrurrozi; Alanjary, M.; Wohlleben, W.; Mast, Y. Complete genome sequence of *Streptomyces* sp. strain BSE7F, a Bali mangrove sediment actinobacterium with antimicrobial activities. *Genome Announc.* **2018**, *6*, e00618-18. [CrossRef] [PubMed]
59. Krause, J.; Ratnakomala, S.; Lisdiyanti, P.; Ort-Winklbauer, R.; Wohlleben, W.; Mast, Y. Complete Genome Sequence of the Putative Phosphonate Producer *Streptomyces* sp. Strain I6, Isolated from Indonesian Mangrove Sediment. *Microbiol. Resour. Announc.* **2019**, *8*, e01580-18. [CrossRef]
60. Tidjani, A.R.; Lorenzi, J.N.; Toussaint, M.; Van Dijk, E.; Naquin, D.; Lespinet, O.; Bontemps, C.; Leblond, P. Massive gene flux drives genome diversity between sympatric *Streptomyces* conspecifics. *MBio* **2019**, *10*, 1–12. [CrossRef] [PubMed]

61. Subramaniam, G.; Thakur, V.; Saxena, R.K.; Vadlamudi, S.; Purohit, S.; Kumar, V.; Rathore, A.; Chitikineni, A.; Varshney, R.K. Complete genome sequence of sixteen plant growth promoting *Streptomyces* strains. *Sci. Rep.* **2020**, *10*, 10294. [CrossRef] [PubMed]
62. Ventura, M.; Canchaya, C.; Tauch, A.; Chandra, G.; Fitzgerald, G.F.; Chater, K.F.; van Sinderen, D. Genomics of Actinobacteria: Tracing the Evolutionary History of an Ancient Phylum. *Microbiol. Mol. Biol. Rev.* **2007**, *71*, 495–548. [CrossRef]
63. Meier-Kolthoff, J.P.; Göker, M. TYGS is an automated high-throughput platform for state-of-the-art genome-based taxonomy. *Nat. Commun.* **2019**, *10*, 2182. [CrossRef]
64. Meier-kolthoff, J.P.; Klenk, H.; Go, M. Taxonomic use of DNA G + C content and DNA–DNA hybridization in the genomic age. *Int. J. Syst. Evol. Microbiol.* **2014**, *64*, 352–356. [CrossRef] [PubMed]
65. Tindall, B.J.; Rosselló-Móra, R.; Busse, H.J.; Ludwig, W.; Kämpfer, P. Notes on the characterization of prokaryote strains for taxonomic purposes. *Int. J. Syst. Evol. Microbiol.* **2010**, *60*, 249–266. [CrossRef] [PubMed]
66. Meier-Kolthoff, J.P.; Auch, A.F.; Klenk, H.-P.; Göker, M. Genome sequence-based species delimitation with confidence intervals and improved distance functions. *BMC Bioinform.* **2013**, *14*, 60. [CrossRef]
67. Luo, X.X.; Kai, L.; Wang, Y.; Wan, C.X.; Zhang, L.L. *Streptomyces luteus* sp. nov., an actinomycete isolated from soil. *Int. J. Syst. Evol. Microbiol.* **2017**, *67*, 543–547. [CrossRef] [PubMed]
68. Mertz, F.P.; Higgens, C.E. *Streptomyces capillispiralis* sp. nov. *Int. J. Syst. Bacteriol.* **1982**, *32*, 116–124. [CrossRef]
69. Eguchi, T.; Takada, N.; Nakamura, S.; Tanaka, T.; Makino, T.; Oshima, Y. *Streptomyces bungoensis* sp. nov. *Int. J. Syst. Bacteriol.* **1993**, *43*, 794–798. [CrossRef]
70. Huang, X.; Zhou, S.; Huang, D.; Chen, J.; Zhu, W. *Streptomyces spongiicola* sp. Nov., An actinomycete derived from marine sponge. *Int. J. Syst. Evol. Microbiol.* **2016**, *66*, 738–743. [CrossRef] [PubMed]
71. Belknap, K.C.; Park, C.J.; Barth, B.M.; Andam, C.P. Genome mining of biosynthetic and chemotherapeutic gene clusters in *Streptomyces* bacteria. *Sci. Rep.* **2020**, *10*, 1–9. [CrossRef]
72. Yamanaka, K.; Oikawa, H.; Ogawa, H.O.; Hosono, K.; Shinmachi, F.; Takano, H.; Sakuda, S.; Beppu, T.; Ueda, K. Desferrioxamine E produced by *Streptomyces griseus* stimulates growth and development of *Streptomyces tanashiensis*. *Microbiology* **2005**, *151*, 2899–2905. [CrossRef] [PubMed]
73. Poralla, K.; Muth, G.; Härtner, T. Hopanoids are formed during transition from substrate to aerial hyphae in *Streptomyces coelicolor* A3(2). *FEMS Microbiol. Lett.* **2000**, *189*, 93–95. [CrossRef]
74. Chater, K.F.; Biró, S.; Lee, K.J.; Palmer, T.; Schrempf, H. The complex extracellular biology of *Streptomyces*. *FEMS Microbiol. Rev.* **2010**, *34*, 171–198. [CrossRef]
75. Waksman, S.A.; Lechevalier, H.A.; Schaffner, C.P. Candicidin and other polyenic antifungal antibiotics. *Bull. World Health Organ.* **1965**, *33*, 219. [PubMed]
76. Tierrafría, V.H.; Ramos-Aboites, H.E.; Gosset, G.; Barona-Gómez, F. Disruption of the siderophore-binding desE receptor gene in *Streptomyces coelicolor* A3(2) results in impaired growth in spite of multiple iron-siderophore transport systems. *Microb. Biotechnol.* **2011**, *4*, 275–285. [CrossRef]
77. van der Meij, A.; Worsley, S.F.; Hutchings, M.I.; van Wezel, G.P. Chemical ecology of antibiotic production by actinomycetes. *FEMS Microbiol. Rev.* **2017**, *41*, 392–416. [CrossRef]
78. Navarro-Muñoz, J.C.; Selem-Mojica, N.; Mullowney, M.W.; Kautsar, S.; Tryon, J.H.; Parkinson, E.I.; De Los Santos, E.L.C.; Yeong, M.; Cruz-Morales, P.; Abubucker, S.; et al. A computational framework for systematic exploration of biosynthetic diversity from large-scale genomic data. *bioRxiv* **2018**, 445270. [CrossRef]
79. El-Gebali, S.; Mistry, J.; Bateman, A.; Eddy, S.R.; Luciani, A.; Potter, S.C.; Qureshi, M.; Richardson, L.J.; Salazar, G.A.; Smart, A.; et al. The Pfam protein families database in 2019. *Nucleic Acids Res.* **2019**, *47*, D427–D432. [CrossRef]
80. Yagüe, P.; Lopez-Garcia, M.T.; Rioseras, B.; Sanchez, J.; Manteca, A. New insights on the development of *Streptomyces* and their relationships with secondary metabolite production. *Curr. Trends Microbiol.* **2012**, *8*, 65–73. [PubMed]
81. Kieser, T.; Bibb, M.J.; Buttner, M.J.; Chater, K.F.; Hopwood, D.A. *Practical Streptomyces Genetics*; The John Innes Foundation: Norwich, UK, 2000; ISBN 0708406238.
82. Shannon, P.; Markiel, A.; Ozier, O.; Baliga, N.S.; Wang, J.T.; Ramage, D.; Amin, N.; Schwikowski, B.; Ideker, T. Cytoscape: A software environment for integrated models of biomolecular interaction networks. *Genome Res.* **2003**, *13*, 2498–2504. [CrossRef]
83. Dührkop, K.; Shen, H.; Meusel, M.; Rousu, J.; Böcker, S. Searching molecular structure databases with tandem mass spectra using CSI:FingerID. *Proc. Natl. Acad. Sci. USA* **2015**, *112*, 12580–12585. [CrossRef]
84. Böcker, S.; Dührkop, K. Fragmentation trees reloaded. *J. Cheminform.* **2016**, *8*, 5. [CrossRef] [PubMed]
85. van Tamelen, E.E.; Dickie, J.P.; Loomans, M.E.; Dewey, R.S.; Strong, F.M. The Chemistry of Antimycin A. X. Structure of the Antimycins1. *J. Am. Chem. Soc.* **1961**, *83*, 1639–1646. [CrossRef]
86. Barrow, C.J.; Oleynek, J.J.; Marinelli, V.; Sun, H.H.; Kaplita, P.; Sedlock, D.M.; Gillum, A.M.; Chadwick, C.C.; Cooper, R. Antimycins, inhibitors of ATP-citrate lyase, from a *Streptomyces* sp. *J. Antibiot.* **1997**, *50*, 729–733. [CrossRef]
87. Hosotani, N.; Kumagai, K.; Nakagawa, H.; Shimatani, T.; Saji, I. Antimycins A10∼A16, Seven New Antimycin Antibiotics Produced by *Streptomyces* spp. SPA-10191 and SPA-8893. *J. Antibiot.* **2005**, *58*, 460–467. [CrossRef]
88. Sidebottom, A.M.; Johnson, A.R.; Karty, J.A.; Trader, D.J.; Carlson, E.E. Integrated Metabolomics Approach Facilitates Discovery of an Unpredicted Natural Product Suite from *Streptomyces coelicolor* M145. *ACS Chem. Biol.* **2013**, *8*, 2009–2016. [CrossRef] [PubMed]

89. Traxler, M.F.; Watrous, J.D.; Alexandrov, T.; Dorrestein, P.C.; Kolter, R. Interspecies Interactions Stimulate Diversification of the *Streptomyces coelicolor* Secreted Metabolome. *MBio* **2013**, *4*, e00459-13. [CrossRef]
90. Blum, S.; Fielder, H.P.; Groth, I.; Kempter, C.; Stephan, H.; Nicholson, G.; Metzger, J.W.; Jung, G. Biosynthetic capacities of actinomycetes. 4. Echinoserine, a new member of the quinoxaline group, produced by *Streptomyces tendae*. *J. Antibiot.* **1995**, *48*, 619–625. [CrossRef]
91. Cox, G.; Sieron, A.; King, A.M.; De Pascale, G.; Pawlowski, A.C.; Koteva, K.; Wright, G.D. A Common Platform for Antibiotic Dereplication and Adjuvant Discovery. *Cell Chem. Biol.* **2017**, *24*, 98–109. [CrossRef] [PubMed]
92. Keller-Schierlein, W.; Mihailović, M.L.; Prelog, V. Stoffwechselprodukte von Actinomyceten. 15. Mitteilung. über die Konstitution von Echinomycin. *Helv. Chim. Acta* **1959**, *42*, 305–322. [CrossRef]
93. Yu, Z.; Vodanovic-Jankovic, S.; Ledeboer, N.; Huang, S.-X.; Rajski, S.R.; Kron, M.; Shen, B. Tirandamycins from *Streptomyces* sp. 17944 inhibiting the parasite Brugia malayi asparagine tRNA synthetase. *Org. Lett.* **2011**, *13*, 2034–2037. [CrossRef] [PubMed]
94. Carlson, J.C.; Li, S.; Burr, D.A.; Sherman, D.H. Isolation and Characterization of Tirandamycins from a Marine-Derived *Streptomyces* sp. *J. Nat. Prod.* **2009**, *72*, 2076–2079. [CrossRef]
95. Kluepfel, D.; Baker, H.A.; Piattoni, G.; Sehgal, S.N.; Sidorowicz, A.; Singh, K.; Vézina, C. Naphthyridinomycin, a new broad-spectrum antibiotic. *J. Antibiot.* **1975**, *28*, 497–502. [CrossRef] [PubMed]
96. Cang, S.; Ohta, S.; Chiba, H.; Johdo, O.; Nomura, H.; Nagamatsu, Y.; Yoshimoto, A. New naphthyridinomycin-type antibiotics, aclidinomycins A and B, from *Streptomyces halstedi*. *J. Antibiot.* **2001**, *54*, 304–307. [CrossRef]
97. Bernan, V.S.; Montenegro, D.A.; Korshalla, J.D.; Maiese, W.M.; Steinberg, D.A.; Greenstein, M. Bioxalomycins, new antibiotics produced by the marine *Streptomyces* sp. LL-31F508: Taxonomy and fermentation. *J. Antibiot.* **1994**, *47*, 1417–1424. [CrossRef]
98. Banskota, A.H.; McAlpine, J.B.; Sørensen, D.; Ibrahim, A.; Aouidate, M.; Piraee, M.; Alarco, A.M.; Farnet, C.M.; Zazopoulos, E. Genomic analyses lead to novel secondary metabolites: Part 3 ECO-0501, a novel antibacterial of a new class. *J. Antibiot.* **2006**, *59*, 533–542. [CrossRef]
99. Stevens, C.L.; Nagarajan, K.; Haskell, T.H. The Structure of Amicetin. *J. Org. Chem.* **1962**, *27*, 2991–3005. [CrossRef]
100. Haneda, K.; Shinose, M.; Seino, A.; Tabata, N.; Tomoda, H.; Iwai, Y.; Omura, S. Cytosaminomycins, new anticoccidial agents produced by *Streptomyces* sp. KO-8119. I. Taxonomy, production, isolation and physico-chemical and biological properties. *J. Antibiot. (Tokyo)* **1994**, *47*, 774–781. [CrossRef]
101. Bu, Y.; Yamazaki, H.; Ukai, K.; Namikoshi, M. Anti-Mycobacterial Nucleoside Antibiotics from a Marine-Derived *Streptomyces* sp. TPU1236A. *Mar. Drugs* **2014**, 6102–6112. [CrossRef]
102. Zhou, S.; Xiao, K.; Huang, D.; Wu, W.; Xu, Y.; Xia, W. Complete genome sequence of *Streptomyces* spongiicola HNM0071T, a marine sponge-associated actinomycete producing staurosporine and echinomycin Marine Genomics Complete genome sequence of *Streptomyces spongiicola* HNM0071 T, a marine sponge-associated act. *Mar. Genomics* **2018**, 1. [CrossRef]
103. Ito, T.; Masubuchi, M. Dereplication of microbial extracts and related analytical technologies. *J. Antibiot.* **2014**, *67*, 353–360. [CrossRef]
104. Gaudêncio, S.P.; Pereira, F. Dereplication: Racing to speed up the natural products discovery process. *Nat. Prod. Rep.* **2015**, *32*, 779–810. [CrossRef]
105. Carrano, L.; Marinelli, F. The relevance of chemical dereplication in microbial natural product screening. *J. Appl. Bioanal.* **2015**, *1*, 55–67. [CrossRef]
106. Chiani, M.; Akbarzadeh, A.; Farhangi, A.; Mazinani, M.; Saffari, Z.; Emadzadeh, K.; Mehrabi, M.R. Optimization of culture medium to increase the production of desferrioxamine B (Desferal) in *Streptomyces pilosus*. *Pakistan J. Biol. Sci.* **2010**, *13*, 546–550. [CrossRef] [PubMed]
107. Chiani, M.; Akbarzadeh, A.; Farhangi, A.; Mehrabi, M.R. Production of Desferoxamine B (Desferal) using Corn Steep Liquor in *Streptomyces pilosus*. *Pakistan J. Biol. Sci.* **2010**, *13*, 1151–1155. [CrossRef]
108. Nicault, M.; Tidjani, A.-R.; Gauthier, A.; Dumarcay, S.; Gelhaye, E.; Bontemps, C.; Leblond, P. Mining the Biosynthetic Potential for Specialized Metabolism of a *Streptomyces* Soil Community. *Antibiotics* **2020**, *9*, 271. [CrossRef]
109. Ishaque, N.M.; Burgsdorf, I.; Limlingan Malit, J.J.; Saha, S.; Teta, R.; Ewe, D.; Kannabiran, K.; Hrouzek, P.; Steindler, L.; Costantino, V.; et al. Isolation, Genomic and Metabolomic Characterization of *Streptomyces tendae* VITAKN with Quorum Sensing Inhibitory Activity from Southern India. *Microorganisms* **2020**, *8*, 121. [CrossRef] [PubMed]
110. AbuSara, N.F.; Piercey, B.M.; Moore, M.A.; Shaikh, A.A.; Nothias, L.-F.; Srivastava, S.K.; Cruz-Morales, P.; Dorrestein, P.C.; Barona-Gómez, F.; Tahlan, K. Comparative Genomics and Metabolomics Analyses of Clavulanic Acid-Producing *Streptomyces* Species Provides Insight Into Specialized Metabolism. *Front. Microbiol.* **2019**, *10*, 2550. [CrossRef]
111. Camesi, A.B.R.; Lukito, A.; Waturangi, D.E.; Kwan, H.J. Screening of Antibiofilm Activity from Marine Bacteria against Pathogenic Bacteria. *Microbiol. Indones.* **2016**, *10*, 87–94. [CrossRef]
112. Artanti, N.; Maryani, F.; Mulyani, H.; Dewi, R.; Saraswati, V.; Murniasih, T. Bioactivities Screening of Indonesian Marine Bacteria Isolated from Sponges. *Ann. Bogor.* **2016**, *20*, 23–28.
113. Cristianawati, O.; Sibero, M.T.; Ayuningrum, D.; Nuryadi, H.; Syafitri, E.; Radjasa, O.K.; Riniarsih, I. Screening of antibacterial activity of seagrass-associated bacteria from the North Java Sea, Indonesia against multidrug-resistant bacteria. *AACL Bioflux* **2019**, *12*, 1054–1064.
114. Nurkanto, A.; Julistiono, H.; Agusta, A.; Sjamsuridzal, W.; Aktivitas, P.; Ampat, R.; Barat, P. Screening Antimicrobial Activity of Actinomycetes Isolated from Raja Ampat, West Papua, Indonesia. *Makara J. Sci.* **2012**, *1*, 21–26. [CrossRef]

115. Mahdiyah, D.; Farida, H.; Riwanto, I.; Mustofa, M.; Wahjono, H.; Laksana Nugroho, T.; Reki, W. Screening of Indonesian peat soil bacteria producing antimicrobial compounds. *Saudi J. Biol. Sci.* **2020**, *27*, 2604–2611. [CrossRef] [PubMed]
116. Fotso, S.; Mahmud, T.; Zabriskie, T.M.; Santosa, D.A.; Sulastri; Proteau, P.J. Angucyclinones from an Indonesian *Streptomyces* sp. *J. Nat. Prod.* **2008**, *71*, 61–65. [CrossRef]
117. Fotso, S.; Mahmud, T.; Zabriskie, T.M.; Santosa, D.A.; Sulastri; Proteau, P.J. Rearranged and unrearranged angucyclinones from Indonesian *Streptomyces* spp. *J. Antibiot.* **2008**, *61*, 449–456. [CrossRef] [PubMed]
118. Fotso, S.; Santosa, D.A.; Saraswati, R.; Yang, J.; Mahmud, T.; Mark Zabriskie, T.; Proteau, P.J. Modified phenazines from an indonesian *Streptomyces* sp. *J. Nat. Prod.* **2010**, *73*, 472–475. [CrossRef]
119. Sheng, Y.; Lam, P.W.; Shahab, S.; Santosa, D.A.; Proteau, P.J.; Zabriskie, T.M.; Mahmud, T. Identification of Elaiophylin Skeletal Variants from the Indonesian *Streptomyces* sp. ICBB 9297. *J. Nat. Prod.* **2015**, *78*, 2768–2775. [CrossRef]
120. Fotso, S.; Zabriskie, T.M.; Proteau, P.J.; Flatt, P.M.; Santosa, D.A.; Sulastri; Mahmud, T.; Limazepines, A.-F. pyrrolo[1,4]benzodiazepine antibiotics from an Indonesian *Micrococcus* sp. *J. Nat. Prod.* **2009**, *72*, 690–695. [CrossRef]
121. Sheng, Y.; Fotso, S.; Serrill, D.; Shahab, S.; Santosa, D.A.; Ishmael, J.E.; Proteau, P.J.; Zabriskie, T.M.; Mahmud, T. Succinylated Apoptolidins from *Amycolatopsis* sp. ICBB 8242. *Org. Lett.* **2015**, *17*, 2526–2529. [CrossRef]
122. Sambrook, J.; Fritsch, E.F.; Maniatis, T. *Molecular Cloning: A Labortaroy Manual*; Cold Spring Harbor Laboratory: New York, NY, USA, 1989; ISBN 0879695773.
123. Garg, N.; Kapono, C.A.; Lim, Y.W.; Koyama, N.; Vermeij, M.J.A.; Conrad, D.; Rohwer, F.; Dorrestein, P.C. Mass spectral similarity for untargeted metabolomics data analysis of complex mixtures. *Int. J. Mass Spectrom.* **2015**, *377*, 719–727. [CrossRef]

marine drugs

MDPI

Article

Applying a Chemogeographic Strategy for Natural Product Discovery from the Marine Cyanobacterium *Moorena bouillonii*

Christopher A. Leber [1], C. Benjamin Naman [1,2], Lena Keller [1,3], Jehad Almaliti [1,4], Eduardo J. E. Caro-Diaz [1,5], Evgenia Glukhov [1], Valsamma Joseph [1,6], T. P. Sajeevan [1,6], Andres Joshua Reyes [7], Jason S. Biggs [7], Te Li [2], Ye Yuan [2], Shan He [2], Xiaojun Yan [2] and William H. Gerwick [1,8,*]

1 Center for Marine Biotechnology and Biomedicine, Scripps Institution of Oceanography, University of California San Diego, La Jolla, CA 92093, USA; cleber@ucsd.edu (C.A.L.); bnaman@nbu.edu.cn (C.B.N.); le.keller85@gmail.com (L.K.); jalmaliti@ucsd.edu (J.A.); eduardo.caro1@upr.edu (E.J.E.C.-D.); eglukhov@ucsd.edu (E.G.); valsamma@cusat.ac.in (V.J.); sajeev@cusat.ac.in (T.P.S.)

2 Li Dak Sum Yip Yio Chin Kenneth Li Marine Biopharmaceutical Research Center, Department of Marine Pharmacy, College of Food and Pharmaceutical Sciences, Ningbo University, Ningbo 315800, China; telinbu@163.com (T.L.); 23yuanye@163.com (Y.Y.); heshan@nbu.edu.cn (S.H.); yanxiaojun@nbu.edu.cn (X.Y.)

3 Department Microbial Natural Products, Helmholtz-Institute for Pharmaceutical Research Saarland (HIPS), Helmholtz Centre for Infection Research (HZI), Campus E8.1, 66123 Saarbrücken, Germany

4 School of Pharmacy, The University of Jordan, Amman 11942, Jordan

5 Department of Pharmaceutical Sciences, School of Pharmacy, University of Puerto Rico—Medical Sciences Campus, San Juan, PR 00921, USA

6 National Centre for Aquatic Animal Health, Cochin University of Science and Technology, Kochi, Kerala 682016, India

7 University of Guam Marine Laboratory, Mangilao, Guam 96923, USA; reyes.andresjoshua@gmail.com (A.J.R.); biggs.js@gmail.com (J.S.B.)

8 Skaggs School of Pharmacy and Pharmaceutical Sciences, University of California San Diego, La Jolla, CA 92093, USA

* Correspondence: wgerwick@health.ucsd.edu

Received: 1 September 2020; Accepted: 8 October 2020; Published: 14 October 2020

Abstract: The tropical marine cyanobacterium *Moorena bouillonii* occupies a large geographic range across the Indian and Western Tropical Pacific Oceans and is a prolific producer of structurally unique and biologically active natural products. An ensemble of computational approaches, including the creation of the ORCA (Objective Relational Comparative Analysis) pipeline for flexible MS^1 feature detection and multivariate analyses, were used to analyze various *M. bouillonii* samples. The observed chemogeographic patterns suggested the production of regionally specific natural products by *M. bouillonii*. Analyzing the drivers of these chemogeographic patterns allowed for the identification, targeted isolation, and structure elucidation of a regionally specific natural product, doscadenamide A (**1**). Analyses of MS^2 fragmentation patterns further revealed this natural product to be part of an extensive family of herein annotated, proposed natural structural analogs (doscadenamides B–J, 2–10); the ensemble of structures reflect a combinatorial biosynthesis using nonribosomal peptide synthetase (NRPS) and polyketide synthase (PKS) components. Compound **1** displayed synergistic in vitro cancer cell cytotoxicity when administered with lipopolysaccharide (LPS). These discoveries illustrate the utility in leveraging chemogeographic patterns for prioritizing natural product discovery efforts.

Keywords: *Moorena bouillonii*; marine natural products; chemogeography; metabolomics

1. Introduction

Natural products discovery programs operate with the general goal of detecting and characterizing chemically unique or biologically active substances. A common obstacle in discovery efforts is the rediscovery of known compounds, suggesting a need for tools and techniques that allow researchers to give priority to samples that possess new or otherwise interesting chemical substances. Various strategies have been employed for the dereplication of known chemicals within samples, and for the prioritization of samples based on chemical composition. In this regard, mass spectrometric analyses, usually in combination with liquid chromatography (e.g., LC-MS), have found great utility in natural products research due to the rapidity, small sample size requirements, and high amount of data generated. As a result, a number of approaches and algorithms have been developed to sift through LC-MS data so as to rapidly detect molecules of greater structural novelty and interest.

PoPCAR (Planes of Principal Component Analysis in R) applies principal component analysis (PCA) to a processed bucket table of sample features, selects outlying samples across different PCA planes, and then leverages the PCA feature loadings to identify the features that make the outlying samples unique [1]. IDBac integrates proteomics and metabolomics data captured via MALDI-TOF MS applied to bacterial colonies on agar plates to classify bacterial strains and distinguish between closely related strains [2]. Global Natural Products Social Molecular Networking (GNPS) is a platform that facilitates the sharing of mass spectral data and provides tools for performing MS^2-based networking analyses [3]. GNPS continues to expand the repertoire of innovative approaches and techniques that it offers, with recent additions including a pipeline for Feature-Based Molecular Networking (FBMN) [4]. FBMN utilizes a processed bucket table of sample MS^1 features in conjunction with MS^2 fragmentation data to produce highly sensitive molecular networks well suited for quantitation and differentiation of isomeric compounds. In addition to these more specific tools, multiple tools are available for the processing and/or statistical analyses of MS-based chemical profile data, including XCMS [5], MZmine [6], and Metaboanalyst [7]. The GNPS classical molecular networking approach [3] is of particular note. While many approaches are sensitive to sample set heterogeneity and rely on specific or consistent sample preparations and data acquisitions in order to provide appropriate results, the classical molecular networking approach is much more flexible, and its outcomes are insulated from imperfect data. This allows classical molecular networking to be used in analyzing datasets that vary across numerous dimensions (instrument type, chromatographic method, sample preparation, etc.), providing many more opportunities for connecting disparate data sources.

The cyanobacterial genus *Moorena* (previously *Lyngbya*, then *Moorea*) is a prolific source of biologically active natural products, with biosynthetic gene clusters accounting for 18% of *Moorena* spp. genomes, on average [8–10]. Consistent with this finding, some 70 different isolated and structurally defined compounds have been reported from *M. bouillonii* (Table S1) [11–44]. These display a broad structural diversity, and include peptides [41], cyclodepsipeptides [16], macrolides [12] and glycosidic macrolides [35], and lipids [43]. These compounds are also notable for their biological activities, including cytotoxins such as bouillonamide [23], lyngbouilloside [35], multiple lyngbyabellins [12,13], and the exquisitely potent apratoxin A [16]. Other *M. bouillonii* compounds have been reported with cannabimimetic properties, such as columbamides A–C [25] and mooreamide A [43], or as modulators of intracellular calcium mobilization such as alotamide A [14]. *M. bouillonii* has a wide distribution across the tropical Western Pacific and Indian Oceans. However, *M. bouillonii* metabolites have only been described from collections made from a limited number of discrete locations, including Papua New Guinea [14,19,23,25,28,33–35,39,41,43], Guam [11,12,15,16,18,20,22,24,29,36,37,42], Palau [11,18,38,40,44], Malaysia [26,27], Palmyra Atoll [13,21], Fiji [31] (The organism in this manuscript is reported as *M. producens*, however the manuscript includes a photo of the organism, which displays a morphology characteristic of shrimp-woven *M. bouillonii*. The 16S rRNA gene-based classification was inconclusive and known compounds previously isolated from *M. bouillonii* were reported.), the Red Sea [17] (The organism in this manuscript is reported as *M. producens*, however the 16S rRNA gene-based classification is inconclusive and known chemistry associated with *M. bouillonii* was reported.), and the islands of southern Japan [30,32]. Collections from these diverse geographical regions differ substantially in their composition of metabolites, suggesting that even though many compounds are already known from *M. bouillonii*, comparing samples of different geographical origin could reveal distributional patterns in chemodiversity that would facilitate the identification of new natural products.

Much of the previous work connecting natural products chemistry and geography has focused on the latitudinal herbivory-defense hypothesis (LHDH). The LHDH suggests that tropical species display more developed defense phenotypes (including chemical defenses) than temperate species, due to higher levels of biotic stressors [45–47]. Studies in both terrestrial organisms [45–48] and marine organisms [49–51] lend support to this hypothesis, but many examples counter to LHDH have also been reported, layering the theory with some degree of controversy while also revealing the complexity of drivers that influence chemical defense [52,53]. Orthogonally, it has become a common strategy to look in underexplored geographical locations in order to find new and unique natural products. This has led natural products discovery efforts to interesting and exotic habitats, including tropical coral reefs [11–44], hypersaline lakes [54], the Arctic [55] and Antarctic [56], hydrothermal vents [57], and the deep sea [58]. In spite of the acknowledgement that sampling in new geographical locations can allow access to new natural products, there are few examples of systematically applying geographical knowledge in order to inform natural product discovery. However, in one study the crude extracts and fractions from 300 geographically and taxonomically diverse cyanobacterial and algal collections were profiled by LC-MS/MS [59]. Analyses by GNPS classical molecular networking revealed geographic hotspots for chemodiversity, thus allowing for a molecular feature to be prioritized based on its chemogeographical distribution. In this case, it led to the characterization of a new metabolite given the common name yuvalamide A. Another example study focused on cyanobacteria from one specific genus, analyzing 10 samples of *Symploca* spp. collected at different times and in different places. This led to the efficient and targeted discovery of a new sample-specific bioactive natural product, samoamide A [60].

In the present study, we illustrate the value of leveraging geographical patterns in chemodiversity to find previously uncharacterized natural products and apply this strategy to the marine filamentous cyanobacterial species *M. bouillonii*. This is a particularly interesting organism because of its wide geographical range and richness in natural products. To enable analyses and inform current discovery efforts based on legacy data, we were inspired to develop a flexible data pipeline described as the Objective Relational Comparative Analysis (ORCA) of chemical profiles from LC-MS data. Analyses of the LC-MS profiles from geographically disparate chemical extracts of *M. bouillonii*, used in conjunction with GNPS classical molecular networking, allowed for the prioritization of a molecular feature that led to the isolation and characterization of a new compound we called laulauamide (**1**). (The discovery, isolation, and structure elucidation of **1** were presented at the 2017 Annual Meeting of the American Society of Pharmacognosy. The name laulauamide was used for a poster presentation, and the associated abstract can be found under abstract P-219 at the following link [http://asp2017.org/wp-content/uploads/2016/12/ASP20201720Annual20Meeting_web.pdf]). Molecular networks along with detailed MS^2 fragmentation analyses revealed the presence of an extensive collection of proposed natural analogs. These display diversification through varied combinations of fatty acid side chains at two locations. Assays for biological activity yielded synergistic cytotoxic activity between **1** and lipopolysaccharide (LPS). Late in the performance of this work, a manuscript appeared from another laboratory that reported the isolation and structure elucidation of the main component of this new natural product family, and assigned it the common name "doscadenamide A" [29], a name we retain so as to not create confusion in the literature record.

2. Results and Discussion

To allow for the comparison of LC-MS traces of extracts from different collections of *M. bouillonii*, a new pipeline was created called the Objective Relational Comparative Analysis (ORCA) pipeline (https://github.com/c-leber/ORCA) (Figure 1). ORCA is a flexible, modular pipeline that includes capabilities for simple and customizable MS^1 feature processing. ORCA can also accept any bucket table of samples vs. features as input, allowing for the comparison of data from any source that can be tabulated in such a manner. To accommodate heterogeneous data and to allow for the comparison of diverse datasets, ORCA MS^1 feature processing starts with an input directory of mzXML files, from which the MS^1 features are picked and integrated based on the mass-to-charge ratio (m/z) and a user-selected variant of retention time (rt). Feature picking is parameterized with the user-defined m/z and rt tolerances, and the peak size and shape parameters. Subsequently, MS^1 features picked from each sample file are consolidated based on the user-defined m/z and rt tolerance parameters and are organized into a samples vs. features bucket table containing feature integration values, with options to apply transformations based on the goals of the downstream analyses.

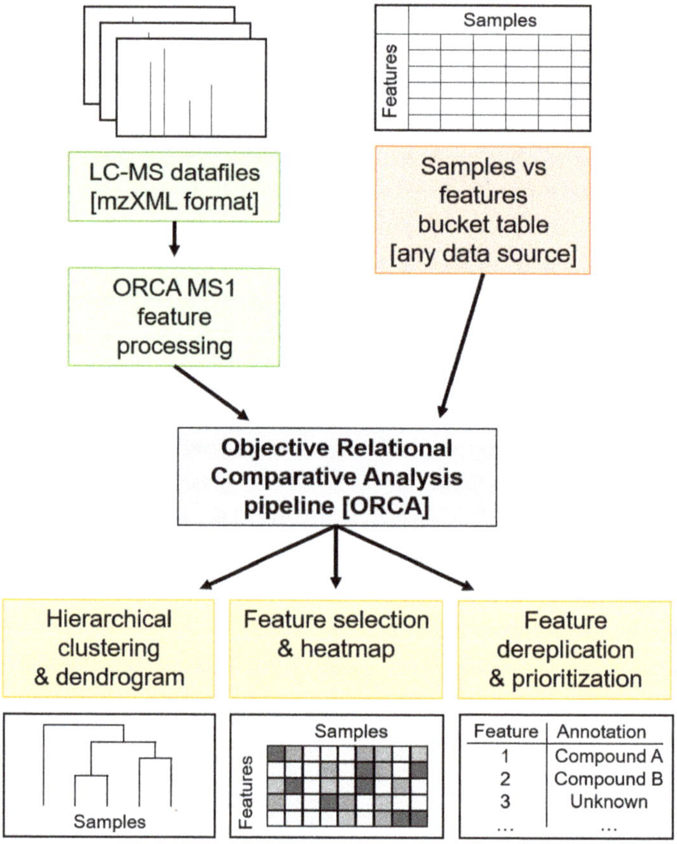

Figure 1. Illustration of the Objective Relational Comparative Analysis (ORCA) pipeline. The pipeline accepts inputs of either LC-MS datafiles in mzXML format, which can then undergo MS^1 feature processing, or an externally created samples vs. features bucket table coming from any data source. Analyses currently offered as a part of the ORCA pipeline include hierarchical clustering, feature selection, and feature dereplication based on user-provided reference data.

After processing of the sample MS^1 features, or the input of an externally generated sample vs. feature bucket table, the vectors of the feature values can then be utilized to initiate a diverse array of analyses, including hierarchical clustering of the samples to gain insights into the relationships between the samples, and univariate feature selection to learn about what specific MS^1 features are driving the differences between groups of samples. These analyses can then be visualized as dendrograms or heat maps, respectively. ORCA can also be used to generate a list of the most prominent MS^1 features across samples and to assign putative identifications from a user-supplied spreadsheet, allowing one to efficiently detect expected peaks across many samples, and to quickly determine the mass spectral signature of new potential isolation targets. ORCA was designed for assessing the relationships between heterogeneous samples and generating hypotheses regarding which features are driving these relationships; this makes ORCA a useful framework for not only learning about chemogeographical patterns, but also for comparing chemical profiles across different growth conditions [61], detecting contamination of botanical extracts [62], identifying chemotaxonomic patterns [63], and many other potential uses.

Crude extracts of field-collected samples of *M. bouillonii* from American Samoa, Guam, Kavaratti (Lakshadweep Islands, India), Saipan, and the Paracel Islands (Xisha) in the South China Sea, as well as an in-house culture from Papua New Guinea, were profiled via LC-MS/MS; the resultant chromatograms were used as inputs for MS^1 feature processing in ORCA. Hierarchical clustering was performed on the MS^1 features and a dendrogram was produced with a cophenetic correlation coefficient of 0.905, indicating that the displayed structure in the dendrogram is highly correlated to the cosine distances between samples, and thus is representative of the data (Figure 2). The structure in the dendrogram suggests clustering of samples according to geographical region, a phenomenon that has previously been observed across other cyanobacterial samples [59] but has not been specifically reported as a pattern for *M. bouillonii*. It is worth noting that, while samples with shared geographical origin are indeed arranged in clusters together in the dendrogram, the branch points for each geographical cluster are quite large, ranging from 0.4763 cosine distance for the two samples from Guam to 0.7248 cosine distance for where the three samples from Saipan converge. This is likely the result of a combination of the high variability and complexity in the composition of the studied samples, as well as the "curse of dimensionality" that artificially enlarges distance values when large numbers of features are being considered [64]. Classical molecular networking analysis using GNPS provided an orthogonal view, supporting the idea of chemogeographical specificity in these *M. bouillonii* samples, as numerous clusters of location-specific nodes are visible in the resultant network (Figure 3 and Figure S1). Furthermore, hierarchical clustering performed on presence-absence data of the MS^2 nodes from GNPS, as visualized with a dendrogram (Figure 4), revealed a chemogeographical clustering similar to that produced from the ORCA MS^1 features (Figure 2). The geographically associated structure in the data, as observable via both ORCA dendrograms, along with the presence of numerous location-specific clusters in the molecular network, led us to generate the hypothesis that the geographically specific distributions of natural products in our samples could be leveraged to identify previously unreported metabolites. The clustering of samples by specific geographical location stimulated further analyses to determine which molecular features were driving the observed geographic clusters, and which peaks were regionally specific. Particular attention was paid to Saipan, as it represented one region from which no new natural products from *M. bouillonii* had been reported in the scientific literature.

One cluster in the GNPS molecular network comprising only nodes originating from the Saipan-collected samples contained a particularly intense node for a feature with m/z 457.785 (Figure 3). Further investigations in ORCA revealed that this feature was present in high abundance in all samples from Saipan but was undetected or detectable at very low levels in the MS^1 spectra of samples from all the other studied locales (Table S2). Additionally, this feature was not dereplicated when queried against all published compounds from *M. bouillonii* at the time (Table S3) and when searched against the MarinLit database (http://pubs.rsc.org/marinlit/). This intriguing chemogeographic pattern prompted prioritization of this feature for isolation and structure elucidation, ultimately resulting in the characterization of a region-specific metabolite. Based on the specific collection site from which the Saipan samples originated (Laulau Bay, Saipan), we originally termed this metabolite "laulauamide". A molecular feature with m/z 721.10 was found to have a very similar geographic distribution. It was detected with high intensity in samples from Saipan, while being undetected or detectable at very low levels in other samples (Table S2), and thus was another strong driver of the clustering of the Saipan samples. Isolation and analytical characterization revealed that this MS feature was the sodiated adduct of the known compound lyngbyapeptin A [41] (Table S3).

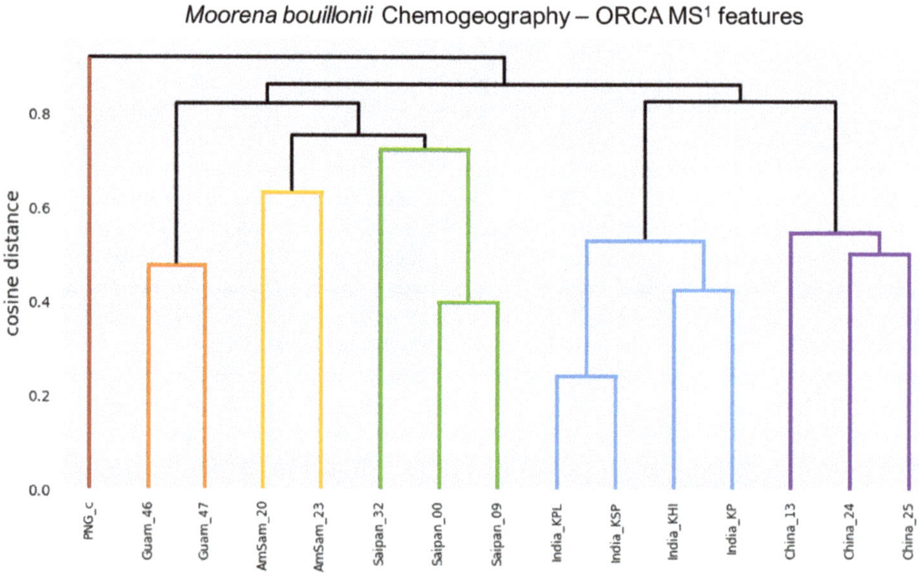

Figure 2. ORCA-generated dendrogram (cophenetic correlation coefficient = 0.905) displaying the results of hierarchical clustering of the MS^1 features from *M. bouillonii* crude extracts. Samples are labeled with aliases comprising a general collection location concatenated to an abbreviated sample code. The structure in the dendrogram suggests that samples collected from the same geographical area are chemically more similar. Colorized for emphasis. Red: Papua New Guinea; Orange: Guam; Gold: American Samoa; Green: Saipan; Blue: Kavaratti (Lakshadweep Islands, India); Purple: Paracel Islands (Xisha) in the South China Sea.

M. bouillonii biomass (1 L sample, 132 g dry biomass yielding 10 g of crude extract) from Saipan's Laulau Bay (denoted as Saipan_32 in Figures 2 and 4) was thoroughly extracted with 2:1 dichloromethane and methanol, and the resulting crude extract was fractionated over silica using vacuum liquid chromatography. LC-MS/MS analysis of the fractions revealed the MS^1 feature of interest to be in highest abundance in two relatively polar fractions. Reverse phase HPLC was used to initially isolate 1.5 mg of this compound from the two fractions. 1D and 2D NMR experiments were utilized to establish the planar structure of **1**, with major contributions from the ^1H-^1H Correlated Spectroscopy (COSY), ^1H-^{13}C Heteronuclear Single Quantum Coherence (HSQC), ^1H-^{13}C Heteronuclear Multiple Bond Coherence (HMBC), HSQC-Total Correlation Spectroscopy (TOCSY), and long-range ^1H-^{13}C Heteronuclear Single Quantum Multiple Bond Coherence (HSQMBC) data.

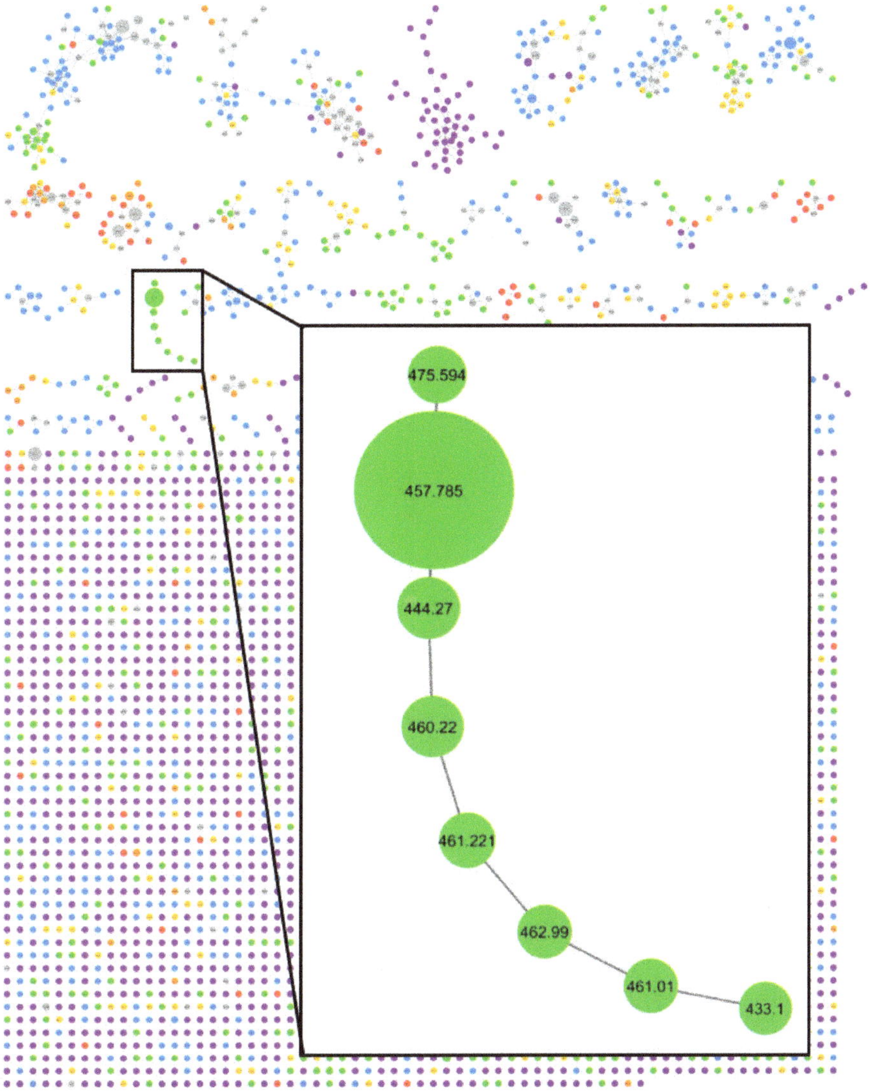

Figure 3. Global Natural Products Social Molecular Networking (GNPS) classical molecular network of fifteen *M. bouillonii* crude extracts with the enlarged inset showing a cluster containing **1** (denoted with precursor mass *m/z* 457.785) and seven other nodes representing potential doscadenamide analogs (based on LR-MS/MS data). The green coloring of the nodes indicates that they represent features only detected in samples from Saipan. Nodes are scaled to summed precursor intensity. Grey nodes represent the MS^2 features that are present in samples from more than one geographical region. Geographical location of samples is colorized as follows: Red: Papua New Guinea; Orange: Guam; Gold: American Samoa; Green: Saipan; Blue: Kavaratti (Lakshadweep Islands, India); Purple: Paracel Islands (Xisha) in the South China Sea.

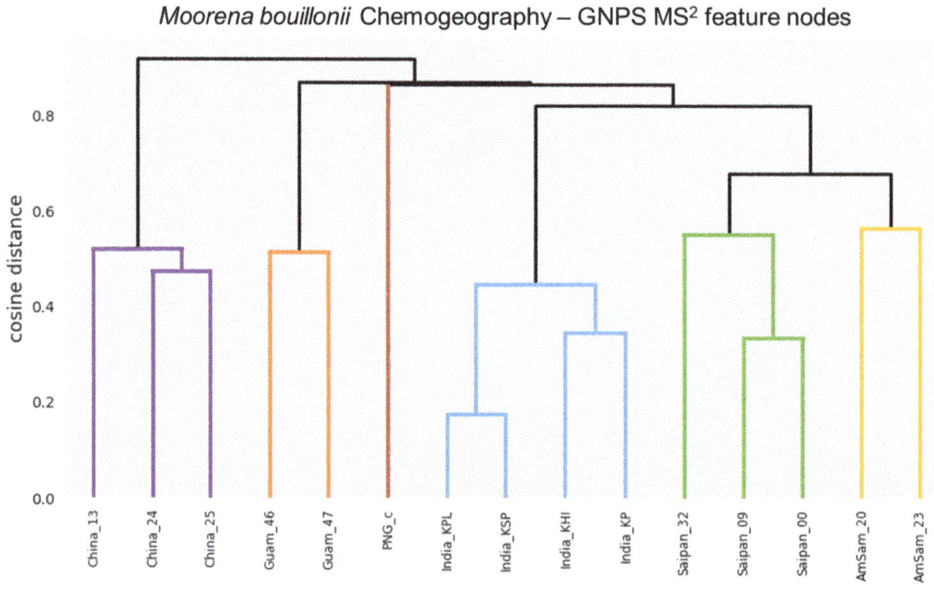

Figure 4. ORCA-generated dendrogram (cophenetic correlation coefficient = 0.960) displaying the results of hierarchical clustering of the *M. bouillonii* crude extracts presence–absence data regarding GNPS nodes. Samples are labeled with aliases comprising a general collection location concatenated to an abbreviated sample code. Similar to Figure 2, the structure in the dendrogram suggests that samples collected from the same geographical area are chemically more similar. Colorized for emphasis. Red: Papua New Guinea; Orange: Guam; Gold: American Samoa; Green: Saipan; Blue: Kavaratti (Lakshadweep Islands, India); Purple: Paracel Islands (Xisha) in the South China Sea.

The ^{1}H and ^{13}C NMR chemical shifts for the two acetylene groups were highly similar, and by HMBC correlations both had an adjacent methylene group at the same shift (δ 2.18, H_2-15 and H_2-24). In one of these two cases, sequential correlations deduced from the ^{1}H-^{1}H COSY data, and supported by the results of a ^{1}H-^{13}C HSQC-TOCSY experiment, provided a spin system involving three additional shielded methylene groups at δ 1.44, 1.39, and 1.75 and 1.42 (H_2-23, H_2-22, and H_2-21). The final of these methylene groups was positioned adjacent to a deshielded methine group at δ 3.75 (H_2-20). By COSY, the methine was determined to be adjacent to a shielded methyl group at δ 1.12 (H_3-27), and its chemical shift was explained by an HMBC correlation placing it adjacent to an ester or amide carbonyl (δ 176.4, C-19). The spin system of the second acetylene-terminating partial structure was highly similar and partially overlapped but terminated with a more shielded methine proton at δ 2.13 (H-11) with an adjacent methyl group (δ 1.11, H_3-18) and amide or ester carbonyl (δ 177.0, C-10). Summarizing, two essentially identical 2-methyl-7-octynoic acid structural units were thus defined from highly similar but non-identical data subsets.

The remainder of the molecule was thus composed of $C_9H_{14}N_2O_2$ with 3 degrees of unsaturation resulting from an enone and one ring structure. Two ^{1}H NMR singlets (δ 5.04, H-2 and 3.84, H_3-9) along with a 9-proton connected spin system remained unassigned. The singlet at 3.84 ppm was assignable to a methoxy group at the β-position of the enone by virtue of its relatively deshielded chemical shift and HMBC correlations to the highly deshielded olefinic carbon at δ 179.2 (C-3). The other singlet was thus assigned to the α-position of this enone as it was attached to a shielded olefinic carbon at δ 94.2 (C-2) and showed an HMBC correlation to the carbonyl carbon at δ 170.0 (C-1). As this partial structure accounted for all oxygen atoms in compound **1**, the shielded nature of this carbonyl necessarily required it to be attached to a nitrogen atom, forming an amide. Based on ^1H and ^{13}C NMR chemical shift data (δ 4.64, H-4; δ 59.2, C-4), one terminus of the remaining spin system was assigned to a methine with an attached nitrogen atom. ^1H-^1H COSY data, in conjunction with the ^1H-^{13}C HSQC-TOCSY, allowed formulation of four sequential methylene groups. The final methylene was also relatively deshielded (δ 3.22 and 3.13, H_2-8; δ 39.3, C-8), consistent with its attachment to a nitrogen atom. At this point, all atoms in the molecular formula of compound **1** were accounted for, except for one proton that was attached to a heteroatom by evaluation of the HSQC data (e.g., only 39 protons were found attached to carbon atoms); this was deduced to be an NH as three of the four oxygen atoms were assigned as carbonyls and one as a methylated enol.

HMBC correlations from the two diastereotopic protons at δ 3.13/3.22 ppm (H_2-8) to the carbonyl at δ 177.0 (C-10) connected these two partial structures. The other 2-methyl-7-octynoic acid was therefore connected to the only remaining heteroatom, the N-atom connected to the δ 170.0 (C-1) carbonyl of the enone functionality. Remaining structural features at this point included the formation of one ring, and placement of a proton on one of the two nitrogen atoms; two possibilities emerged (**1a** and **1b**) (Figure 5).

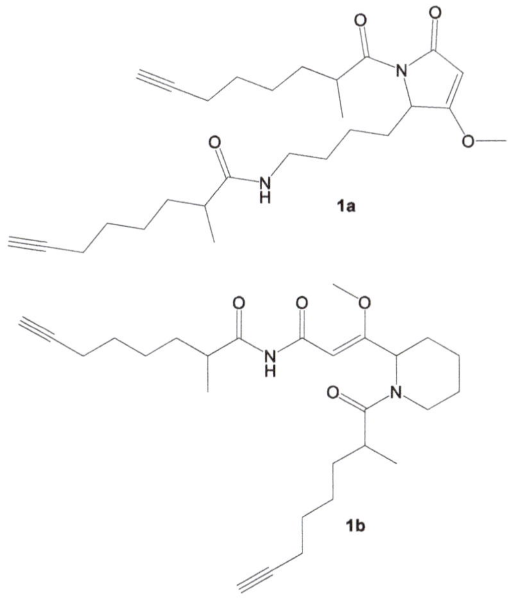

Figure 5. Competing structural hypotheses for the two-dimensional structure of compound **1**.

Both structural possibilities had features that were attractive and unattractive from a predicted biosynthetic perspective. In **1a**, the fundamental assembly of the PKS derived octynoic acid; its passage to an NRPS to incorporate a lysine residue, followed by a ketide extension, *O*-methylation of the β-enol, and cyclization to a pyrrolidone ring, is well precedented within cyanobacterial natural products [65–67]. However, the acylation of a second octynoic acid residue to the lysine side chain nitrogen is an unprecedented event. Alternative structure **1b** has the attractiveness of a regular, predicted PKS(4)-NRPS(glycine)-PKS(3)-NRPS(glycine)-PKS architecture; however, it is quite awkward in requiring several unusual adjustments to the oxidation state of the carbon atoms, and creation of the second 2-methyl-7-octynoic acid residue via a completely different set of biosynthetic steps from the first one.

Modeling of these two alternative cyclization products for ^{13}C NMR shifts (see Figures S2 and S3 for the predicted ^{13}C NMR shifts for **1a** and **1b**, respectively) and comparison with those experimentally measured for **1** revealed that both possibilities were reasonably good fits, but the predicted values for 1a tended to be closer to the shifts experimentally derived for compound **1**. For both C-2, the methyl enol carbon (**1a** δ 95.5, **1b** δ 101.4, **1** δ 94.2), and C-3, the deshielded olefinic carbon (**1a** δ 180.7, **1b** δ 171.5, **1** δ 179.2), the fit for alternative **1a** was considerably better. Only at C-6 was the cyclization product proposed in **1b** favored (1a δ 24.3, **1b** δ 19.6, **1** δ 20.4). A deeper look into the long-range ^{1}H-^{13}C HSQMBC data was undertaken. The key proton distinguishing these two possible structures, H-4 at δ 4.64, showed correlations to several resonances, including two of the three carbonyl resonances (δ 170.0, C-1; δ 176.4, C-19) and the β-oxygenated enone (δ 179.2, C-3); these correlations were compatible with structure **1a** (one 2-bond and two 3-bond correlations), while in structure **1b** these correlations would result from one 2-bond, one 4-bond, and one 6-bond ^{1}H-^{13}C coupling. Furthermore, analysis of the HMBC correlations observed for H-4 and H_2-8, both from the lysine-derived residue, showed mutual signals with only C-5 at δ 29.0 and C-6 at δ 20.4 that would be consistent with either proposed structure. There were no shared correlations observed between these protons and the equally 3-bond proximal carbonyl in **1b**, nor 3-bond correlations from H-4 to C-8 and H-8 to C-4 that would be reasonably expected to be observed from **1b**, lending further support for **1a** as being the correct structure of **1**.

Compound **1** contains three stereocenters—two associated with the two 2-methyl-7-octynoic acid side chains, and one contained in the central heterocycle. A racemic standard of 2-methyloctanoic acid was derivatized with (*S*)-(+)-2-phenylglycine methyl ester. A chiral standard of (*S*)-2-methyloctanoic was generated via the zirconium-catalyzed asymmetric carbo-alumination (ZACA) reaction [68] of 1-octene to stereoselectively install a methyl group at the C-2 position, followed by an oxidation to 2-methyloctanoic acid and derivatization with (*S*)-(+)-2-phenylglycine methyl ester. Configuration of both 2-methyloctynoic acid moieties of compound **1** was established to be *R* through catalytic hydrogenation, acid hydrolysis, derivatization with (*S*)-(+)-2-phenylglycine methyl ester, and comparison via LC-MS to the generated standards of 2-methyloctanoic acid coupled with the same chiral auxiliary group (Figure S4). Ozonolysis with an oxidative work-up [69], followed by acid hydrolysis, was used to open the heterocyclic ring structure and liberate lysine from compound **1**. The lysine was then derivatized with Marfey's reagent (L-FDAA) and compared to racemic and L-lysine standards derivatized with the same Marfey's reagent, indicating an *S* configuration of this residue (Figure S5). The fully elucidated structure of compound **1** was thus determined as in Figure 6.

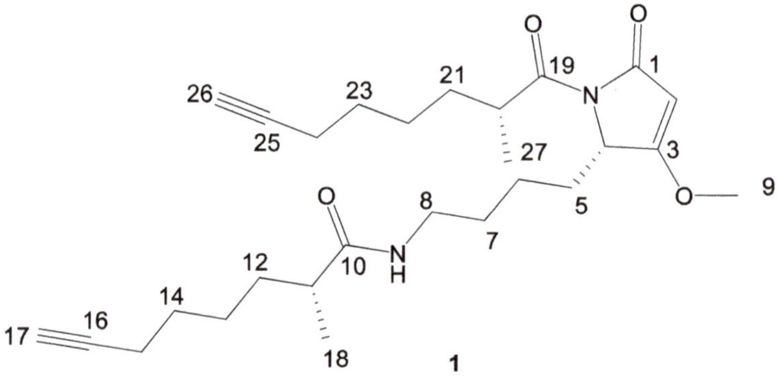

1

Figure 6. Complete structure of compound **1**.

Low-resolution LC-MS/MS fragmentation data for **1** consistently showed three peaks at *m/z* 321, 303, and 168 (Figure S6), which we predicted to represent a side-chain loss, a side-chain loss plus the loss of an amine, and the loss of both side chains plus an amine, respectively. To better understand the fragmentations of compound **1** and use this information for identifying analogs based on repeating the MS^2 fragmentation patterns, high-resolution MS^2 fragmentation data were acquired for compound **1**. Numerous fragment peaks were recorded, including peaks observed at

m/z 321.2171, 303.1901, and 168.1016. These values match very well to the calculated monoisotopic masses of the predicted fragment structures shown in Figure 7 (m/z 321.217, 303.183, 168.102; allowing for hydrogen rearrangements), lending support to our fragmentation hypothesis, and providing a starting point for understanding and proposing the structures of analogs via their fragmentation patterns.

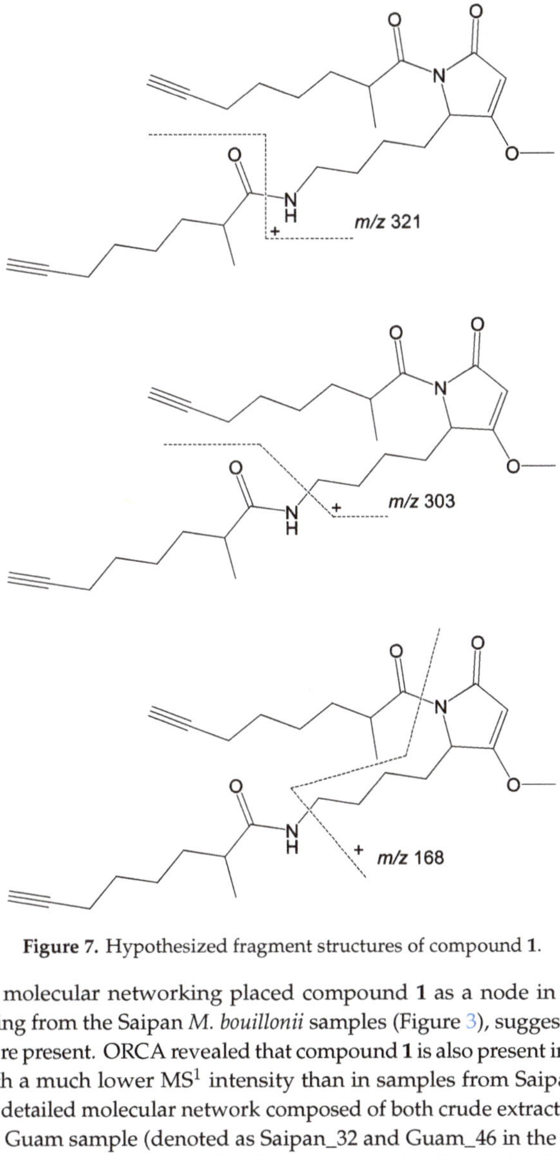

Figure 7. Hypothesized fragment structures of compound **1**.

GNPS classical molecular networking placed compound **1** as a node in a cluster with seven other nodes originating from the Saipan *M. bouillonii* samples (Figure 3), suggesting several naturally occurring analogs were present. ORCA revealed that compound **1** is also present in samples from Guam, though detected with a much lower MS^1 intensity than in samples from Saipan. This inspired the generation of a more detailed molecular network composed of both crude extracts and fractions from a Saipan sample and a Guam sample (denoted as Saipan_32 and Guam_46 in the above dendrograms), revealing an even larger cluster of potential analogs that contained 33 nodes, including compound **1** (Figure S7). Some nodes in the cluster had very similar masses, which could be the result of an artifact from the particular parameter set selected for the analysis, an artifact of the low resolution MS data analyzed, or be an indicator of isomeric analogs; therefore, further analysis was needed.

Analysis using the GNPS in browser network visualizer suggested that there was a common connection between many of the potential analogs (23 out of 33, including **1**), namely the presence of an

MS^2 fragment peak at *m/z* 168 (Figure S7). To facilitate further analysis of MS^2 spectra and the presence of potential analogs, the ORCA MS^2 auxiliary pipeline was developed. MS^2 scans from the Saipan and Guam crude extract and fractions were binned based on precursor mass, and then filtered to only precursor masses with scans that included a *m/z* 168 fragment peak. Clustering scans from each relevant precursor mass by cosine distance, paired with manual analysis, allowed the structures of 9 analogs (**2–10**) to be proposed (Figure 8; see Figures S8–S26 for the proposed structures, consensus spectra, and predicted fragment structures). It must be noted that alternative structural proposals are conceivable for these analogs; however, given the literature precedent for cyanobacteria to produce families of natural products with the same array of variations in desaturation and oxidation as proposed here, e.g., [66,70,71], and the predictable MS^2 fragmentation spectra observed, these proposals represent the most parsimonious and best supported structural hypotheses. Ambiguities in the remaining related MS^2 spectra prevent the definitive assignment of carbon chain isomers and positional isomers, and the proposal of additional analogs, but suggest a process of combinatorial biosynthesis in generating this expansive natural product family. While quantities of these minor metabolites in our samples were not sufficient for isolation and further characterization, the total synthesis published alongside the characterization of **1** [29] is very amenable to incorporating alternative side chains, and this could be used for generating these proposed analogs for further study.

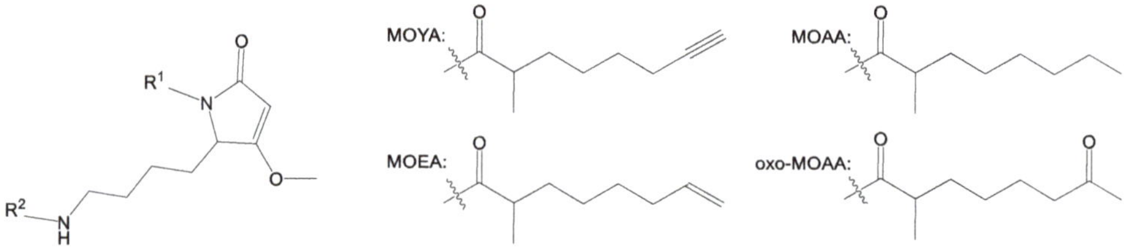

1 doscadenamide A: R^1 = MOYA, R^2 = MOYA; **2** doscadenamide B: R^1 = MOEA, R^2 = MOEA;
3 doscadenamide C: R^1 = MOYA, R^2 = MOEA; **4** doscadenamide D: R^1 = MOEA, R^2 = MOYA;
5 doscadenamide E: R^1 = MOYA, R^2 = MOAA; **6** doscadenamide F: R^1 = MOAA, R^2 = MOYA;
7 doscadenamide G: R^1 = MOEA, R^2 = MOAA; **8** doscadenamide H: R^1 = MOAA, R^2 = MOEA;
9 doscadenamide I: R^1 = MOYA, R^2 = oxo-MOAA; **10** doscadenamide J: R^1 = oxo-MOAA, R^2 = MOYA

Figure 8. The doscadenamides: compound **1**, along with its analogs whose proposed structures were annotated via informative patterns in the MS^2 fragmentation data (see Figures S9–S26). Each analog consists of a heterocyclic core with two fatty acid side chains with the following possibilities: MOYA = 2-methyl octynoic acid; MOEA = 2-methyl octenoic acid; MOAA = 2-methyl octanoic acid; oxo-MOAA = 2-methyl 7-oxo octanoic acid.

Compound **1** contains unusual structural features that, while having precedent in other cyanobacterial natural products, have not previously been seen together. Terminal alkynes can be found in several other natural products from *Moorena* spp., including jamaicamide B [66], carmabin A [71], and vatiamides A, C, and E [72], but having two is notable. While ribosomally synthesized and post-translationally modified peptides (RiPPs) and NRPS-derived natural products with amino acid subunits are common in cyanobacteria, lysine is not often seen, especially in the natural products of marine cyanobacteria [73,74]. The heterocycle in **1**, composed of an acetate extended amino acid, has been observed in the malyngamides [65], jamaicamides [66], gallinamides [67], and other cyanobacterial natural products, but again, never has it been reported involving a lysine residue. Two curiosities of the biosynthesis of compound **1**, namely the origin of the two 2-methyl octynoic acid residues and the formation of the heterocycle, can be explained by analogy to what is known about the biosynthesis of the jamaicamides [66]. To generate 2-methyl octynoic acid, a fatty-acid desaturase analogous to JamB could act upon an octanoic acid precursor, or a smaller precursor that has been PKS-extended to the appropriate size. The placement of the methyl group in the 2 position suggests incorporation via

S-adenosyl methionine (SAM). Formation of the heterocycle likely occurs as the result of an acetate extension of the carboxyl group of lysine, followed by a Claisen-like condensation and cyclization directed by a cyclase analogous to JamQ. As noted above in the discussion of structural possibilities **1a** and **1b**, what is less clear is how 2-methyl octynoic acid is appended to the terminus of the lysine side chain; the peptide bond formed is far from unusual, but its placement suggests enzymatic activity occurring beyond the otherwise linear PKS-NRPS assembly of the molecule.

To further evaluate the relationships of the structural features found together in compound **1** to the known natural product chemical space, we applied a Small Molecule Accurate Recognition Technology (SMART) [75] analysis to search for structurally similar molecules based on HSQC spectra. SMART did not yield any similar compounds with a cosine value higher than 0.84, further revealing the structural uniqueness of compound **1**. We also utilized the structure similarity search function in SciFinder (https://scifinder.cas.org/), which yielded only the sintokamides (Figure S27). The sintokamides share a similar heterocycle and are halogenated natural products from sponges [76]. While not suggested by either structure similarity query, tetramic acids [77] and prostaglandins (PGE_2, for example) [78] (Figure S27) are two chemical classes that possess some distant level of structural similarity to compound **1**, and this inspired additional bioactivity testing efforts, as described below.

Structural similarity to tetramic acids inspired in silico antibiotic screening (http://chemprop.csail.mit.edu/) [79]. The known antibacterials C_{12}-tetramic acid and C_{14}-tetramic acid scored over five times greater than the highest scoring doscadenamide (Table S4), providing little incentive to further evaluate the doscadenamides for antibiotic activity.

Compound **1** was assayed for cytotoxicity against human NCI-H460 cells and yielded an $IC_{50} > 22$ μM, suggesting negligible cytotoxicity. This lack of cytotoxicity, plus some distant structural similarity to prostaglandins, inspired the screening of compound **1** in a Griess assay for anti-inflammation (as well as cytotoxicity) toward murine macrophages RAW264.7 cells at a range of 7–55 μM. Curiously, rather than producing inflammatory or anti-inflammatory effects, compound **1** yielded dose-dependent synergistic cytotoxicity with lipopolysaccharide (LPS). This anomalous result was confirmed through multiple replicates of the assay (Figures S28–S30).

The doscadenamides were discovered based on global scale patterns in *M. bouillonii* chemical diversity. This illustrates that cyanobacteria harbor intraspecific chemogeographic patterns, and that these patterns can be utilized to direct discovery efforts towards new, regionally specific natural product families. There are many tools available for pursuing chemogeographic and other metabolite patterns in sample sets that can inform discovery efforts, each with their own strengths and limitations. While tools like the ORCA pipeline and GNPS classical molecular networking may be of limited utility in terms of quantitative analyses and effective separation of isomeric features, their flexibility in handling heterogeneous sample sets allows for comparative analyses between samples that could otherwise not be conducted. Furthermore, the intrinsic imperfection of real-world data and the deficiencies inherent to various tools and approaches encourages that an ensemble of tools and approaches be applied. By using ORCA in conjunction with GNPS, we were able to generate convergent results that increased confidence in our conclusions. Converging results from ORCA and GNPS were also helpful in giving confidence to the parameters selected for our analyses; parameter selection is often a challenge when applying computational techniques and requires deep knowledge of the dataset as well as manual validation. The chemogeographic patterns in *M. bouillonii* natural products that are qualitatively presented in this manuscript highlight the opportunity to further explore *M. bouillonii* natural products chemistry and how compounds and compound families are distributed ubiquitously vs. regionally, at different geographical scales. Studying *M. bouillonii* metabolomics in a more controlled, semi-quantitative fashion would allow these patterns to be evaluated more deeply and will be the focus of a future manuscript.

Doscadenamide A (**1**), when considered in isolation, is a structurally intriguing compound. Being composed of a heterocyclized, acetate-extended amino acid core appended with terminal alkyne containing side chains, it blends structural features common among cyanobacterial natural products with a flair of the unusual: the inclusion of lysine, the dual terminal alkynes, and the acylation of the lysine side chain with one of those terminal alkyne containing side chains. In considering the doscadenamides as a family of cyanobacterial natural products, it is likely they are produced via a seemingly combinatorial addition of different acyl groups to a consistent core structure. From a biosynthetic perspective, this suggests a low level of fidelity in the assembly process. Connecting this family of compounds to the biosynthetic gene cluster responsible for their production would elevate our understanding of how cyanobacteria diversify their natural product arsenals. Since the aforementioned procedure for the total synthesis of compound **1** [29] is amenable to incorporating alternative sidechains, this could be used for generating the nine proposed natural structural analogs reported here (**2**–**10**), as well as for evaluating their activities as quorum sensing modulators [29] and their cytotoxic synergism with LPS.

3. Materials and Methods

3.1. General Experimental Procedures

Optical rotation was measured using a JASCO P-2000 polarimeter (Easton, MD, USA), UV/Vis data were obtained using a Beckman DU800 spectrophotometer (Brea, CA, USA), and IR spectra were recorded on a ThermoScientific Nicolet 6700 FT-IR spectrometer (Waltham, MA, USA). NMR experiments were conducted using a JEOL ECZ 500 NMR spectrometer (Akishima, Tokyo, Japan) equipped with a 3 mm inverse probe (H3X), a Bruker AVANCE III 600 MHz NMR with a 1.7 mm dual tune TCI cryoprobe (Billerica, MA, USA), and a Varian VX500 (Palo Alto, CA, USA). NMR data were processed using Mestrenova (Mestrelab, Santiago de Compostela, Spain) and TopSpin (Bruker, Billerica, MA, USA). NMR data were recorded in $CDCl_3$ and referenced to the solvent peak (7.260, 77.160). For the low-resolution LC-MS/MS analysis, a ThermoFinnigan Surveyor HPLC System (San Jose, CA, USA) with a Phenomenex Kinetex 5 μm C18 100 × 4.6 mm column (Torrance, CA, USA) coupled to a ThermoFinnigan LCQ Advantage Max Mass Spectrometer (San Jose, CA, USA) in positive ion mode was used. Samples were analyzed using one of two linear gradients from 30% CH_3CN + 0.1% formic acid to 99% CH_3CN + 0.1% formic acid in H_2O + 0.1% formic acid at a flow rate of either 0.6 mL/min or 0.7 mL/min over 32 min or 30 min, respectively. Samples were run at a concentration of 1 mg/mL, with concentrations increased up to 4 mg/mL in situations where the peak intensities were insufficient. For the HiRes-ESI-MS analysis, an Agilent 6230 time-of-flight mass spectrometer (TOFMS) (Santa Clara, CA, USA) with Jet Stream ESI source was used. For HiResMS^2 fragmentation data, a ThermoScientific Orbitrap XL mass spectrometer (Waltham, MA, USA) with direct infusion of the sample into the Thermo IonMax electrospray interface was used.

Compound isolation was performed using two semi-preparative HPLCs: a Thermo Scientific Dionex UltiMate 3000 HPLC (Waltham, MA, USA) system with automated fraction collector, a Waters HPLC system with 1500 series pumps (Milford, MA, USA), and a 996 photodiode array detector with manual fraction collection. HPLC separation was performed using a Phenomenex Kinetex 5 μm C18 10 × 150 mm column (Torrance, CA, USA) and reverse phase gradients of acetonitrile in H_2O, with both solvents containing 0.1% (*v*/*v*) formic acid. HPLC grade organic solvents and Millipore Milli-Q system (Burlington, MA, USA) purified water were used.

All reagents, catalysts, and solvents used for the synthetic experiments were purchased in their purest and driest form. All experiments were carried out under an inert atmosphere (Ar) unless otherwise specified.

National Cancer Institute (NCI) H460 hypotriploid human cells [American Type Culture Collection (ATCC) HTB-177] and RAW 264.7 murine macrophages (ATCC TIB-71) were purchased from the ATCC (Manassas, VA, USA).

3.2. Sample Collection

Fifteen benthic filamentous tropical marine cyanobacterial samples were hand-collected via self-contained underwater breathing apparatus (SCUBA) or snorkeling in American Samoa, Guam, Kavaratti (Lakshadweep Islands, India), Papua New Guinea, Saipan, and the Paracel Islands (Xisha) in the South China Sea between the years 2005 and 2018. Samples from all locations besides Papua New Guinea were preserved in 1:1 seawater and either ethyl or isopropyl alcohol, transported back to laboratories, and stored frozen until extraction. The sample from Papua New Guinea was transported back to the laboratory in a culture flask and propagated in seawater (SW) BG-11 media [80]. For additional metadata about these samples, see Table S5.

3.3. Sample Preparation

Cyanobacterial biomass was exhaustively extracted with 2:1 dichloromethane and methanol, concentrated under vacuum, and resuspended in methanol or acetonitrile at a concentration of 1 mg/mL. Samples were prepared for LC-MS/MS analysis via elution through C18 solid phase extraction (SPE) cartridges.

3.4. ORCA Pipeline

Code, data files, and supporting documentation on use and workings of the ORCA pipeline are available at https://github.com/c-leber/ORCA, while the parameter sets used for the various analyses reported in this study are available in Tables S6–S8. ORCA was written in Python [81] and is built off the following Python packages: pandas (0.25.2) [82,83], numpy (1.16.5) [84,85], pyteomics (4.1.2) [86,87], scipy (1.3.1) [88], networkx (2.4) [89], matplotlib (3.0.3) [90], sklearn (0.21.3) [91], and seaborn (0.9.0) [92]. ORCA is available in the form of a Jupyter Notebook [93,94], to facilitate customization and interactive experimentation. Prior to analyses in ORCA, proprietary LC-MS datafiles were converted to mzXML using MSCONVERT (https://bio.tools/msconvert) [95], which is a part of the ProteoWizard Library [96]. MSCONVERT was also used to convert proprietary LC-MS/MS datafiles to mzML for the ORCA MS^2 Auxiliary pipeline, and to mzXML or mzML for GNPS.

3.5. GNPS Classical Molecular Networking

Molecular networks were created using the online workflow (https://ccms-ucsd.github.io/GNPSDocumentation/) on the GNPS website (http://gnps.ucsd.edu) and were visualized using Cytoscape (3.7.2) (https://cytoscape.org/) [97] and the GNPS in-browser network visualizer. For full accounting of the networking parameter sets, see Tables S9–S11.

3.6. Compound Isolation

M. bouillonii biomass from Laulau Bay, Saipan, was thoroughly extracted with 2:1 dichloromethane and methanol, yielding 10 g crude extract from 132 g (1 L) biomass. A portion of the crude extract was fractionated over silica with vacuum liquid chromatography and a standardized solvent system protocol (Table S12). Two relatively polar fractions (fractions F and G) were found to contain the bulk of compound **1**. Reverse phase HPLC was used to isolate 2.6 mg of this compound from these two fractions. A gradient method from 37% to 50% CH_3CN + 0.1% formic acid in H_2O + 0.1% formic acid over 60 min at a flow rate of 4 mL/min resulted in the elution of compound **1** starting at a retention time of approximately 38 min.

3.7. Planar Structure Characterization

Compound **1**: white solid, $[\alpha]_D^{26}$ +17.7 (*c* 0.1, MeOH); UV/Vis (Figure S31); IR (Figure S32). NMR data Table S13; ^1H, ^{13}C, COSY, HSQC, HMBC, HSQC-TOCSY, and long-range HSQMBC spectra (Figures S33–S39); HR ESIMS (observed *m/z* $[M + Na]^+$ at 479.2877, $C_{27}H_{40}N_2O_4$, calculated 479.2880).

3.8. Structure Elucidation—Standard Preparation and Derivatization for Configurational Characterization

Methods for ZACA methylalumination-oxidation [68], catalytic hydrogenation [98], ozonolysis [69,99], acid hydrolysis [69,98,99], peptide coupling [98,100], and derivatization with Marfey's reagent [98,99] were adapted from the literature.

3.8.1. Synthesis of (S)-2-methyloctanoic Acid

To a solution of trimethylaluminum (891 μL, 1.782 mmol) and (+)-$(NMI)_2ZrCl_2$ (23.84 mg, 0.036 mmol) in 1.5 mL of CH_2Cl_2 was added a solution of oct-1-ene (100 mg, 0.891 mmol) in 1.5 mL of CH_2Cl_2. After stirring overnight at 23 °C, the mixture was treated with a vigorous stream of O_2 for 1 h at 0 °C and then stirred for 5 h under an atmosphere of O_2 at room temperature. The reaction mixture was quenched with 1 M HCl, extracted with CH_2Cl_2, washed with brine, dried over $MgSO_4$ and concentrated. The residue was purified via silica flash column chromatography (20% ethyl acetate/hexanes) to yield (*S*)-2-methyloctan-1-ol (50 mg, 0.347 mmol, 39% yield) as a clear oil. The crude product was used in the next step without further purification.

To a solution of (*S*)-2-methyloctan-1-ol (50 mg, 0.347 mmol) in acetonitrile (1.4 mL) was added *N*-methyl morpholine *N*-oxide (NMO) solution in H_2O (468 mg, 3.47 mmol) and tetrapropylammonium perruthenate (TPAP) (12.18 mg, 0.035 mmol) sequentially at room temperature and the mixture was stirred for 2 h. The mixture was then concentrated, and the residue passed through a pad of silica gel using hexanes:diethyl ether (3:1) containing 0.1% acetic acid. The eluted solvent was concentrated to yield (*S*)-2-methyloctanoic acid (48 mg, 0.303 mmol, 88% yield). $[\alpha]_D^{26}$ +10.0 (c 1.05, MeOH); ^{1}H NMR (500 MHz, $CDCl_3$) δ 2.46 (ddq, J = 9.7, 6.8, 3.1 Hz, 1H), 1.69 (m, 2H), 1.44 (m, 2H), 1.37–1.24 (m, 6H), 1.19 (m, 3H), 0.89 (m, 3H); ^{13}C NMR (126 MHz, $CDCl_3$) δ 183.2, 39.6, 33.7, 31.9, 29.4, 27.3, 22.8, 17.1, 14.3. HRESIMS *m/z* $[M + H]^+$ 159.1394 (calc. for $C_9H_{19}O_2$, 159.1385).

3.8.2. Derivatization of 2-methyloctanoic Acid with 2-phenylglycine Methyl Ester

To generate a 1:1 standard mixture of both possible diastereomers of 2-methyloctanoic acid, 6.0 mg (37.9 μmol) of racemic 2-methyloctanoic acid was combined with 1-[bis(dimethylamino)methylene]-1H-1,2,3-triazolo[4,5-b]pyridinium 3-oxid hexafluorophosphate (HATU) (14.4 mg, 37.9 μmol), (*S*)-(+)-2-phenylglycine methyl ester hydrochloride (7.6 mg, 37.9 μmol) and *N*,*N*-diisopropylethylamine (DIPEA) (30 μL) in dimethylformamide (DMF) (300 μL). This was stirred overnight at room temperature and ambient atmosphere. The reaction mixture was then diluted with 1.0 mL of EtOAc, washed with saturated aqueous NH_4Cl (3 × 1.0 mL), concentrated under vacuum, and prepared for LC-MS analysis. To generate a chiral standard, 1.8 mg (11.4 μmol) of (*S*)-2-methyloctanoic acid was combined with HATU (4.3 mg, 11.4 μmol), (*S*)-(+)-2-phenylglycine methyl ester hydrochloride (2.3 mg, 11.4 μmol) and DIPEA (30 μL) in DMF (300 μL), and stirred overnight at room temperature and ambient atmosphere. The reaction mixture was then diluted with 1.0 mL of EtOAc, washed with saturated aqueous NH_4Cl (3 × 1.0 mL), concentrated under vacuum, and prepared for LC-MS analysis. The diastereomeric ratio of the chiral standard was 3:1 by area-under-curve analysis.

3.8.3. Derivatization of Lysine with Marfey's Reagent (FDAA)

To generate a racemic standard, 0.8 mg (4 μmol) of racemic lysine hydrochloride and 0.1 M $NaHCO_3$ (200 μL) were added to a solution of L-FDAA (4.4 mg, 16 μmol) in acetone (600 μL). The reaction mixture was sealed in a vial with ambient atmosphere, stirred at 90 °C for 5 min, neutralized with 6 M HCl, concentrated under vacuum, and prepared for LC-MS analysis. To generate a chiral standard, 1.0 mg (6 μmol) of L-lysine monohydrate and 0.1 M $NaHCO_3$ (200 μL) were added to a solution of L-FDAA (6.5 mg, 24 μmol) in acetone (600 μL). The reaction mixture was sealed in a vial with ambient atmosphere, stirred at 90 °C for 5 min, neutralized with 6 M HCl, concentrated under vacuum, and prepared for LC-MS analysis.

3.8.4. Derivatization of Compound 1

Compound **1** (0.5 mg) was combined with 1.0 mg of Pd/C in 1 mL EtOH and stirred under an atmosphere of H_2 for 8 h. The mixture was filtered through glass wool, rinsed with EtOH (3 × 1.0mL), and concentrated in vacuo.

Hydrogenated compound **1** (0.25 mg) was dissolved in 1 mL CH_2Cl_2, into which a stream of ozone gas was bubbled at −78 °C for 25 min. The reaction was concentrated under vacuum, and the residue was treated with 1 mL of 1:2 35% H_2O_2:HCOOH at 70 °C and ambient atmosphere for 20 min. The reaction was again concentrated in vacuo, followed by the addition of 1 mL 6 M HCl. The reaction mixture was stirred in a sealed vial with ambient atmosphere overnight at 110 °C, and then concentrated under vacuum. To the residue, a solution of L-FDAA (0.6 mg, 2 µmol) in acetone (200 µL) and 0.1 M $NaHCO_3$ (200 µL) were added. The reaction mixture was sealed in a vial with ambient atmosphere, stirred at 90 °C for 5 min, neutralized with 6 M HCl, concentrated in vacuo, and prepared for LC-MS analysis.

Hydrogenated compound **1** (0.25 mg) was dissolved in 1 mL 6 M HCl. This reaction mixture was stirred in a sealed vial with ambient atmosphere overnight at 110 °C, and then concentrated under vacuum. The residue was combined with HATU (0.4 mg, 1 µmol), (*S*)-(+)-2-phenylglycine methyl ester hydrochloride (0.2 mg, 1 µmol), and DIPEA (20 µL) in DMF (200 µL) and stirred for 6 h at room temperature and at ambient atmosphere. The reaction mixture was then diluted with 1.0 mL of EtOAc, washed with saturated aqueous NH_4Cl (3 × 1.0 mL), concentrated under vacuum, and prepared for LC-MS analysis.

3.9. ORCA MS^2 Auxiliary Pipeline

Code, data files, and supporting documentation on the use and workings of the ORCA MS^2 Auxiliary pipeline are available at https://github.com/c-leber/ORCA. MS^2 spectra were binned with the bin_OOM parameter set to 0, and the cutoff parameter for the hierarchical clustering of the MS^2 scans for a particular precursor mass was set to 0.15. The MS^2 scans were filtered to only include scans for precursor masses, which contained fragment peaks with *m*/*z* 168, resulting in 78 precursor masses. These precursor masses were individually analyzed via the hierarchical clustering of scan fragmentation patterns followed by the generation of consensus spectra for each cluster. Consensus spectra were manually inspected to detect interpretable fragmentation patterns similar to those of compound **1**.

3.10. Bioassays

Methods for the NCI-H460 cytotoxicity assay [101] and the Griess assay [102,103] were adapted from the literature.

3.10.1. Cytotoxicity Assay of Compound 1 with NCI-H460 Cell Line

NCI-H460 hypotriploid human cells (ATCC HTB-177) were grown in monolayers to near confluence in flasks and then seeded into wells at 3.33 × 10^4 cells/mL of Roswell Park Memorial Institute (RPMI) medium with standard fetal bovine serum (FBS), 180 µL/well, and incubated for 24 h at 37 °C in 96-well plates. Cells were exposed to compound **1** at ten half log concentrations, the highest being 21.9 µM with 1% dimethyl sulfoxide (DMSO) present, while the lowest was 0.7 nM. Plates were incubated for an additional 48 h and then stained with 3-(4,5-dimethylthiazol-2-yl)-2,5-diphenyltetrazolium bromide (MTT), for 25 min, after which the optical densities were recorded at 630 and 570 nm for each well on a SpectraMax M2 microplate reader with SoftMax® Pro Microplate Data Acquisition and Analysis Software (Molecular Devices, LLC, Version No. M2, Sunnyvale, CA, USA). The test samples were compared with a negative control of 1% DMSO and a positive control of doxorubicin (0.1 µg/mL and 1 µg/mL), both in RPMI medium. Due to the limited availability of compound **1**, fully toxic concentrations were not reached; hence, the resultant dose–response curve was incomplete. Nevertheless, the IC_{50} value for compound **1** is greater than 21.9 µM.

3.10.2. Griess Assay and Cytotoxicity of Compound **1** in RAW 264.7 Cells

RAW 264.7 murine macrophages (ATCC TIB-71) were seeded at 5 × 10^4 cells in 96-well plates in Dulbecco's Modified Eagle Medium (DMEM; Gibco, Carlsbad, CA, USA) supplemented with 10% endotoxin-low FBS (HyClone, characterized, Endotoxin: ≤ 25 EU/mL), 190 μL/well, and incubated for 24 h at 37 °C. Compound **1** at concentrations of 55, 28, 14, or 7 μM was applied in triplicate, and after 1 h lipopolysaccharide (LPS from Escherichia coli 026:B6, =10,000 EU/mg, Sigma-Aldrich, Oakville, ON, Canada) was added (0.5 or 1.5 μg/mL) to all wells except those for the LPS-free controls and those for evaluating the pro-inflammatory effects of compound **1**. LPS alone was used as a negative control, whereas the same LPS concentration with 1% DMSO served as the positive control in the Griess assay. After 24 h, Griess reactions (Section 3.10.3) were used to assess NO generation as a proxy for inflammation, and MTT staining (Section 3.10.1) was used to assess cell viability. Doxorubicin at 3.3 μg/mL was used as a positive control for assessing cell viability. Cell survival was calculated as a percentage compared to wells with 1% or 1.5% EtOH and no LPS. A NO concentration standard curve was prepared in Microsoft Excel based on eight serial dilutions of a nitrite standard (0–100 μM) with DMEM. One-way ANOVA and Tukey's method were used to test for significance in the cell survival results from the assay; high mortality in certain conditions made statistical analyses of the inflammation data inappropriate. Statistical analyses were applied using GraphPad Prism version 8.0.0 for Windows. Batch variability in LPS potency and RAW 264.7 murine macrophage sensitivity, as well as limited availability of compound **1** necessitated using differing reagent concentrations across the biological replicates.

3.10.3. Griess Reaction

Supernatant from each sample well (50 μL) was added to the experimental wells in triplicate. A 1:1 mixture of 1% sulfanilamide solution in 5% phosphoric acid and 0.1% *N*-1-napthylethylenediamine dihydrochloride (100 μL) was added to each well and the plate was incubated in the dark for 20 min. Optical density was measured at 570 nm on a SpectraMax M2 microplate reader. The raw data were exported to a Microsoft Excel work sheet and the concentration of nitrite in the samples was determined by comparison to the standard curve using regression analysis.

3.10.4. In silico Antibiotic Screening

The simplified molecular-input line-entry system (SMILES) structures of compound **1**, proposed analogs **2–10**, C_{12}-tertramic acid, and C_{14}-tetramic acid were submitted to Chemprop Predict (http://chemprop.csail.mit.edu/predict) [79], using the Antibiotics model checkpoint.

Supplementary Materials: The following are available online at http://www.mdpi.com/1660-3397/18/10/515/s1, Figure S1: Molecular network of *M. bouillonii* crude extracts; Figure S2: Predicted ^{13}C shifts for candidate structure **1a**; Figure S3: Predicted ^{13}C shifts for candidate structure **1b**; Figure S4: Compound **1** derived 2-methyoctanoic acid compared to standards; Figure S5: Compound **1** derived lysine compared to standards; Figure S6: Doscadenamide A (**1**) consensus MS^2 spectrum; Figure S7: Molecular network cluster of compound **1** and analogs, highlighting *m/z* 168 frag. peak; Figure S8: Structure of compound **1** with structure proposals for analogs (**2–10**); Figure S9: Doscadenamide B (**2**) consensus MS^2 spectrum; Figure S10: Doscadenamide B (**2**) proposed fragmentation; Figure S11: Doscadenamide C (**3**) consensus MS^2 spectrum; Figure S12: Doscadenamide C (**3**) proposed fragmentation; Figure S13: Doscadenamide D (**4**) consensus MS^2 spectrum; Figure S14: Doscadenamide D (**4**) proposed fragmentation; Figure S15: Doscadenamide E (**5**) consensus MS^2 spectrum; Figure S16: Doscadenamide E (**5**) proposed fragmentation; Figure S17: Doscadenamide F (**6**) consensus MS^2 spectrum; Figure S18: Doscadenamide F (**6**) proposed fragmentation; Figure S19: Doscadenamide G (**7**) consensus MS^2 spectrum; Figure S20: Doscadenamide G (**7**) proposed fragmentation; Figure S21: Doscadenamide H (**8**) consensus MS^2 spectrum; Figure S22: Doscadenamide H (**8**) proposed fragmentation; Figure S23: Doscadenamide I (**9**) consensus MS^2 spectrum; Figure S24: Doscadenamide I (**9**) proposed fragmentation; Figure S25: Doscadenamide J (**10**) consensus MS^2 spectrum; Figure S26: Doscadenamide J (**10**) proposed fragmentation; Figure S27: Representative structures from compound families similar to the doscadenamides; Figure S28: Results of compound **1** in Griess assay—biological replicate 1; Figure S29: Results of compound **1** in Griess assay—biological replicate 2; Figure S30: Results of compound **1** in Griess assay—biological replicate 3; Figure S31: UV/Vis absorbance spectrum (200–400 nm) for compound **1**; Figure S32: IR spectrum for compound **1**; Figure S33: ^1H NMR spectrum for compound **1**; Figure S34: ^{13}C NMR spectrum for compound **1**; Figure S35: ^{1}H-^{1}H COSY spectrum for compound **1**; Figure S36: ^{1}H-^{13}C HSQC spectrum for compound **1**; Figure S37: ^{1}H-^{13}C HMBC spectrum for compound **1**; Figure S38: ^{1}H-^{13}C HSQC-TOCSY spectrum for compound **1**; Figure S39: ^{1}H-^{13}C Long-range HSQMBC spectrum for compound **1**; Table S1: Known compounds isolated from *M. bouillonii*; Table S2: Average relative abundances and feature selection scores for top 10 Saipan MS^1 features; Table S3: Putative identifications for top 30 MS^1 features in the *M. bouillonii* crude extract dataset; Table S4: In silico antibiotic screening results for the doscadenamides and tetramic acids; Table S5: *M. bouillonii* crude extract sample metadata; Table S6: ORCA parameter set for MS^1 feature dendrogram; Table S7: ORCA parameter set for GNPS MS^2 feature presence/absence dendrogram; Table S8: ORCA parameter set for MS^1 feature selection; Table S9: GNPS parameter set for *M. bouillonii* crude extract molecular network; Table S10: GNPS parameter set for *M. bouillonii* crude extract MS^2 feature bucket table; Table S11: GNPS parameter set for Saipan and Guam crude extracts and fractions molecular network; Table S12: VLC fractionation solvent systems; and Table S13: ^{1}H and ^{13}C NMR data for doscadenamide A (**1**) in $CDCl_3$.

Author Contributions: Conceptualization, C.A.L. and W.H.G.; methodology, C.A.L., C.B.N., L.K., J.A. and E.J.E.C.-D.; software, C.A.L.; validation, C.A.L.; formal analysis, C.A.L.; investigation, C.A.L., C.B.N., L.K., J.A., E.J.E.C.-D. and E.G.; resources, C.A.L., C.B.N., J.A., E.J.E.C.-D., E.G., V.J., T.P.S., A.J.R., J.S.B., T.L., Y.Y., S.H., X.Y. and W.H.G.; data curation, C.A.L.; writing—original draft preparation, C.A.L. and W.H.G.; writing—review and editing, C.A.L., C.B.N., L.K., J.A., E.J.E.C.-D., E.G., V.J., T.P.S., A.J.R., J.S.B., T.L., Y.Y., S.H., X.Y. and W.H.G.; visualization, C.A.L.; supervision, W.H.G.; project administration, C.A.L.; funding acquisition, W.H.G. and C.B.N. All authors have read and agreed to the published version of the manuscript.

Funding: This study was supported by the National Institutes of Health (NIH) (grant GM107550 to W.H.G.) and the Gordon and Betty Moore Foundation (grant GBMF7622 to W.H.G.). This study was further supported in part by the National Key Research and Development Program of China, funded through MOST (the Ministry of Science and Technology of China; grant 2018YFC0310900 to X.Y. and C.B.N.), NSFC (the National Natural Science Foundation of China; grant 81850410553 to C.B.N.), and Ningbo STI (Ningbo Science and Technology Bureau; grant 010-20171JCGY01172 to C.B.N.). A portion of this study was supported by the University Grants Commission, Government of India under Indo-US 21st Century Knowledge Initiative Project (Grant No. 194-1/2009(IC) dated 7/2/2015) to V.J. and T.P.S. C.A.L. was supported by the UCSD Regents Pre-Doctoral Fellowship, the Robert L. Cody Memorial Pre-Doctoral Fellowship, the Kaplan Trust CMBB Pre-Doctoral Fellowship, and the NIH Training Program in Marine Biotechnology (T32GM067550). L.K. was supported by the Deutsche Forschungsgemeinschaft (Grant KE 2172/3-1 and KE 2172/4-1).

Acknowledgments: We acknowledge F.M. Brunner and C.P. Kubiak (UCSD Department of Chemistry & Biochemistry) for facilitating acquisition of IR data, and Y. Su, and L. Gross for HiRes mass spectrometry support at the UCSD Molecular Mass Spectrometry Facility. We thank B. Duggan and A. Mrse for NMR support, and M.P. Christy (Scripps Institution of Oceanography, UCSD) for support with the synthesis of standards. We also acknowledge the government of Sansha city, China, for permission to collect and study several of the marine samples used in this research and the sample collection assistance from L. Zhenhua, L. Daning and H. Da of the Xisha Marine Science Comprehensive Experimental Station, South China Sea Institute of Oceanology, Chinese Academy of Sciences. We acknowledge the support of I.S. Bright Singh of the National Centre for Aquatic Animal Health, Cochin University of Science and Technology, India, and the Department of Science and Technology, Kavaratti, Lakshadweep Islands, India for the required research permits. C.L. acknowledges travel support from the LBG foundation.

Conflicts of Interest: William H. Gerwick declares a competing financial interest as a cofounder of NMR Finder LLC. Otherwise, the authors declare no conflict of interest. The funders had no role in the design of the study; in the collection, analyses, or interpretation of data; in the writing of the manuscript, or in the decision to publish the results.

References

1. Chanana, S.; Thomas, C.S.; Braun, D.R.; Hou, Y.; Wyche, T.P.; Bugni, T.S. Natural Product Discovery Using Planes of Principal Component Analysis in R (PoPCAR). *Metabolites* **2017**, *7*, 34. [CrossRef]
2. Clark, C.M.; Costa, M.S.; Sanchez, L.M.; Murphy, B.T. Coupling MALDI-TOF mass spectrometry protein and specialized metabolite analyses to rapidly discriminate bacterial function. *Proc. Natl. Acad. Sci. USA* **2018**, *115*, 4981–4986. [CrossRef]
3. Wang, M.; Carver, J.J.; Phelan, V.V.; Sanchez, L.M.; Garg, N.; Peng, Y.; Nguyen, D.D.; Watrous, J.; Kapono, C.A.; Luzzatto-Knaan, T.; et al. Sharing and community curation of mass spectrometry data with Global Natural Products Social Molecular Networking. *Nat. Biotechnol.* **2016**, *34*, 828–837. [CrossRef]
4. Nothias, L.F.; Petras, D.; Schmid, R.; Dührkop, K.; Rainer, J.; Sarvepalli, A.; Protsyuk, I.; Ernst, M.; Tsugawa, H.; Fleischauer, M.; et al. Feature-based Molecular Networking in the GNPS Analysis Environment. *Nat. Methods* **2020**, *17*, 905–908. [CrossRef]

5. Gowda, H.; Ivanisevic, J.; Johnson, C.H.; Kurczy, M.E.; Benton, H.P.; Rinehart, D.; Nguyen, T.; Ray, J.; Kuehl, J.; Arevalo, B.; et al. Interactive XCMS Online: Simplifying Advanced Metabolomic Data Processing and Subsequent Statistical Analyses. *Anal. Chem.* **2014**, *86*, 6931–6939. [CrossRef] [PubMed]
6. Pluskal, T.; Castillo, S.; Villar-Briones, A.; Orešič, M. MZmine 2: Modular framework for processing, visualizing, and analyzing mass spectrometry-based molecular profile data. *BMC Bioinform.* **2010**, *11*, 395. [CrossRef] [PubMed]
7. Chong, J.; Soufan, O.; Li, C.; Caraus, I.; Li, S.; Bourque, G.; Wishart, D.S.; Xia, J. MetaboAnalyst 4.0: Towards more transparent and integrative metabolomics analysis. *Nucleic Acids Res.* **2018**, *46*, W486–W494. [CrossRef] [PubMed]
8. Tronholm, A.; Engene, N. Moorena gen. nov., a valid name for "Moorea Engene & al." nom. inval. (Oscillatoriaceae, Cyanobacteria). *Notulae Algarum* **2019**, *122*, 1–2.
9. Engene, N.; Rottacker, E.C.; Kaštovský, J.; Byrum, T.; Choi, H.; Ellisman, M.H.; Komárek, J.; Gerwick, W.H. *Moorea producens* gen. nov., sp. nov. and *Moorea bouillonii* comb. nov., tropical marine cyanobacteria rich in bioactive secondary metabolites. *Int. J. Syst. Evol. Micr.* **2012**, *62*, 1171–1178. [CrossRef] [PubMed]
10. Leao, T.; Castelão, G.; Korobeynikov, A.; Monroe, E.A.; Podell, S.; Glukhov, E.; Allen, E.E.; Gerwick, W.H.; Gerwick, L. Comparative genomics uncovers the prolific and distinctive metabolic potential of the cyanobacterial genus *Moorea*. *Proc. Natl. Acad. Sci. USA* **2017**, *114*, 3198–3203. [CrossRef] [PubMed]
11. Williams, P.G.; Luesch, H.; Yoshida, W.Y.; Moore, R.E.; Paul, V.J. Continuing Studies on the Cyanobacterium *Lyngbya sp.*: Isolation and Structure Determination of 15-Norlyngbyapeptin A and Lyngbyabellin D. *J. Nat. Prod.* **2003**, *66*, 595–598. [CrossRef]
12. Matthew, S.; Salvador, L.A.; Schupp, P.J.; Paul, V.J.; Luesch, H. Cytotoxic Halogenated Macrolides and Modified Peptides from the Apratoxin-Producing Marine Cyanobacterium *Lyngbya bouillonii* from Guam. *J. Nat. Prod.* **2010**, *73*, 1544–1552. [CrossRef]
13. Choi, H.; Mevers, E.; Byrum, T.; Valeriote, F.A.; Gerwick, W.H. Lyngbyabellins K-N from two Palmyra atoll collections of the marine cyanobacterium *Moorea bouillonii*. *Eur. J. Org. Chem.* **2012**, *2012*, 5141–5150. [CrossRef]
14. Soria-Mercado, I.E.; Pereira, A.; Cao, Z.; Murray, T.F.; Gerwick, W.H. Alotamide A, a novel neuropharmacological agent from the marine cyanobacterium *Lyngbya bouillonii*. *Org. Lett.* **2009**, *11*, 4704–4707. [CrossRef]
15. Luesch, H.; Yoshida, W.Y.; Moore, R.E.; Paul, V.J. Apramides A–G, Novel Lipopeptides from the Marine Cyanobacterium *Lyngbya majuscula*. *J. Nat. Prod.* **2000**, *63*, 1106–1112. [CrossRef]
16. Luesch, H.; Yoshida, W.Y.; Moore, R.E.; Paul, V.J.; Corbett, T.H. Total Structure Determination of Apratoxin A, a Potent Novel Cytotoxin from the Marine Cyanobacterium *Lyngbya majuscula*. *J. Am. Chem. Soc.* **2001**, *123*, 5418–5423. [CrossRef]
17. Thornburg, C.C.; Cowley, E.S.; Sikorska, J.; Shaala, L.A.; Ishmael, J.E.; Youssef, D.T.A.; McPhail, K.L. Apratoxin H and Apratoxin A Sulfoxide from the Red Sea Cyanobacterium *Moorea producens*. *J. Nat. Prod.* **2013**, *76*, 1781–1788. [CrossRef]
18. Luesch, H.; Yoshida, W.Y.; Moore, R.E.; Paul, V.J. New apratoxins of marine cyanobacterial origin from guam and palau. *Bioorg. Med. Chem.* **2002**, *10*, 1973–1978. [CrossRef]
19. Gutiérrez, M.; Suyama, T.L.; Engene, N.; Wingerd, J.S.; Matainaho, T.; Gerwick, W.H. Apratoxin D, a Potent Cytotoxic Cyclodepsipeptide from Papua New Guinea Collections of the Marine Cyanobacteria *Lyngbya majuscula* and *Lyngbya sordida*. *J. Nat. Prod.* **2008**, *71*, 1099–1103. [CrossRef]
20. Matthew, S.; Schupp, P.J.; Luesch, H. Apratoxin E, a Cytotoxic Peptolide from a Guamanian Collection of the Marine Cyanobacterium *Lyngbya bouillonii*. *J. Nat. Prod.* **2008**, *71*, 1113–1116. [CrossRef]
21. Tidgewell, K.; Engene, N.; Byrum, T.; Media, J.; Doi, T.; Valeriote, F.A.; Gerwick, W.H. Evolved Diversification of a Modular Natural Product Pathway: Apratoxins F and G, Two Cytotoxic Cyclic Depsipeptides from a Palmyra Collection of *Lyngbya bouillonii*. *Chembiochem* **2010**, *11*, 1458–1466. [CrossRef] [PubMed]
22. Cai, W.; Salvador-Reyes, L.A.; Zhang, W.; Chen, Q.Y.; Matthew, S.; Ratnayake, R.; Seo, S.J.; Dolles, S.; Gibson, D.J.; Paul, V.J.; et al. Apratyramide, a Marine-Derived Peptidic Stimulator of VEGF-A and Other Growth Factors with Potential Application in Wound Healing. *ACS Chem. Biol.* **2018**, *13*, 91–99. [CrossRef]
23. Tan, L.T.; Okino, T.; Gerwick, W.H. Bouillonamide: A Mixed Polyketide-Peptide Cytotoxin from the Marine Cyanobacterium *Moorea bouillonii*. *Mar. Drugs* **2013**, *11*, 3015–3024. [CrossRef] [PubMed]

24. Rubio, B.K.; Parrish, S.M.; Yoshid, W.; Schupp, P.J.; Schils, T.; Williams, P.G. Depsipeptides from a Guamanian marine cyanobacterium, *Lyngbya bouillonii*, with selective inhibition of serine proteases. *Tetrahedron Lett.* **2010**, *51*, 6718–6721. [CrossRef]
25. Kleigrewe, K.; Almaliti, J.; Tian, I.Y.; Kinnel, R.B.; Korobeynikov, A.; Monroe, E.A.; Duggan, B.M.; Di Marzo, V.; Sherman, D.H.; Dorrestein, P.C.; et al. Combining Mass Spectrometric Metabolic Profiling with Genomic Analysis: A Powerful Approach for Discovering Natural Products from Cyanobacteria. *J. Nat. Prod.* **2015**, *78*, 1671–1682. [CrossRef]
26. Lopez, J.A.V.; Petitbois, J.G.; Vairappan, C.S.; Umezawa, T.; Matsuda, F.; Okino, T. Columbamides D and E: Chlorinated Fatty Acid Amides from the Marine Cyanobacterium *Moorea bouillonii* Collected in Malaysia. *Org. Lett.* **2017**, *19*, 4231–4234. [CrossRef]
27. Mehjabin, J.J.; Wei, L.; Petitbois, J.G.; Umezawa, T.; Matsuda, F.; Vairappan, C.S.; Morikawa, M.; Okino, T. Biosurfactants from Marine Cyanobacteria Collected in Sabah, Malaysia. *J. Nat. Prod.* **2020**, *83*, 1925–1930. [CrossRef]
28. Pereira, A.R.; McCue, C.F.; Gerwick, W.H. Cyanolide A, a Glycosidic Macrolide with Potent Molluscicidal Activity from the Papua New Guinea Cyanobacterium *Lyngbya bouillonii*. *J. Nat. Prod.* **2010**, *73*, 217–220. [CrossRef]
29. Liang, X.; Matthew, S.; Chen, Q.Y.; Kwan, J.C.; Paul, V.J.; Luesch, H. Discovery and Total Synthesis of Doscadenamide A: A Quorum Sensing Signaling Molecule from a Marine Cyanobacterium. *Org. Lett.* **2019**, *21*, 7274–7278. [CrossRef] [PubMed]
30. Nakamura, F.; Maejima, H.; Kawamura, M.; Arai, D.; Okino, T.; Zhao, M.; Ye, T.; Lee, J.; Chang, Y.; Fusetani, N.; et al. Kakeromamide A, a new cyclic pentapeptide inducing astrocyte differentiation isolated from the marine cyanobacterium *Moorea bouillonii*. *Bioorg. Med. Chem. Lett.* **2018**, *28*, 2206–2209. [CrossRef]
31. Sweeney-Jones, A.M.; Gagaring, K.; Antonova-Koch, J.; Zhou, H.; Mojib, N.; Soapi, K.; Skolnick, J.; McNamara, C.W.; Kubanek, J. Antimalarial Peptide and Polyketide Natural Products from the Fijian Marine Cyanobacterium *Moorea producens*. *Mar. Drugs* **2020**, *18*, 167. [CrossRef]
32. Sumimoto, S.; Iwasaki, A.; Ohno, O.; Sueyoshi, K.; Teruya, T.; Suenaga, K. Kanamienamide, an Enamide with an Enol Ether from the Marine Cyanobacterium *Moorea bouillonii*. *Org. Lett.* **2016**, *18*, 4884–4887. [CrossRef]
33. Klein, D.; Braekman, J.C.; Daloze, D.; Hoffmann, L.; Demoulin, V. Laingolide, a novel 15-membered macrolide from *Lyngbya bouillonii* (cyanophyceae). *Tetrahedron Lett.* **1996**, *37*, 7519–7520. [CrossRef]
34. Klein, D.; Braekman, J.C.; Daloze, D.; Hoffmann, L.; Castillo, G.; Demoulin, V. Madangolide and Laingolide A, Two Novel Macrolides from *Lyngbya bouillonii* (Cyanobacteria). *J. Nat. Prod.* **1999**, *62*, 934–936. [CrossRef]
35. Tan, L.T.; Márquez, B.L.; Gerwick, W.H. Lyngbouilloside, a Novel Glycosidic Macrolide from the Marine Cyanobacterium *Lyngbya bouillonii*. *J. Nat. Prod.* **2002**, *65*, 925–928. [CrossRef]
36. Luesch, H.; Yoshida, W.Y.; Moore, R.E.; Paul, V.J.; Mooberry, S.L. Isolation, Structure Determination, and Biological Activity of Lyngbyabellin A from the Marine Cyanobacterium *Lyngbya majuscula*. *J. Nat. Prod.* **2000**, *63*, 611–615. [CrossRef]
37. Luesch, H.; Yoshida, W.Y.; Moore, R.E.; Paul, V.J. Isolation and Structure of the Cytotoxin Lyngbyabellin B and Absolute Configuration of Lyngbyapeptin A from the Marine Cyanobacterium *Lyngbya majuscula*. *J. Nat. Prod.* **2000**, *63*, 1437–1439. [CrossRef]
38. Luesch, H.; Yoshida, W.Y.; Moore, R.E.; Paul, V.J. Structurally diverse new alkaloids from Palauan collections of the apratoxin-producing marine cyanobacterium *Lyngbya* sp. *Tetrahedron* **2002**, *58*, 7959–7966. [CrossRef]
39. Klein, D.; Braekman, J.C.; Daloze, D.; Hoffmann, L.; Demoulin, V. Lyngbyaloside, a Novel 2,3,4-Tri-O-methyl-6-deoxy-α-mannopyranoside Macrolide from *Lyngbya bouillonii* (Cyanobacteria). *J. Nat. Prod.* **1997**, *60*, 1057–1059. [CrossRef]
40. Luesch, H.; Yoshida, W.Y.; Harrigan, G.G.; Doom, J.P.; Moore, R.E.; Paul, V.J. Lyngbyaloside B, a New Glycoside Macrolide from a Palauan Marine Cyanobacterium, *Lyngbya* sp. *J. Nat. Prod.* **2002**, *65*, 1945–1948. [CrossRef]
41. Klein, D.; Braekman, J.C.; Daloze, D.; Hoffmann, L.; Castillo, G.; Demoulin, V. Lyngbyapeptin A, a modified tetrapeptide from *Lyngbya bouillonii* (Cyanophyceae). *Tetrahedron Lett.* **1999**, *40*, 695–696. [CrossRef]
42. Luesch, H.; Yoshida, W.Y.; Moore, R.E.; Paul, V.J. Lyngbyastatin 2 and Norlyngbyastatin 2, Analogues of Dolastatin G and Nordolastatin G from the Marine Cyanobacterium *Lyngbya majuscula*. *J. Nat. Prod.* **1999**, *62*, 1702–1706. [CrossRef] [PubMed]

43. Mevers, E.; Matainaho, T.; Allara, M.; Di Marzo, V.; Gerwick, W.H. Mooreamide A: A cannabinomimetic lipid from the marine cyanobacterium *Moorea bouillonii*. *Lipids* **2014**, *49*, 1127–1132. [CrossRef] [PubMed]
44. Luesch, H.; Williams, P.G.; Yoshida, W.Y.; Moore, R.E.; Paul, V.J. Ulongamides A–F, New β-Amino Acid-Containing Cyclodepsipeptides from Palauan Collections of the Marine Cyanobacterium *Lyngbya* sp. *J. Nat. Prod.* **2002**, *65*, 996–1000. [CrossRef] [PubMed]
45. Levin, D.A. Alkaloid-bearing plants: An ecogeographic perspective. *Am. Nat.* **1976**, *110*, 261–284. [CrossRef]
46. Coley, P.D.; Aide, T.M. Comparison of herbivory and plant defenses in temperate and tropical broad-leaved forests. In *Plant–Animal Interaction: Evolutionary Ecology in Tropical and Temperate Regions*; Wiley-Interscience: New York, NY, USA, 1991; pp. 25–49.
47. Coley, P.D.; Barone, J.A. Herbivory and plant defenses in tropical forests. *Annu. Rev. Ecol. Syst.* **1996**, *27*, 305–335. [CrossRef]
48. Rasmann, S.; Agrawal, A.A. Latitudinal patterns in plant defense: Evolution of cardenolides, their toxicity and induction following herbivory. *Ecol. Lett.* **2011**, *14*, 476–483. [CrossRef]
49. Bakus, G.J.; Green, G. Toxicity in sponges and holothurians: A geographic pattern. *Science* **1974**, *185*, 951–953. [CrossRef]
50. Hay, M.E.; Fenical, W. Marine plant-herbivore interactions: The ecology of chemical defense. *Annu. Rev. Ecol. Syst.* **1988**, *19*, 111–145. [CrossRef]
51. Bolser, R.C.; Hay, M.E. Are tropical plants better defended? Palatability and defenses of temperate vs tropical seaweeds. *Ecology* **1996**, *77*, 2269–2286. [CrossRef]
52. Anstett, D.N.; Nunes, K.A.; Baskett, C.; Kotanen, P.M. Sources of Controversy Surrounding Latitudinal Patterns in Herbivory and Defense. *Trends Ecol. Evol.* **2016**, *31*, 789–802. [CrossRef] [PubMed]
53. Kooyers, N.J.; Blackman, B.K.; Holeski, L.M. Optimal defense theory explains deviations from latitudinal herbivory defense hypothesis. *Ecology* **2017**, *98*, 1036–1048. [CrossRef]
54. Shang, Z.; Winter, J.M.; Kauffman, C.A.; Yang, I.; Fenical, W. Salinipeptins: Integrated Genomic and Chemical Approaches Reveal D-Amino Acid-Containing Ribosomally Synthesized and Post-Translationally Modified Peptides from a Great Salt Lake *Streptomyces* sp. *ACS Chem. Biol.* **2019**, *14*, 415–425. [CrossRef] [PubMed]
55. Marcolefas, E.; Leung, T.; Okshevsky, M.; McKay, G.; Hignett, E.; Hamel, J.; Aguirre1, G.; Blenner-Hassett, O.; Boyle, B.; Lévesque, R.C.; et al. Culture-Dependent Bioprospecting of Bacterial Isolates From the Canadian High Arctic Displaying Antibacterial Activity. *Front. Microbiol.* **2019**, *10*, 1836. [CrossRef] [PubMed]
56. Bory, A.; Shilling, A.J.; Allen, J.; Azhari, A.; Roth, A.; Shaw, L.N.; Kyle, D.E.; Adams, J.H.; Amsler, C.D.; McClintock, J.B.; et al. Bioactivity of Spongian Diterpenoid Scaffolds from the Antarctic Sponge Dendrilla antarctica. *Mar. Drugs* **2020**, *18*, 327. [CrossRef]
57. Zhou, H.; He, Y.; Tian, Y.; Cong, B.; Yang, H. Bacilohydrin A, a New Cytotoxic Cyclic Lipopeptide of Surfactins Class Produced by *Bacillus* sp. SY27F from the Indian Ocean Hydrothermal Vent. *Nat. Prod. Commun.* **2019**, *14*, 141–146. [CrossRef]
58. Zhang, S.; Gui, C.; Shao, M.; Kumar, P.S.; Huang, H.; Ju, J. Antimicrobial tunicamycin derivatives from the deep sea-derived Streptomyces xinghaiensis SCSIO S15077. *Nat. Prod. Res.* **2020**, *34*, 1499–1504. [CrossRef]
59. Luzzatto-Knaan, T.; Garg, N.; Wang, M.; Glukhov, E.; Peng, Y.; Ackermann, G.; Amir, A.; Duggan, B.M.; Ryazanov, S.; Gerwick, L.; et al. Digitizing mass spectrometry data to explore the chemical diversity and distribution of marine cyanobacteria and algae. *eLife* **2017**, *6*, e24214. [CrossRef]
60. Naman, C.B.; Rattan, R.; Nikoulina, S.E.; Lee, J.; Miller, B.W.; Moss, N.A.; Armstrong, L.; Boudreau, P.D.; Debonsi, H.M.; Valeriote, F.A.; et al. Integrating molecular networking and biological assays to target the isolation of a cytotoxic cyclic octapeptide, samoamide A, from an American Samoan marine cyanobacterium. *J. Nat. Prod.* **2017**, *80*, 625–633. [CrossRef]
61. Crnkovic, C.M.; May, D.S.; Orjala, J. The impact of culture conditions on growth and metabolomic profiles of freshwater cyanobacteria. *J. Appl. Phycol.* **2018**, *30*, 375–384. [CrossRef]
62. Pallarés, N.; Tolosa, J.; Mañes, J.; Ferrer, E. Occurrence of Mycotoxins in Botanical Dietary Supplement Infusion Beverages. *J. Nat. Prod.* **2019**, *82*, 403–406. [CrossRef] [PubMed]
63. Engene, N.; Tronholm, A.; Paul, V.J. Uncovering cryptic diversity of *Lyngbya*: The new tropical marine cyanobacterial genus *Dapis* (Oscillatoriales). *J. Phycol.* **2018**, *54*, 435–446. [CrossRef]
64. Jayaram, B.; Klawonn, F. Can unbounded distance measures mitigate the curse of dimensionality? *Int. J. Data Min. Model. Manag.* **2012**, *4*, 361–383. [CrossRef]

65. Milligan, K.E.; Márquez, B.; Williamson, R.T.; Davies-Coleman, M.; Gerwick, W.H. Two New Malyngamides from a Madagascan *Lyngbya majuscula*. *J. Nat. Prod.* **2000**, *63*, 965–968. [CrossRef] [PubMed]
66. Edwards, D.J.; Marquez, B.L.; Nogle, L.M.; McPhail, K.; Goeger, D.E.; Roberts, M.A.; Gerwick, W.H. Structure and Biosynthesis of the Jamaicamides, New Mixed Polyketide-Peptide Neurotoxins from the Marine Cyanobacterium *Lyngbya majuscula*. *Chem. Biol.* **2004**, *11*, 817–833. [CrossRef] [PubMed]
67. Linington, R.G.; Clark, B.R.; Trimble, E.E.; Almanza, A.; Ureña, L.D.; Kyle, D.E.; Gerwick, W.H. Antimalarial Peptides from Marine Cyanobacteria: Isolation and Structural Elucidation of Gallinamide A. *J. Nat. Prod.* **2009**, *72*, 14–17. [CrossRef] [PubMed]
68. Negishi, E.; Tan, Z.; Liang, B.; Novak, T. An efficient and general route to reduced polypropionates via Zr-catalyzed asymmetric C-C bond formation. *Proc. Natl. Acad. Sci. USA* **2004**, *101*, 5782–5787. [CrossRef]
69. Pereira, A.; Etzbach, L.; Engene, N.; Müller, R.; Gerwick, W.H. Molluscicidal Metabolites from an Assemblage of Palmyra Atoll Cyanobacteria. *J. Nat. Prod.* **2011**, *74*, 1175–1181. [CrossRef]
70. Boudreau, P.D.; Byrum, T.; Liu, W.T.; Dorrestein, P.C.; Gerwick, W.H. Viequeamide A, a Cytotoxic Member of the Kulolide Superfamily of Cyclic Depsipeptides from a Marine Button Cyanobacterium. *J. Nat. Prod.* **2012**, *75*, 1560–1570. [CrossRef]
71. Hooper, G.J.; Orjala, J.; Schatzman, R.C.; Gerwick, W.H. Carmabins A and B, New Lipopeptides from the Caribbean Cyanobacterium *Lyngbya majuscula*. *J. Nat. Prod.* **1998**, *61*, 529–533. [CrossRef]
72. Moss, N.A.; Seiler, G.; Leão, T.F.; Castro-Falcón, G.; Gerwick, L.; Hughes, C.C.; Gerwick, W.H. Nature's Combinatorial Biosynthesis Produces Vatiamides A–F. *Angew. Chem. Int. Ed.* **2019**, *58*, 9027–9031. [CrossRef] [PubMed]
73. Gerwick, W.H.; Tan, L.T.; Sitachitta, N. Nitrogen-containing metabolites from marine cyanobacteria. In *The Alkaloids: Chemistry and Biology*, 1st ed.; Cordell, G.A., Ed.; Academic Press: Cambridge, MA, USA, 2001; Volume 57, pp. 75–184. [CrossRef]
74. Tidgewell, K.; Clark, B.R.; Gerwick, W.H. The Natural Products Chemistry of Cyanobacteria. In *Comprehensive Natural Products II: Chemistry and Biology*, 1st ed.; Mander, L.N., Liu, H.-W., Eds.; Elsevier: Amsterdam, The Netherlands, 2010; Volume 2, pp. 144–188. [CrossRef]
75. Zhang, C.; Idelbayev, Y.; Roberts, N.; Tao, Y.; Nannapaneni, Y.; Duggan, B.M.; Min, J.; Lin, E.C.; Gerwick, E.C.; Cottrell, G.W.; et al. Small Molecule Accurate Recognition Technology (SMART) to Enhance Natural Products Research. *Sci. Rep.* **2017**, *7*, 14243. [CrossRef]
76. Sadar, M.D.; Williams, D.E.; Mawji, N.R.; Patrick, B.O.; Wikanta, T.; Chasanah, E.; Irianto, H.E.; Van Soest, R.; Andersen, R.J. Sintokamides A to E, Chlorinated Peptides from the Sponge Dysidea sp. that Inhibit Transactivation of the N-Terminus of the Androgen Receptor in Prostate Cancer Cells. *Org. Lett.* **2008**, *10*, 4947–4950. [CrossRef]
77. Lowery, C.A.; Park, J.; Gloeckner, C.; Meijler, M.M.; Mueller, R.S.; Boshoff, H.I.; Ulrich, R.L.; Barry, C.E.; Bartlett, D.H.; Kravchenko, V.V.; et al. Defining the Mode of Action of Tetramic Acid Antibacterials Derived from Pseudomonas aeruginosa Quorum Sensing Signals. *J. Am. Chem. Soc.* **2009**, *131*, 14473–14479. [CrossRef]
78. Ricciotti, E.; FitzGerald, G.A. Prostaglandins and Inflammation. *Arterioscler. Thromb. Vasc. Biol.* **2011**, *31*, 986–1000. [CrossRef] [PubMed]
79. Stokes, J.M.; Yang, K.; Swanson, K.; Jin, W.; Cubillos-Ruiz, A.; Donghia, N.M.; MacNair, C.R.; French, S.; Carfrae, L.A.; Bloom-Ackermann, Z.; et al. A Deep Learning Approach to Antibiotic Discovery. *Cell* **2020**, *181*, 475–483. [CrossRef]
80. Moss, N.A.; Leao, T.; Glukhov, E.; Gerwick, L.; Gerwick, W.H. Collection, Culturing, and Genome Analyses of Tropical Marine Filamentous Benthic Cyanobacteria. In *Methods in Enzymology*, 1st ed.; Tawfik, D.S., Ed.; Academic Press: Cambridge, MA, USA, 2018; Volume 604, pp. 3–43. [CrossRef]
81. Van Rossum, G.; Drake, F.L., Jr. *Python Reference Manual, Release 2.0.1*; PythonLabs: Amsterdam, The Netherlands, 1995; Available online: https://docs.python.org/2.0/ref/ref.html (accessed on 14 October 2020).
82. McKinney, W. Data Structures for Statistical Computing in Python. In Proceedings of the 9th Python in Science Conference (SciPy2010), Austin, TX, USA, 28 June–3 July 2010; pp. 51–56. [CrossRef]
83. Pandas-Dev/Pandas, Version v0.25.2, 2018, Zenodo. Available online: https://doi.org/10.5281/zenodo.3509135 (accessed on 14 October 2020).
84. Oliphant, T.E. *A Guide to NumPy*, 2nd ed.; Trelgol Publishing: USA, 2006; Available online: https://web.mit.edu/dvp/Public/numpybook.pdf (accessed on 14 October 2020).

85. van der Walt, S.; Colbert, S.C.; Varoquaux, G. The NumPy Array: A Structure for Efficient Numerical Computation. *Comput. Sci. Eng.* **2011**, *13*, 22–30. [CrossRef]
86. Goloborodko, A.A.; Levitsky, L.I.; Ivanov, M.V.; Gorshkov, M.V. Pyteomics—A Python Framework for Exploratory Data Analysis and Rapid Software Prototyping in Proteomics. *J. Am. Soc. Mass Spectr.* **2013**, *24*, 301–304. [CrossRef] [PubMed]
87. Levitsky, L.I.; Klein, J.; Ivanov, M.V.; Gorshkov, M.V. Pyteomics 4.0: Five years of development of a Python proteomics framework. *J. Proteome Res.* **2019**, *18*, 709–714. [CrossRef] [PubMed]
88. Virtanen, P.; Gommers, R.; Oliphant, T.E.; Haberland, M.; Reddy, T.; Cournapeau, D.; Burovski, E.; Peterson, P.; Weckesser, W.; Bright, J.; et al. SciPy 1.0: Fundamental algorithms for scientific computing in Python. *Nat. Methods* **2020**, *17*, 261–272. [CrossRef]
89. Hagberg, A.A.; Schult, D.A.; Swart, P.J. Exploring network structure, dynamics, and function using NetworkX. In Proceedings of the 7th Python in Science Conference (SciPy2008), Pasadena, CA, USA, 19–24 August 2008; pp. 11–15.
90. Hunter, J.D. Matplotlib: A 2D graphics environment. *Comput. Sci. Eng.* **2007**, *9*, 90–95. [CrossRef]
91. Pedregosa, F.; Varoquaux, G.; Gramfort, A.; Michel, V.; Thirion, B.; Grisel, O.; Blondel, M.; Prettenhofer, P.; Weiss, R.; Dubourg, V.; et al. Scikit-learn: Machine Learning in Python. *J. Mach. Learn. Res.* **2011**, *12*, 2825–2830.
92. Mwaskom/Seaborn, v0.9.0. 2018. Available online: https://doi.org/10.5281/zenodo.1313201 (accessed on 14 October 2020).
93. Pérez, F.; Granger, B.E. IPython: A System for Interactive Scientific Computing. *Comput. Sci. Eng.* **2007**, *9*, 21–29. [CrossRef]
94. Kluyver, T.; Ragan-Kelley, B.; Pérez, F.; Granger, B.; Bussonnier, M.; Frederic, J.; Kelley, K.; Hamrick, J.; Grout, J.; Corlay, S.; et al. Jupyter Notebooks—A publishing format for reproducible computational workflows. In *Positioning and Power in Academic Publishing: Players, Agents and Agendas*; Loizides, F., Scmidt, B., Eds.; IOS Press: Amsterdam, The Netherlands, 2016; pp. 87–90. [CrossRef]
95. Holman, J.D.; Tabb, D.L.; Mallick, P. Employing ProteoWizard to Convert Raw Mass Spectrometry Data. *Curr. Protoc. Bioinform.* **2014**, *46*, 1–9. [CrossRef]
96. Chambers, M.C.; Maclean, B.; Burke, R.; Amodei, D.; Ruderman, D.L.; Neumann, S.; Gatto, L.; Fischer, B.; Pratt, B.; Egertson, J. A cross-platform toolkit for mass spectrometry and proteomics. *Nat. Biotechnol.* **2012**, *30*, 918–920. [CrossRef]
97. Shannon, P.; Markiel, A.; Ozier, O.; Baliga, N.S.; Wang, J.T.; Ramage, D.; Amin, N.; Schwikowski, B.; Ideker, T. Cytoscape: A software environment for integrated models of biomolecular interaction networks. *Genome Res.* **2003**, *13*, 2498–2504. [CrossRef]
98. Iwasaki, A.; Ohno, O.; Sumimoto, S.; Ogawa, H.; Nguyen, K.A.; Suenaga, K. Jahanyne, an Apoptosis-Inducing Lipopeptide from the Marine Cyanobacterium *Lyngbya* sp. *Org. Lett.* **2015**, *17*, 652–655. [CrossRef]
99. Linington, R.G.; González, J.; Ureña, L.D.; Romero, L.I.; Ortega-Barría, E.; Gerwick, W.H. Venturamides A and B: Antimalarial Constituents of the Panamanian Marine Cyanobacterium *Oscillatoria* sp. *J. Nat. Prod.* **2007**, *70*, 397–401. [CrossRef]
100. Yoshimura, A.; Kishimoto, S.; Nishimura, S.; Otsuka, S.; Sakai, Y.; Hattori, A.; Kakeya, H. Prediction and Determination of the Stereochemistry of the 1,3,5-Trimethyl-Substituted Alkyl Chain in Verucopeptin, a Microbial Metabolite. *J. Org. Chem.* **2014**, *79*, 6858–6867. [CrossRef]
101. Tao, Y.; Li, P.; Zhang, D.; Glukhov, E.; Gerwick, L.; Zhang, C.; Murray, T.F.; Gerwick, W.H. Samholides, Swinholide-Related Metabolites from a Marine Cyanobacterium cf. *Phormidium* sp. *J. Org. Chem.* **2018**, *83*, 3034–3046. [CrossRef]

102. Choi, H.; Mascuch, S.J.; Villa, F.A.; Byrum, T.; Teasdale, M.E.; Smith, J.E.; Preskitt, L.B.; Rowley, D.C.; Gerwick, L.; Gerwick, W.H. Honaucins A-C, potent inhibitors of inflammation and bacterial quorum sensing: Synthetic derivatives and structure-activity relationships. *Chem. Biol.* **2012**, *19*, 589–598. [CrossRef] [PubMed]
103. Green, L.C.; Wagner, D.A.; Glogowski, J.; Skipper, P.L.; Wishnok, J.S.; Tannenbaum, S.R. Analysis of nitrate, nitrite, and [N-15]-labeled nitrate in biological-fluids. *Anal. Biochem.* **1982**, *126*, 131–138. [CrossRef]

marine drugs

MDPI

Article

Sustainable Low-Volume Analysis of Environmental Samples by Semi-Automated Prioritization of Extracts for Natural Product Research (SeaPEPR)

Riyanti [1,2,3,†], Michael Marner [3,†], Christoph Hartwig [3], Maria A. Patras [3], Stevy I. M. Wodi [4], Frets J. Rieuwpassa [4], Frans G. Ijong [4,5], Walter Balansa [4,*] and Till F. Schäberle [1,3,6,*]

1 Institute for Insect Biotechnology, Justus-Liebig-University of Giessen, 35392 Giessen, Germany; riyanti@bio.uni-giessen.de
2 Faculty of Fisheries and Marine Science, Jenderal Soedirman University, Purwokerto 53122, Indonesia
3 Fraunhofer Institute for Molecular Biology and Applied Ecology (IME), Branch for Bioresources, 35392 Giessen, Germany; Michael.Marner@ime.fraunhofer.de (M.M.); Christoph.Hartwig@ime.fraunhofer.de (C.H.); Maria.Patras@ime.fraunhofer.de (M.A.P.)
4 Department of Fisheries and Marine Science, Politeknik Negeri Nusa Utara, Tahuna Sangihe Islands, North Sulawesi 95812, Indonesia; wodiimelda@gmail.com (S.I.M.W.); frets.jr@gmail.com (F.J.R.); ijongfrans@yahoo.com (F.G.I.)
5 Faculty of Fisheries and Marine Science, Sam Ratulangi University, Manado 95115, Indonesia
6 German Center for Infection Research (DZIF), Partner Site Giessen-Marburg-Langen, 35392 Giessen, Germany
* Correspondence: walterbalansa@polnustar.ac.id (W.B.); till.f.schaeberle@agrar.uni-giessen.de (T.F.S.); Tel.: +49-641-99-37140 (T.F.S.)
† These authors contributed equally.

Received: 23 October 2020; Accepted: 11 December 2020; Published: 17 December 2020

Abstract: The discovery of novel natural products (NPs) that will serve as lead structures has to be an ongoing effort to fill the respective development pipelines. However, identification of NPs, which possess a potential for application in e.g., the pharma or agro sector, must be as cost effective and fast as possible. Furthermore, the amount of sample available for initial testing is usually very limited, not least because of the fact that the impact on the environment, i.e., the sampled biosystem, should be kept minimal. Here, our pipeline SeaPEPR is described, in which a primary bioactivity screening of crude extracts is combined with the analysis of their metabolic fingerprint. This enabled prioritization of samples for subsequent microfractionation and dereplication of the active compounds early in the workflow. As a case study, 76 marine sponge-derived extracts were screened against a microbial screening panel. Thereunder, human pathogenic bacteria (*Escherichia coli* ATCC35218 and *Staphylococcus aureus* ATCC33592) and yeast (*Candida albicans* FH2173), as well as the phytopathogenic fungus *Septoria tritici* MUCL45407. Overall, nine extracts revealed activity against at least one test organism. Metabolic fingerprinting enabled assigning four active extracts into one metabolic group; therefore, one representative was selected for subsequent microfractionation. Dereplication of the active fractions showed a new dibrominated aplysinopsin and a hypothetical chromazonarol stereoisomer derivative. Furthermore, inhibitory activity against the common plant pest *Septoria tritici* was discovered for NPs of marine origin.

Keywords: natural products; dereplication; antibiotics; marine sponges; plant pathogen

1. Introduction

Natural products (NPs) are the oldest form of medicine utilized by humans. Technologies and methods improved and NPs remained one of the most important source for the development of medicinal drugs. Today, NPs and their derivatives make up a significant percentage of approved drugs worldwide. Especially in the antibiotics sector, almost all lead structures were identified from bio-resources (~75% either unaltered or semi-synthetically modified; 1981–2014) [1,2]. Although being a traditional source for antimicrobial compounds, the pool of NP-derived structural novelty is not exhausted as exemplified by the discovery of teixobactin [3] and darobactin [4].

Besides clinical application, specialized natural products are drivers of socio-economic stability by finding application in food preservation, livestock and aquaculture treatment, as well as crop protection [5]. In all fields, humans benefit from the evolutionary shaped intrinsic antimicrobial activity of NPs. In the 1940s, the "Waksman antibiotic discovery platform" was the first systematical approach to identify antimicrobial NPs and led to the isolation of the first aminoglycosides [6].

However, high rediscovery rates make classical discovery campaigns unattractive and pose an unreasonable financial risk for the private sector. This might partly be circumvented by implementing chemo-informatics in systematic, routine processes. Data mining processes such as automatic annotation of bucket matrices [7] or MS/MS networks [8] against public databases help to identify signals and interest, even in gigantic datasets.

Besides discovery of novelty, repurposing of already known structures to different fields of application seems an encouraging approach, but high expense or no commercial availability of many natural products reduce feasibility substantially. In this context, SeaPEPR represents a methodology allowing a preliminary determination of specific bioactivity of single compounds within crude environmental extracts. Application allows us to evaluate the bio-economical value of large sets of low volume sample on the metabolite level in a standardized manner and finally facilitates decision making on downstream processes such as isolation of unknown metabolites or repurposing studies.

Here, we chose a promising and likewise challenging bio-resource as a case study to present our approach of crude environmental extract analysis. Sponges, as sessile filter feeders without physical defense, are believed to depend on chemical defense or deterrence mechanisms mediated NPs, biosynthesized either by themselves or by associated microorganisms. Due to ethical reasons, straightforward isolation and characterization of compounds by harvesting sponges from nature should be discouraged. Limited availability of material usually prohibits extensive information retrieval from a given environmental sample. Frequently, scaffolds initially discovered in environmental samples are subject to delicate chemical synthesis without a clear product application. MS/MS coupled microfractionation of environmental extracts facilitates semi-automatic dereplication and allows attributing bioactivity observed in crude extract primary screens to single compounds without the necessity of cost and time-consuming isolation or synthesis.

2. Results

2.1. Sample Collection and Extract Generation

Sponges are a well-known bioresource for bioactive molecules and can be regarded as a complex environmental sample, since the holobiont (consisting of the sponge and its associated microbes) is extracted as a whole. Furthermore, the taxonomic classification of sponges, which is based on both, genetic barcoding and morphology, is time consuming and challenging. In this project, 76 sponge samples from seven different dive sites at the coastal area of Sangihe and Siau Island (Pacific Ocean, Indonesia) were obtained (Figure 1). At each diving site, around 11–15 sponge samples were collected, except sponge sample T_5, which was the only one obtained from the site named Towo. Hence, it can be expected that the sample set represents a survey of the biodiversity around the islands. How this translates into chemical diversity was investigated in the following. As starting material, 5 mg of dried sponge, which is approximately equivalent to the size of a thumbnail, was used. From all samples, crude extracts were prepared. The extraction yield (based on dry mass) using methanol was between 12 and 86% (Figure S1).

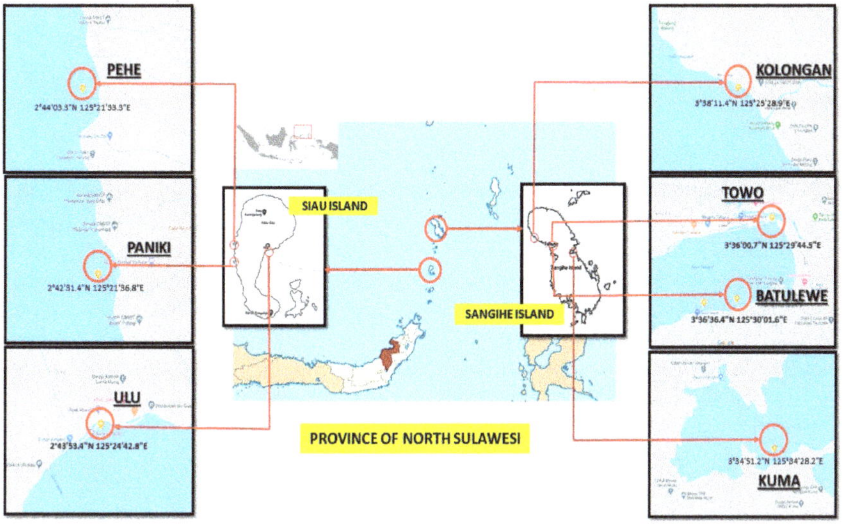

Figure 1. Sampling sides of sponge specimen. Samples were retrieved by SCUBA in a depth of 4–20 m below the surface.

The generated extracts represent the material further analyzed for NP discovery. The general workflow of SeaPEPR is depicted in Figure 2.

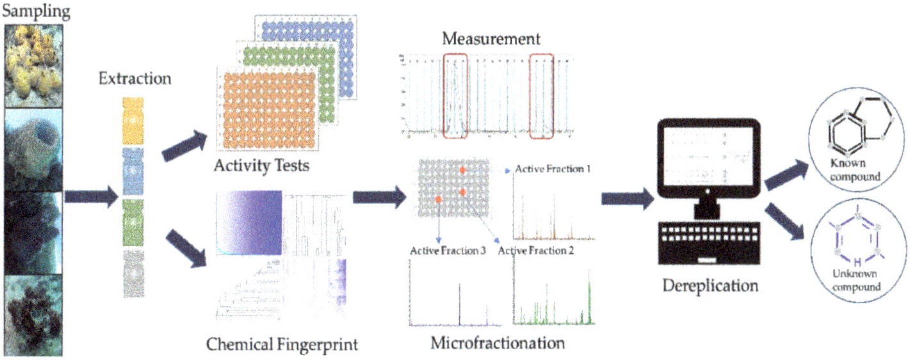

Figure 2. Schematic overview of the SeaPEPR pipeline. In a first step, crude environmental extracts are subject of bioactivity assessment. At the same time, the chemical diversity of the entire set of samples is determined by cosine similarity calculation ("chemical fingerprints"). Prioritized samples are microfractionated to identify the causative agent responsible for the initially observed bioactivity. If desired, dereplicated compounds of interest can be selected for isolation.

2.2. Bioactivity Assessment—Microbroth Dilution Assays

In order to determine the antimicrobial potency, the generated extracts were screened against a diverse panel of pathogenic microorganisms including *Escherichia coli* ATCC35218, *Staphylococcus aureus* ATCC33592, *Pseudomonas aeruginosa* ATCC27853, as well as *Candida albicans* FH2173 and the phytopathogenic fungus *Septoria tritici* MUCL45407. In total, seven of the 76 tested sponge extracts exhibited growth inhibitory effects of at least 85% across 3 dilution steps against one or more test strains and were thereby considered bioactive: Essentially, samples KOL_8, KOL_16, KOL_18, and ULU_13 were active against *S. aureus*, *C. albicans*, and *S. tritici*, PEHE_5 against *S. aureus* and *S. tritici*, and extracts

PANIKI_4 and ULU_16 showed activity only against *S. tritici*. In addition, two extracts (ULU_11 and ULU_17) showed weak activity against *C. albicans* by inhibiting the cell viability of the test strain only in the highest concentrations. No growth inhibition of the selected Gram-negative test strains was observed.

2.3. Prioritization—Metabolic Fingerprinting

Results from metabolic fingerprinting and bioactivity screening were combined to allow prioritization of samples and are summarized in Figure 3. The detailed grouping results with pairwise similarities are presented in Table S1. While a total of 45 distinct metabolic groups was generated, extracts sharing the same activity pattern (KOL_8, KOL_16, KOL_18, and ULU_13) were assigned to the same group (Figure 3), strongly suggesting a similar metabolite composition of the extracts (see also Figure 4). Similarly, extracts ULU_11 and ULU_17 formed one group, while extracts PEHE_5, PANIKI_4, and ULU_16 appeared to consist of unique metabolite mixtures. From each metabolic group containing bioactive extracts, one representative was selected for microfractionation. Samples selected for microfractionation are marked.

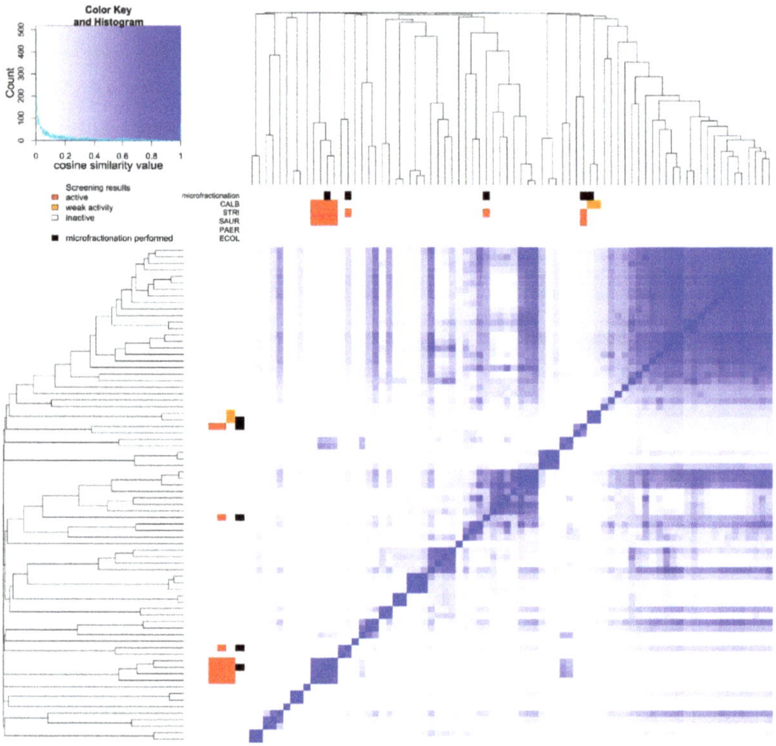

Figure 3. Cosine similarity heatmap of all 76 extracts. Blue color indicates a high degree of similarity among compared extracts (see color key histogram). Flags in sidebar mark selected samples for microfractionation (black) and screening results (red = active, orange = weak activity, white = inactive) of the respective extract against the indicator strains (CALB = *C. albicans*, STRI = *S. tritici*, SAUR = *S. aureus*, PAER = *P. aeruginosa*, ECOL = *E. coli*).

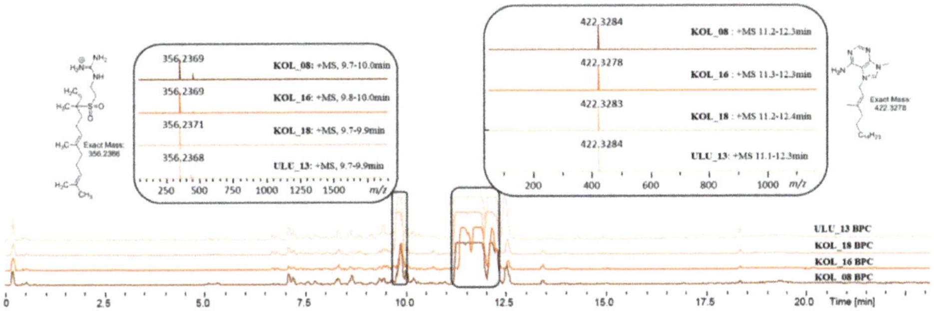

Figure 4. Base peak chromatogram (BPC) of the extracts KOL_08, KOL_16, KOL_18, and ULU_13 obtained from different *Agelas nakamurai* organisms. Most intense peaks within the similar BPCs correspond to the agelasines groups (box, top right) and agelasidine A (box, top left).

2.4. Dereplication of Bioactive Compounds—Microfractionation

2.4.1. KOL_18 (TSRR0002_D-07) *Agelas nakamurai*

Extract KOL_18 was selected as representative of the group of the four extracts exhibiting an identical bioactivity pattern and similar metabolite composition (Figure 4). Based on the primary activity of the crude extract against *S. aureus*, the corresponding crude extract (1 mg/mL in MeOH) was fractionated in 1 and 2 μL injection volume replicates and rescreened against the same indicator strain. The active fractions were reproduced in both dilutions. The two activity zones, namely fractions 80–81 and 83–84 (Figure S2), could be assigned to partly co-eluting isomeric compounds with an *m/z* 422.3283 $[M]^+$, corresponding to the molecular formula $[C_{26}H_{40}N_5]^+$. The compounds showed an UV absorption at 220 and 272 nm. Based on the MS/MS fragmentation pattern, the compounds could be assigned as members of the agelasine A-F family (Figure 5) [9]; since MS/MS fragmentation does not allow for distinction between the different isomeric structures of the diterpene unit. As the name indicates, agelasines are known metabolites of the sponge *Agelas nakamurai*.

The same extract was fractionated against *S. tritici* (injection volume 2 and 5 μL). Both of the replicates showed activity, corresponding to the above-described agelasines. The 5 μL injection volume replicate showed an additional activity zone, namely fraction 69 (Figure S3), which could be assigned to a compound of *m/z* 356.2370 $[M + H]^+$, corresponding to the molecular formula $C_{18}H_{33}N_3O_2S_1$. The compound shows UV absorption at 220 nm. Based on the MS/MS fragmentation pattern (Figure S3d), the compound was dereplicated as agelasidine A [10] (Figure 5), also a known metabolite of *A. nakamurai* [11]. The extract was also fractionated against *C. albicans* (2 mg/mL solution, injection volume 2 and 5 μL). Both injection replicates showed activity in the fractions corresponding to the above described agelasines (A-F) and agelasidine A (Figure S4).

Molecular networking analysis revealed the presence of several derivatives (minor compounds) including oxo-agelasines (A-F) of *m/z* 436.3073 $[M]^+$ with a molecular formula of $C_{26}H_{38}N_5O_1$, hydroxy-agelasines of *m/z* 438.3231 $[M]^+$ with a molecular formula of $C_{26}H_{40}N_5O_1$, and dihydro-hydroxy-agelasines of *m/z* 440.3389 $[M]^+$ with a molecular formula of $C_{26}H_{42}N_5O_1$, each present in the extract as a complex mixture of isomers (Figures S5 and S6).

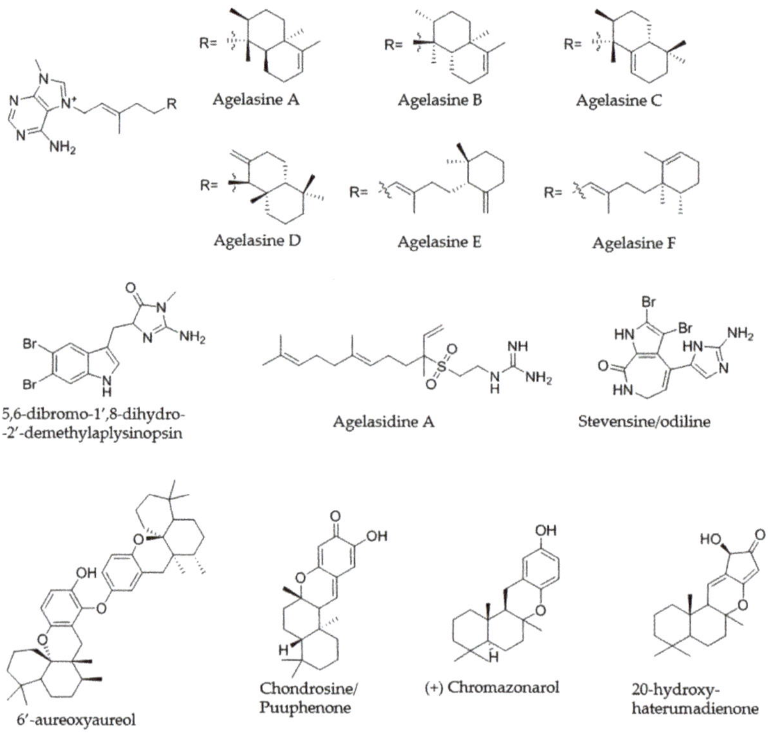

Figure 5. Chemical structures of the dereplicated compounds responsible for the activity of the microfractionated samples.

2.4.2. PEHE_5 (TSRR0002_F-08) *Haliclona* sp.

Based on the results of the primary screening against *S. aureus*, the corresponding crude extract (1 mg/mL in MeOH) was fractionated in 2 and 5 μL injection volume replicates and rescreened against the same indicator strain. Only the 5 μL replicate showed active fractions, namely fractions 47–48 and fraction 108 (Figures S7 and S8).

Activity of fractions 47-48 was assigned to a compound of *m/z* 398.9449 $[M + H]^+$ showing the specific isotope pattern of a dibrominated compound (Figure S7b) corresponding to a molecular formula of $C_{13}H_{13}Br_2N_4O_1$. The compound shows UV absorption maxima at 220 and 292 nm. The fragmentation pattern is indicative of a dibrominated triptamine framework as structural subunit. A substructure search on SciFinder retrieved no hits corresponding to the assigned molecular formula, however, one candidate, namely 5,6-dibromo-2′-demethylaplysinopsin ($C_{13}H_{11}Br_2N_4O_1$ - one additional degree of unsaturation compared to the compound in the extract), was found to fit the fragmentation pattern observed for the compound in the extract. Therefore, the active compound was putatively assigned the structure of 5,6-dibromo-1′,8-dihydro-2′-demethylaplysinopsin [12] (Figure 5), which is in agreement with the molecular formula, fragmentation pattern, and observed UV spectrum. Aplysinopsins are a family of indole alkaloids isolated from sponges [13], scleractinian corals [14,15] and sea anemones [16]. The tentative 5,6-dibromo-1′,8-dihydro-2′-demethylaplysinopsin is, to our knowledge, not reported in literature.

Activity of fraction 108 was assigned to a mixture of co-eluting compounds of *m/z* 627.4414 $[M + H]^+$, *m/z* 315.2321 $[M + H]^+$, *m/z* 329.2115 $[M + H]^+$ (Figure S8b–d; proposed structures in Figure 5), corresponding to the molecular formulae $C_{42}H_{58}O_4$, $C_{21}H_{30}O_2$, and $C_{21}H_{28}O_3$, respectively. The compounds showed UV absorption maxima at 223 and 299 nm. The MS/MS fragmentation pattern of all three compounds showed a base peak ion of *m/z* 191.1798, corresponding to the molecular formula of $C_{14}H_{23}^+$, which was assigned to the retro Diels–Alder fragmentation product ion of sesquiterpene hydroquinone frameworks. Based on the MS/MS data for $C_{21}H_{30}O_2$, no distinction between the two literature known isomeric sponge metabolites, aureol and chromazonarol [17,18], could be made. The same holds true for $C_{42}H_{58}O_4$ (putatively 6′-aureoxyaureol or 6′-aureoxychromazonarol). The bissesquiterpene 6′-aureoxyaureol was reported together with several dibrominated aplysinopsin derivatives in *Smenospongia* sp., whereas the hypothetical chromazonarol stereoisomer was not described [19]. Finally, literature query of $C_{21}H_{28}O_3$, produced a range of hits corresponding to algal metabolites, while only one compound, chondrosine (a.k.a. puupehenone) [20], was previously reported from sponges. The structures of 6′-aureoxyaureol, chondrosine, and chromazonarol (Figure 5) were chosen as representative examples for each of the ions of *m/z* 627.4414, *m/z* 329.2115, and *m/z* 315.2321, respectively.

The same extract was fractionated against *S. tritici* (injection volume 2 and 5 μL), however, no active fractions could be observed.

2.4.3. ULU_16 (TSRR0002_H-07) *Neopetrosia* sp.

To investigate the observed antifungal activity of ULU_16, the extract was fractionated in 2 and 5 μL injection volume replicates and rescreened against *S. tritici*. The activity zone was reproduced in the two replicates and could be assigned to a compound of *m/z* 385.9249 $[M + H]^+$ showing the specific isotope pattern of a dibrominated compound (Figure S9) with the molecular formula $C_{11}H_9Br_2N_5O_1$. The compound showed UV absorption maxima at 220 and 340 nm. Based on the MS/MS fragmentation pattern, the compound was dereplicated as stevensine, also known as odiline (Figure 5), a metabolite reported in various sponge species [21].

2.4.4. PANIKI_4 (TSRR0002_D-12) *Halichondria* sp.

The microfractionated extract PANIKI_4 (injection volume 1 and 2 μL, 1 mg/mL) was rescreened against *S. tritici*. Only the 2 μL injection volume replicate produced one active zone (Figure S10), which could be assigned to a compound of *m/z* 317.2112 $[M + H]^+$ corresponding to the molecular formula of $C_{20}H_{28}O_3$. The fragmentation pattern of the compound does not allow for clear assignment of substructural frameworks. The UV absorption maximum was detected at 220 nm. A database search of the molecular formula retrieved a sesquiterpene compound, namely 20-hydroxyhaterumadienone (Figure 5), as plausible candidate for tentative structure assignment. 20-hydroxyhaterumadienone is a cytotoxic compound reported from *Dysidea* sp. [22].

2.4.5. ULU_11 (TSRR0002_H-03)

The extract ULU_11 was selected as a representative of extracts exhibiting weak *C. albicans* activity and highly similar metabolite composition (together with ULU_17, Figure 3). The crude extract was fractionated in 2 and 5 μL injection volume replicates and rescreened against *C. albicans*. However, no active fractions could be identified.

3. Discussion

In this study, we used a set of 76 sponge samples to present our Semi-automated Prioritization of Extracts for natural Product Research (SeaPEPR) pipeline. Primary bioactivity assessment led to the identification of nine sponge extracts exhibiting bioactivity against at least one of the selected indicator strains. Simultaneously, unsupervised chemical diversity visualization by cosine similarity heat map construction facilitated the overall data interpretation and prioritization of extracts for downstream processes.

During prioritization, four bioactive extracts (KOL_08, KOL_16, KOL_18, and ULU_13) were grouped together, indicating highly similar metabolite composition. In fact, orthogonal data obtained from sponge identification by morphological features, such as spicule identification (Figure 6, Table S2), indicated taxonomic uniformity of the organisms (i.e., all specimens were identified as *A. nakamurai* based on spicule morphology). In this case, taxonomic uniformity translated into chemical uniformity. Consequently, agelasines and agelasidines (dereplicated in the active fractions of the representative extract KOL_18) were found in all members of this metabolic group (Figure 3).

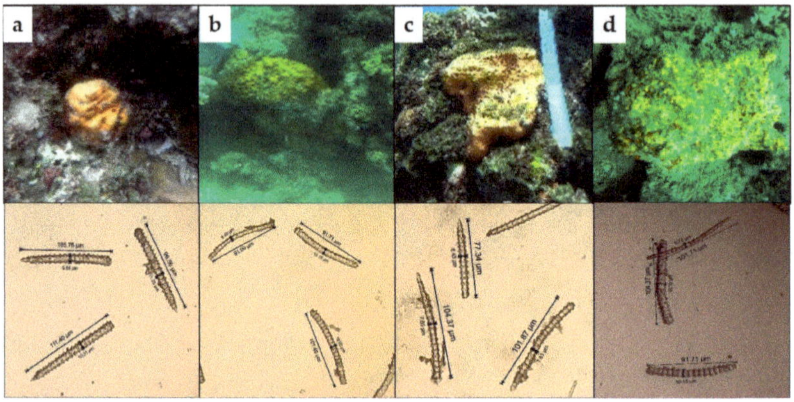

Figure 6. Underwater pictures and isolated spicules of the *Agelas nakamurai* cf specimens (**a**) Sample KOL_8, (**b**) Sample KOL_16, (**c**) Sample KOL_18, and (**d**) Sample ULU_13. It can be seen that the specimens are thick encrusting orange sponges and the type of spicule is megascleres acanthostyle for all four samples. This suggested the assignment as *Agelas nakamurai* cf.

On the other hand, PEHE_5 and PANIKI_4 were initially taxonomically classified as members of the genus *Haliclona*. In contrast, the metabolite fingerprinting of these two sponges clearly indicated distinctiveness of organisms. A focused investigation on morphological level finally revealed that PANIKI_4 belongs to the genus *Halichondria*. Six other sponges were morphologically identified as *Haliclona* sp. However, only two pairs of high metabolic similarity could be observed in the heat map, indicating different *Haliclona* species. Within this genus, speciation seems to be tightly linked to chemical diversification, as *Haliclona* extracts did not cluster, but were distributed throughout the heat map. It is known that besides species affiliation of the holobiont, the chemical profile could also be shaped by the associated microbial communities [23], the habitat [24], as well as stress associated to predation and wounding [25].

Both observations, chemical uniformity within a species (*A. nakamurai*) and interspecies metabolic diversity (*Haliclona* sp.) can be explained by the well-accepted assumption that taxonomic, thus genetic, diversity is often expressed by chemical diversity. Broad chemical diversity is generally desired in natural product discovery campaigns and thereby careful selection of the source material is crucial. In this context, the prioritization of extracts based on the similarity of their chemical composition helps to maximize metabolite diversity in downstream processes. Especially for samples for which reliable species identification in the field (e.g., sponges) is challenging, chemotyping (e.g., cosine similarity heatmaps) as interface between primary screenings and follow up experiments seems useful to decrease workload. Besides, it has to be kept in mind that even different intra-species samples have the potential for the detection of new and even novel compounds, since analysis of the same species could result in different metabolomes due to the dynamic environmental factors [26]. Independent from the sample set, it demands a straightforward downstream pipeline to mine the vast amount of data. While other microfractionation platforms are suitable to acquire detailed information about extracts obtained from precisely selected samples such as different medicinal plants [27,28], one benefit of the herein presented pipeline is the potential to characterize extracts (and not necessarily the source organism) in detail without processing replicates and yet account for most drivers of metabolic diversity. After prioritization, extract components (ions) are directly linked to the observed bioactivity. Other elegant strategies (e.g., bioactive molecular networking [29]) establish this connection by calculation of the Pearson correlation between the relative abundance of ions across chromatographic fractions (usually 18–20) and the observed bioactivity. Our alternative dereplication approach aims to screen fractions containing only a very limited number of, if not single, ions or ions all belonging to the same molecular feature against the indicators strain (Figures S3, S7–S10). Because fraction collection in assay plates is coupled to MS/MS, a direct, experimental connected between candidate molecule and bioactivity can be established. By using this workflow, five out of initially 76 extracts were prioritized based on bioactivity and unique metabolic fingerprint, before the causative metabolites were determined by microfractionation.

Bioactivity of extracts obtained from *A. nakamurai* could be assigned to agelasines and agelasidine A. Synthetic access to the agelasines was already established [30] and broad compound profiling was carried out: Reported bioactivities include Na,K-ATPase inhibition [9], cyto- and ichthyotoxicitiy, antiprotozoal [31], and antifouling activity, as well as growth inhibition of *M. tuberculosis*, Gram-positive and negative pathogenic bacteria [32], as well as yeast (reviewed by Gordaliza) [33]. Likewise, agelasidines were observed to exhibit activity against *S. aureus* and *C. albicans* [11]. Broad screening of aplysinopsins demonstrated a modulating activity against the glycine-gated chloride channel receptor [13], antineoplastic, antiplasmodial, anti-bacterial, as well as anti-fungal activities. The latter included growth inhibition of *Penicillium atrovenetum* and *Trichophyton mentagrophytes* (reviewed by Bialonska and Zjawiony) [12]. Besides aplysidine A, a mix of several cytotoxic [17,18] sesquiterpene hydroquinones was dereplicated in the extract PEHE_5 obtained from *Haliclona* sp. The bioactivity of *Neopetrosia* sp. extract ULU_16 was attributed to stevensine (odiline). Reported activity of stevensine comprises fish deterrence [34] and weak antimicrobial growth inhibition (e.g., *Deleya marina*, a common fouling bacterium) [35]. The compound 20-hydroxyhaterumadienone (here dereplicated from PANIKI_4 a putative *Halichondria* sp.) is known to possess cytotoxic effects [22,36], and exhibit weak interaction with human lipoxygenase (5-hLO) [37].

While these results indicate a generally robust transfer of primarily observed growth inhibitory effects to microfractionated assays, two extracts did not show bioactivity in any fraction. These findings emphasize a general challenge in bioactivity driven NP research (in contrast to cheminformatics inclined discovery projects [38]): Microbial crude extracts are composed of a mixture of various substances at dramatically different concentrations and potencies. It is important to realize that almost each substance (or a combination of several metabolites) becomes unspecifically toxic at high concentrations, hence producing a positive assay read out. As discrimination between specific and unspecific effects might come at the price of insensitivity, we chose a trade off in favor of false positive instead of false negative results. Consequently, initially moderately active crude extracts (e.g., ULU_11 against *C. albicans*) might not produce positive microfractionation read outs. Given suitable chromatography parameters, members of compound families are separated and tested individually at lower overall concentration. In the case of PEHE_5, the microfractionated extract was unsuccessfully rescreened against *S. tritici*. Potentially, the sum of compounds present in the extract (di-brominated aplysinopsins; aureol/chromazonal) possessed additive, however unspecific, growth inhibition of the test strain, while individual compounds did not show the effect. Although the reduction of unspecific effects caused by high concentration of compounds seems to be an advantage, separation and individual testing of metabolites might also prohibit identification of synergistic effects.

Another limitation of rapid MS/MS-based annotation approaches, including the herein presented methodology, is the reduced identification confidence of target molecules (as defined by the Metabolite Annotation Task Group of the Metabolomics Society) [39,40] compared to full structure and stereochemistry assignment studies. In that sense, no distinction between the isomeric sponge metabolites aureol and chromazonarol or between putatively 6′-aureoxyaureol and 6′-aureoxychromazonarol could be made. Besides these challenges, SeaPEPR has proven its value as prioritization strategy allowing data-based decision making on follow-up projects early in the discovery process. This study gave insight into the metabolites of four morphologically seemingly different specimens of *A. nakamurai*, preventing an otherwise very daunting task of molecular structure elucidation.

If a compound exhibits the desired properties such as structural novelty, repurposing potential, or just the isolation of more material for further in detail investigation of observed bioactivities, the metabolite should undergo further analysis, including confirmation of the 3-dimensional structure and extensive activity profiling. For repurposing studies of small molecules, the required amount (~ 1 mg) to carry out experiments required for hit characterization might be generated by straightforward chemical synthesis as shown for the agelasines [30]. While an unknown and likewise bioactive metabolite is scientifically most intriguing, it initially requires more sample material; hence, detailed metadata should be recorded in the field (Table S2) to allow resupply. Collection of specimens with the same chemotype might be challenging, but not per se, as observed by the robust metabolic fingerprint of *A. nakamurai* across sampling sites (>60 km distance between Kolongan and Ulu sampling sites). Before isolation from animal tissue is conducted, metabolite access via fermentation of the cultivable microbiome should be investigated. If this route is obstructed, authorities should decide case by case whether a targeted isolation campaign from animal tissue, towards new and urgently needed antibiotic or agrochemical lead structures, is ethically justifiable. Selection of promising projects might be facilitated by data obtained from prioritization processes, such as SeaPEPR.

Finally, yet importantly, to the best of our knowledge, no bioactivity against the common plant pest *S. tritici* was reported for any of the herein dereplicated sponge compounds. The ascomycete *S. tritici*, which is the causative agent of blotch disease on wheat, is responsible for serious losses in cereal yields and quality in Western European countries. In 2014, an estimated $1.3 billion worth of fungicides was used to control *Septoria*-induced crop rust [41]. Resistance development, strict EU regulations, and increased public awareness against the use of petrochemicals drive the continuous demand for new agents with potency against *S. tritici*. The herein presented data indicate that marine-derived natural products pose potential solutions for current challenges in plant pest control.

4. Materials and Methods

4.1. Sponge Collection

Sponges were collected from Paniki (2°42′31.4″ N, 125°21′36.8″ E), Pehe (2°44′03.3″ N, 125°21′33.3″ E), and Ulu (2°43′53.4″ N, 125°24′42.8″ E) of Siau Islands Regency and from Batulewehe (3°36′00.7″ N, 125°29′44.5″ E), Kolongan (3°38′11.4″ N, 125°25′28.9″ E), and Kuma (3°34′51.2″ N, 125°34′28.2″ E) of Sangihe Islands Regency North Sulawesi Indonesia at a depth between ~4 and ~20 m during May 2019. After morphological description and underwater documentation by photograph (GoPro Hero 4.0, except for specimens from Kolongan which were taken by GroPro Hero 7.0), each specimen was cut and kept individually in a plastic bag. Samples were transferred to the laboratory in Politeknik Negeri Nusa Utara Tahuna Indonesia where the specimens were stored at −16 °C until used. From each specimen, a small portion (1 cm^3) was taken for taxonomic identification using slightly modified bleach digestion method [42,43]. All specimens were individually sliced into small pieces, dried in the oven at 45 °C for 3 days and blended to give either powder or mash of sponges. This drying step was performed, since the infrastructure available at the islands is limited and the material prepared in this way was then ready to be sent by normal post. Sponges of 2 to 5 g were packed individually in a small plastic bag separately secured in 76 sample bottles and sent to Justus-Liebig-University Giessen, Germany on October 2019.

4.2. Sample Extraction

From the sponge samples, a portion of 5 mg dry weight was solved in 500 μL of methanol. The sample was cut in small pieces and subsequently macerated in a shaker (140 rpm, 30 °C overnight). In a next step, the debris was pelleted by centrifugation in a table top centrifuge at full speed for 5 min. The supernatant was taken and the remaining material (pellet) was extracted one more time with

500 μL methanol. The supernatants were combined and evaporated under a flow of N_2, before storage at −20 °C. The dry weight of the extract was determined and extraction efficiency was calculated. The crude extract was dissolved in dimethyl sulfoxide (DMSO, final concentration 1 mg/mL) for the antimicrobial assays and in methanol (1 mg/mL) for LC-HRMS measurement.

4.3. Antimicrobial Bioassays

Antimicrobial activity of the crude sponge extracts was determined by micro broth dilution assays in 384 well microtiter plates (Greiner, Kremsmünster, Austria). A Cybi Liquid handling system (Analytic Jena, Jena, Germany) was used to distribute 0.5, 0.25, and 0.125 μL (in duplicate, corresponding to 10.0, 5.0, and 2.5 μg/mL extract concentration) of each extract to the assay plates. A dilution series of gentamycin (64–0.002 μg/mL, Sigma Aldrich, St. Louis, MS, USA) was added to the antibacterial assays as positive control, while wells containing only medium or only bacterial suspension were used as sterile and growth control respectively. Pre-cultures of *E. coli* ATCC35218, *S. aureus* ATCC33592, and *P. aeruginosa* ATCC27853 were incubated (overnight, 37 °C, 180 rpm) in cation adjusted Mueller Hinton II medium (Becton Dickinson, Sparks, NV, USA) before the cell density was adjusted to 2×10^4 cells/mL and 50 μL bacterial suspension was added to each well (except the sterile control) using a multi-well dispenser (Multidrop; Thermo Labsystems, Waltham, MA, USA). After incubation (18 h, 37 °C, 180 rpm, 80% rH), cell growth was assessed by turbidity measurement with a microplate spectrophotometer at 600 nm (LUMIstar® Omega BMG Labtech, Ortenberg, Germany).

The pre culture of *C. albicans* FH2173 was incubated for two days at 27 °C. Cell density was diluted to 1×10^5 cells/mL in Mueller Hinton II medium before the assay plates were incubated for 48 h at 37 °C, 180 rpm, and 80% rH. For *S. tritici* MUCL45407, a previously prepared spore solution was used to adjust the assay inoculum to 1×10^5 spores/mL in YM medium (yeast extract 4 g $\times$ L^{-1}, malt extract 4 g $\times$ L^{-1}, sucrose 4 g $\times$ L^{-1}). *Septoria* assay plates were incubated for 72 h at 24 °C, 180 rpm, and 80% rH. Nystatin (Sigma Aldrich) was used as positive control for both, yeast and mold assays. Cell viability was evaluated via ATP quantification (BacTiter-Glo™, Promega, Madison, WI, USA) according to the manufacturer's instructions.

4.4. UPLC-HRMS/MS and Microfractionation

UHPLC-HR-MS analysis was performed on a 1290 UHPLC system (Agilent, Santa Clara, CA, USA) equipped with DAD, ELSD, and maXis II™ (Bruker, Billerica, MA, USA) ESI-qTOF-UHRMS with the following gradient: 0 min: 95% A; 0.30 min: 95% A; 18.00 min: 4.75% A; 18.10 min: 0% A; 22.50 min: 0% A; 22.60 min: 95% A; 25.00 min: 95% A (A: H2O, 0.1% formic acid (FA); B: Acetonitrile, 0.1% FA; Flow: 600 μL/min). Column oven temperature: 45°C. Column: Acquity UPLC BEH C18 1.7 μm (2.1x100 mm) with Acquity UPLC BEH C18 1.7 μm VanGuard Pre-Column (2.1 × 5 mm).

For microfractionation, the flow path was changed, so that 90% of the flow was collected with a custom made fraction collector (Zinsser–Analytik, Eschborn, Germany) while the rest was analyzed in MS/MS mode in maXis II™. Collision induced fragmentation was performed at 28.0–35.05 eV using argon at 10^{-2} mbar.

Depending on the potency observed in the primary screening, microfractionation assay plates were prepared by injecting 1 and 2 μL or 2 and 5 μL of extract. A total of 159 fractions were generated per extract and collected on one 384 well plate (fraction length is 7 s, starting immediately after injection) (Figure S11). Plates were dried in vacuo using a HT12-II centrifugal concentrator (Genevac, Ipswitch, Suffolk, GB) at 35 °C before screening. Microfractionation assay volume of *S. aureus* and *C. albicans* was 20 μL, while volume of *S. tritici* assays was 50 μL.

4.5. Metabolic Fingerprinting

MS Data processing was performed with DataAnalysis 4.4 (Bruker, Billerica, MA, USA) using recalibration with sodium formate (Sigma Aldrich), RecalculateLinespectra (threshold 10,000), and FindMolecularFeatures (0.5–25 min, S/N = 0). Bucketing was performed using ProfileAnalysis 2.3

(Bruker, Billerica, MA, USA) (30–1080 s, *m/z* 100–1600, Advanced Bucketing with Δ12 s and Δ5 ppm, no transformation, Bucketing basis = H^+). The bucket table was subsequently used as input for analysis via R.R (version 3.6.0) [44] with libraries readr [45], coop [46], gplots [47], data.table [48], parallelDist [49], and devtools [50] were used. For heatmap-generation with several sidebars, a variation of heatmap.2 by Griffith [51] was used. The script used in this publication is deposited on GitHub [repository https://github.com/christoph-hartwig-ime-br/cosine-V3; https://dx.doi.org/10.5281/zenodo.4320539]. For sample comparison, the cosine similarities (dot product of vectors) between samples were calculated. Samples were sorted according to clustering results and pairwise similarities were used to determine metabolic groups. If the pairwise similarity between subsequent clustered samples is 0.7 or higher, they were assigned to one metabolic group.

4.6. Dereplication

MS and MS/MS Data analysis was performed with DataAnalysis 4.4 (Bruker, Billerica, MA, USA). Molecular formula assignment was done manually for all compounds present in the active fractions, allowing a mass accuracy tolerance of ± 2 ppm. Annotation of the MS/MS spectra was performed manually for all the compounds present in active fractions, whenever no hits against our pure compound library were observed. Molecular formula searches were performed on AntiBase 2017 [52], Dictionary of Natural Products [53] and SciFinder® [54].

4.7. Molecular Networking

The UHPLC-QTOF-MS/MS data of the prioritized extracts were visualized and subsequently analyzed using molecular networking. Established parameters [8,55] were used for the experiment. MSConvert (ProteoWizard package32) was used to convert the raw data (*.d files) into plain text (*.mgf) files, wherein all detected fragment ions are expressed as a list of mass/intensity value pairs sorted according to their parent ions (peak picking: vendor MS level = 1-2; threshold type = absolute intensity, value = 1000, orientation = most-intense). The networking algorithm itself, thus the calculation of cosine similarity values between parent ion vectors, was computed offline, using an in house server [38].

5. Conclusions

In summary, a combination of (i) phenotypic activity screening assays and (ii) metabolic fingerprinting allowed a fast prioritization and dereplication of samples with the desired bioactivity for further processing. Applying our SeaPEPR pipeline, we were able to dereplicate the active component(s) of crude extracts responsible for the antimicrobial activities observed in primary screens. Thereby, a new dibrominated aplysinopsin and a hypothetical chromazonarol stereoisomer derivative were dereplicated. Furthermore, inhibitory activity against the common plant pest *S. tritici* was discovered for natural products of marine origin. The pipeline represents a valuable tool for further bioprospecting projects, since only low sample volumes are needed that in turn renders extensive collection of limited bioresources for screening purposes (e.g., slow-growing macroorganisms like sponges) obsolete.

Supplementary Materials: The following are available online at http://www.mdpi.com/1660-3397/18/12/649/s1, Pairwise similarities of clustered samples and resulting metabolic grouping; Morphological description and underwater documentation; Microfractionation bioassays and dereplication results.

Author Contributions: T.F.S.: conceptualization, study design and acquisition; F.G.I. and W.B.: study design and acquisition. S.I.M.W., F.J.R., W.B. collected sponge specimens and performed identification. R., M.M., M.A.P., C.H., performed experiments, analyzed and/or interpreted data. All authors have read and agreed to the published version of the manuscript.

Funding: This research was funded by the LOEWE program of the state of Hesse. Riyanti obtained a fellowship from the Indonesia Endowment Fund for Education (LPDP), grant number 20160222305487. W.B. was supported by the Indonesian Ministry of Research Technology and Higher Education for the Basic Research Grant No.01/PL30/P3M/P-DSR/2019. The Federal Ministry of Education and Research (BMBF) supported the work in the lab of T.F.S. with the grant 16GW0117K.

Acknowledgments: The authors thank Junhui Cho (Justus-Liebig-University Giessen) for his help in extract generation and Herjumes Atjin (Ucil) (Politeknik Negeri Nusa Utara) for sample collecting.

Conflicts of Interest: The authors declare no conflict of interest.

References

1. Newman, D.J.; Cragg, G.M. Natural products as sources of new drugs from 1981 to 2014. *J. Nat. Prod.* **2016**, *79*, 629–661. [CrossRef]
2. Newman, D.J.; Cragg, G.M. Natural products as sources of new drugs over the last 25 years. *J. Nat. Prod.* **2007**, *70*, 461–477. [CrossRef] [PubMed]
3. Ling, L.L.; Schneider, T.; Peoples, A.J.; Spoering, A.L.; Engels, I.; Conlon, B.P.; Mueller, A.; Schäberle, T.F.; Hughes, D.E.; Epstein, S.; et al. A new antibiotic kills pathogens without detectable resistance. *Nature* **2015**, *517*, 455–459. [CrossRef] [PubMed]
4. Imai, Y.; Meyer, K.J.; Iinishi, A.; Favre-Godal, Q.; Green, R.; Manuse, S.; Caboni, M.; Mori, M.; Niles, S.; Ghiglieri, M.; et al. A new antibiotic selectively kills Gram-negative pathogens. *Nature* **2019**, *576*, 459–464. [CrossRef] [PubMed]
5. Meek, R.W.; Vyas, H.; Piddock, L.J.V. Nonmedical uses of antibiotics: Time to restrict their use? *PLoS Biol.* **2015**, *13*, e1002266. [CrossRef] [PubMed]
6. Schatz, A.; Bugle, E.; Waksman, S.A. Streptomycin, a substance exhibiting antibiotic activity against Gram-positive and Gram-negative bacteria. *Proc. Soc. Exp. Biol. Med.* **1944**, *55*, 66–69. [CrossRef]
7. Forner, D.; Berrué, F.; Correa, H.; Duncan, K.; Kerr, R.G. Chemical dereplication of marine actinomycetes by liquid chromatography–high resolution mass spectrometry profiling and statistical analysis. *Anal. Chim. Acta* **2013**, *805*, 70–79. [CrossRef] [PubMed]
8. Yang, J.Y.; Sanchez, L.M.; Rath, C.M.; Liu, X.; Boudreau, P.D.; Bruns, N.; Glukhov, E.; Wodtke, A.; de Felicio, R.; Fenner, A.; et al. Molecular networking as a dereplication strategy. *J. Nat. Prod.* **2013**, *76*, 1686–1699. [CrossRef]
9. Nakamura, H.; Wu, H.; Ohizumi, Y.; Hirata, Y. Agelasine-A, -B, -C and -D, novel bicyclic diterpenoids with a 9-methyladeninium unit possessing inhibitory effects on Na, K-ATPase from the Okinawa sea sponge *Agelas* sp. *Tetrahedron Lett.* **1984**, *25*, 2989–2992. [CrossRef]
10. Nakamura, H.; Wu, H.; Kobayashi, J.; Kobayashi, M.; Ohizumi, Y.; Hirata, Y. Agelasidines. Novel hypotaurocyamine derivatives from the Okinawan sea sponge *Agelas nakamurai* Hoshino. *J. Org. Chem.* **1985**, *50*, 2494–2497. [CrossRef]
11. Stout, E.P.; Yu, L.C.; Molinski, T.F. Antifungal diterpene alkaloids from the Caribbean sponge *Agelas citrina*: Unified configurational assignments of agelasidines and agelasines. *Eur. J. Org. Chem.* **2012**, *2012*, 5131–5135. [CrossRef] [PubMed]
12. Bialonska, D.; Zjawiony, J.K. Aplysinopsins-marine indole alkaloids: Chemistry, bioactivity and ecological significance. *Mar. Drugs* **2009**, *7*, 166–183. [CrossRef] [PubMed]
13. Balansa, W.; Islam, R.; Gilbert, D.F.; Fontaine, F.; Xiao, X.; Zhang, H.; Piggott, A.M.; Lynch, J.W.; Capon, R.J. Australian marine sponge alkaloids as a new class of glycine-gated chloride channel receptor modulator. *Bioorg. Med. Chem* **2013**, *21*, 4420–4425. [CrossRef] [PubMed]
14. Mancini, I.; Guella, G.; Zibrowius, H.; Pietra, F. On the origin of quasi-racemic aplysinopsin cycloadducts, (bis)indole alkaloids isolated from scleractinian corals of the family Dendrophylliidae. Involvement of enantiodefective Diels–Alderases or asymmetric induction in artifact processes involving adventitious catalysts? *Tetrahedron* **2003**, *59*, 8757–8762. [CrossRef]
15. Guella, G.; Mancini, I.; Zibrowius, H.; Pietra, F. Aplysinopsin-type alkaloids from *Dendrophyllia* sp., a scleractinian coral of the family Dendrophylliidae of the philippines, facile photochemical (Z/E) photoisomerization and thermal reversal. *Helv. Chim. Acta* **1989**, *72*, 1444–1450. [CrossRef]
16. Murata, M.; Miyagawa-Kohshima, K.; Nakanishi, K.; Naya, Y. Characterization of compounds that induce symbiosis between sea anemone and anemone fish. *Science* **1986**, *234*, 585–587. [CrossRef]
17. Cimino, G.; De Stefano, S.; Minale, L. ent-Chromazonarol, a chroman-sesquiterpenoid from the sponge *Disidea pallescens*. *Experientia* **1975**, *31*, 1117–1118. [CrossRef]
18. Gordaliza, M. Cytotoxic terpene quinones from marine sponges. *Mar. Drugs* **2010**, *8*, 2849–2870. [CrossRef]

19. Prawat, H.; Mahidol, C.; Kaweetripob, W.; Wittayalai, S.; Ruchirawat, S. Iodo–sesquiterpene hydroquinone and brominated indole alkaloids from the Thai sponge *Smenospongia* sp. *Tetrahedron* **2012**, *68*, 6881–6886. [CrossRef]
20. Ravi, B.N.; Perzanowski, H.P.; Ross, R.A.; Erdman, T.R.; Scheuer, P.J.; Finer, J.; Clardy, J. Recent research in marine natural products: The puupehenones. *Pure Appl. Chem.* **1979**, *51*, 1893–1900. [CrossRef]
21. Albizati, K.F.; Faulkner, D.J. Stevensine, a novel alkaloid of an unidentified marine sponge. *J. Org. Chem.* **1985**, *50*, 4163–4164. [CrossRef]
22. Katsuhiro, U.; Takayuki, O.; Atsushi, S. Cytotoxic haterumadienone congeners from the Okinawan marine sponge *Dysidea* sp. *Heterocycles* **2007**, *72*, 655–663.
23. Noyer, C.; Thomas, O.P.; Becerro, M.A. Patterns of chemical diversity in the Mediterranean sponge *Spongia lamella*. *PLoS ONE* **2011**, *6*, e20844. [CrossRef] [PubMed]
24. El-Demerdash, A.; Atanasov, A.G.; Horbanczuk, O.K.; Tammam, M.A.; Abdel-Mogib, M.; Hooper, J.N.; Sekeroglu, N.; Al-Mourabit, A.; Kijjoa, A. Chemical diversity and biological activities of marine sponges of the genus *Suberea*: A systematic review. *Mar. Drugs* **2019**, *17*, 115. [CrossRef] [PubMed]
25. Koopmans, M.; Martens, D.; Wijffels, R.H. Towards commercial production of sponge medicines. *Mar. Drugs* **2009**, *7*, 787–802. [CrossRef] [PubMed]
26. Malve, H. Exploring the ocean for new drug developments: Marine pharmacology. *J. Pharm. Bioallied Sci.* **2016**, *8*, 83–91. [CrossRef]
27. Bohni, N.; Cordero-Maldonado, M.L.; Maes, J.; Siverio-Mota, D.; Marcourt, L.; Munck, S.; Kamuhabwa, A.R.; Moshi, M.J.; Esguerra, C.V.; de Witte, P.A.M.; et al. Integration of microfractionation, qNMR and zebrafish screening for the in vivo bioassay-guided isolation and quantitative bioactivity analysis of natural products. *PLoS ONE* **2013**, *8*, e64006. [CrossRef]
28. Mohotti, S.; Rajendran, S.; Muhammad, T.; Strömstedt, A.A.; Adhikari, A.; Burman, R.; de Silva, E.D.; Göransson, U.; Hettiarachchi, C.M.; Gunasekera, S. Screening for bioactive secondary metabolites in Sri Lankan medicinal plants by microfractionation and targeted isolation of antimicrobial flavonoids from *Derris scandens*. *J. Ethnopharmacol.* **2020**, *246*, 112158. [CrossRef]
29. Nothias, L.-F.; Nothias-Esposito, M.; da Silva, R.; Wang, M.; Protsyuk, I.; Zhang, Z.; Sarvepalli, A.; Leyssen, P.; Touboul, D.; Costa, J.; et al. Bioactivity-based molecular networking for the discovery of drug leads in natural product bioassay-guided fractionation. *J. Nat. Prod.* **2018**, *81*, 758–767. [CrossRef]
30. Roggen, H.; Gundersen, L.-L. Synthetic studies directed towards agelasine analogs—Synthesis, tautomerism, and alkylation of 2-substituted N-methoxy-9-methyl-9H-purin-6-amines. *Eur. J. Org. Chem.* **2008**, *2008*, 5099–5106. [CrossRef]
31. Roggen, H.; Charnock, C.; Burman, R.; Felth, J.; Larsson, R.; Bohlin, L.; Gundersen, L.-L. Antimicrobial and antineoplastic activities of agelasine analogs modified in the purine 2-position. *Arch. Pharm. Chem. Life Sci.* **2011**, *344*, 50–55. [CrossRef] [PubMed]
32. Balansa, W.; Wodi, S.I.M.; Rieuwpassa, F.J.; Ijong, F.G. Agelasines B, D and antimicrobial extract of a marine sponge *Agelas* sp. from Tahuna Bay, Sangihe Islands, Indonesia. *Biodiversitas* **2020**, *21*, 699–706. [CrossRef]
33. Gordaliza, M. Terpenyl-purines from the sea. *Mar. Drugs* **2009**, *7*, 833–849. [CrossRef] [PubMed]
34. Wilson, D.M.; Puyana, M.; Fenical, W.; Pawlik, J.R. Chemical defense of the Caribbean reef sponge *Axinella corrugata* against predatory fishes. *J. Chem. Ecol.* **1999**, *25*, 2811–2823. [CrossRef]
35. Newbold, R.W.; Jensen, P.R.; Fenical, W.; Pawlik, J.R. Antimicrobial activity of Caribbean sponge extracts. *Aquat. Microb. Ecol.* **1999**, *19*, 279–284. [CrossRef]
36. Katsuhiro, U.; Tomoyuki, U.; Oktavianus, S.E.R.; Masaki, K.; Daisuke, U. Haterumadienone: A new puupehenone congener from an Okinawan marine sponge, *Dysidea* sp. *Chem. Lett.* **2005**, *34*, 1530–1531. [CrossRef]
37. Robinson, S.J.; Hoobler, E.K.; Riener, M.; Loveridge, S.T.; Tenney, K.; Valeriote, F.A.; Holman, T.R.; Crews, P. Using enzyme assays to evaluate the structure and bioactivity of sponge-derived meroterpenes. *J. Nat. Prod.* **2009**, *72*, 1857–1863. [CrossRef]
38. Marner, M.; Patras, M.A.; Kurz, M.; Zubeil, F.; Förster, F.; Schuler, S.; Bauer, A.; Hammann, P.; Vilcinskas, A.; Schäberle, T.F.; et al. Molecular networking-guided discovery and characterization of stechlisins, a group of cyclic lipopeptides from a *Pseudomonas* sp. *J. Nat. Prod.* **2020**, *83*, 2607–2617. [CrossRef]
39. Salek, R.M.; Steinbeck, C.; Viant, M.R.; Goodacre, R.; Dunn, W.B. The role of reporting standards for metabolite annotation and identification in metabolomic studies. *GigaScience* **2013**. [CrossRef]

40. Creek, D.J.; Dunn, W.B.; Fiehn, O.; Griffin, J.L.; Hall, R.D.; Lei, Z.; Mistrik, R.; Neumann, S.; Schymanski, E.L.; Sumner, L.W. Metabolite identification: Are you sure? And how do your peers gauge your confidence? *Metabolomics* **2014**, *10*, 350–353. [CrossRef]
41. Torriani, S.F.F.; Melichar, J.P.E.; Mills, C.; Pain, N.; Sierotzki, H.; Courbot, M. *Zymoseptoria tritici*: A major threat to wheat production, integrated approaches to control. *Fungal Genet. Biol.* **2015**, *79*, 8–12. [CrossRef] [PubMed]
42. Hooper, J.N.A.; Van Soest, R.W.M. Systema Porifera. A Guide to the Classification of Sponges. In *Systema Porifera a Guide to the Classification of Sponges*; Hooper, J.N.A., Van Soest, R.W.M., Willenz, P., Eds.; Springer: Boston, MA, USA, 2002; pp. 1–7. ISBN 978-0-306-47260-2.
43. Hooper, J. Sponguide: Guide to Sponge Collection and Identification. Available online: https://www.researchgate.net/publication/242495363_Sponguide_Guide_to_Sponge_Collection_and_Identification (accessed on 20 April 2020).
44. R Core Team. The R Project for Statistical Computing. Available online: https://www.r-project.org/ (accessed on 12 December 2020).
45. Wickham, H.; Hester, J.; Francois, R. readr: Read Rectangular Text Data. Available online: https://CRAN.R-project.org/package=readr (accessed on 12 December 2020).
46. Schmidt, D.; Heckendorf, C. coop: Co-Operation: Fast Covariance, Correlation, and Cosine Similarity Operations. Available online: https://CRAN.R-project.org/package=coop (accessed on 12 December 2020).
47. Warnes, G.R.; Bolker, B.; Bonebakker, L.; Gentleman, R.; Huber, W.; Liaw, A.; Lumley, T.; Maechler, M.; Magnusson, A.; Moeller, S.; et al. Gplots: Various R Programming Tools for Plotting Data. Available online: https://CRAN.R-project.org/package=gplots (accessed on 12 December 2020).
48. Dowle, M.; Srinivasan, A.; Gorecki, J.; Chirico, M.; Stetsenko, P.; Short, T.; Lianoglou, S.; Antonyan, E.; Bonsch, M.; Parsonage, H.; et al. Data.Table: Extension of "Data.Frame". Available online: https://CRAN.R-project.org/package=data.table (accessed on 12 December 2020).
49. Eckert, A.; Godoy, L.; KS, S. parallelDist: Parallel Distance Matrix Computation using Multiple Threads. Available online: https://CRAN.R-project.org/package=parallelDist (accessed on 12 December 2020).
50. Wickham, H.; Hester, J.; Chang, W.; RStudio, R. Core team devtools: Tools to Make Developing R Packages Easier. Available online: https://CRAN.R-project.org/package=devtools (accessed on 12 December 2020).
51. Griffith, O. L Heatmap.3.R. GitHub. Available online: https://github.com/obigriffith/biostar-tutorials (accessed on 12 December 2020).
52. Laatsch, H. *AntiBase: The Natural Compound Identifier*; Wiley-Vch: Weinheim, Germany, 2017; ISBN 978-3-527-34359-1.
53. Dictionary of Natural Products 29.1 Chemical Search. Available online: http://dnp.chemnetbase.com/faces/chemical/ChemicalSearch.xhtml;jsessionid=DB01289ACAA79C222859E1CD8A98A894 (accessed on 12 December 2020).
54. SciFinder. Redistributed with Permission. Copyright © 2020 American Chemical Society (ACS). All rights reserved.
55. Allard, P.-M.; Péresse, T.; Bisson, J.; Gindro, K.; Marcourt, L.; Pham, V.C.; Roussi, F.; Litaudon, M.; Wolfender, J.-L. Integration of molecular networking and in-silico MS/MS fragmentation for natural products dereplication. *Anal. Chem.* **2016**, *88*, 3317–3323. [CrossRef] [PubMed]

marine drugs

Article

Genome Mining for Antimicrobial Compounds in Wild Marine Animals-Associated Enterococci

Janira Prichula [1], Muriel Primon-Barros [1], Romeu C. Z. Luz [1], Ícaro M. S. Castro [1], Thiago G. S. Paim [1], Maurício Tavares [2], Rodrigo Ligabue-Braun [3], Pedro A. d'Azevedo [1], Jeverson Frazzon [4], Ana P. G. Frazzon [5], Adriana Seixas [3] and Michael S. Gilmore [6,7,*]

1 Gram-Positive Cocci Laboratory, Federal University of Health Sciences of Porto Alegre (UFCSPA), Porto Alegre 90050-170, RS, Brazil; janirap@ufcspa.edu.br (J.P.); murielp@ufcspa.edu.br (M.P.-B.); romeulu@ufcspa.edu.br (R.C.Z.L.); icaromsc@ufcspa.edu.br (Í.M.S.C.); thiagopucrs@gmail.com (T.G.S.P.); pedroaze@ufcspa.edu.br (P.A.d.)

2 Centro de Estudos Costeiros, Limnológicos e Marinhos (CECLIMAR), Universidade Federal do Rio Grande do Sul (UFRGS), Campus Litoral Norte, Imbé 95625-000, RS, Brazil; mauricio.tavares@ufrgs.br

3 Department of Pharmacosciences, UFCSPA, Porto Alegre 90050-170, RS, Brazil; rodrigolb@ufcspa.edu.br (R.L.-B.); adrianaseixas@ufcspa.edu.br (A.S.)

4 Food Science Institute, UFRGS, Porto Alegre 90035-003, RS, Brazil; jeverson.frazzon@ufrgs.br

5 Department of Microbiology, Immunology and Parasitology, UFRGS, Porto Alegre 90050-170, RS, Brazil; ana.frazzon@ufrgs.br

6 Massachusetts Eye and Ear Infirmary, Department of Ophthalmology, Harvard Medical School, Boston, MA 02114, USA

7 Department of Microbiology, Harvard Medical School, Boston, MA 02115, USA

* Correspondence: michael_gilmore@meei.harvard.edu

Citation: Prichula, J.; Primon-Barros, M.; Luz, R.C.Z.; Castro, Í.M.S.; Paim, T.G.S.; Tavares, M.; Ligabue-Braun, R.; d'Azevedo, P.A.; Frazzon, J.; Frazzon, A.P.G.; et al. Genome Mining for Antimicrobial Compounds in Wild Marine Animals-Associated Enterococci. *Mar. Drugs* **2021**, *19*, 328. https://doi.org/10.3390/md19060328

Academic Editor: Max Crüsemann

Received: 1 May 2021
Accepted: 3 June 2021
Published: 6 June 2021

Abstract: New ecosystems are being actively mined for new bioactive compounds. Because of the large amount of unexplored biodiversity, bacteria from marine environments are especially promising. Further, host-associated microbes are of special interest because of their low toxicity and compatibility with host health. Here, we identified and characterized biosynthetic gene clusters encoding antimicrobial compounds in host-associated enterococci recovered from fecal samples of wild marine animals remote from human-affected ecosystems. Putative biosynthetic gene clusters in the genomes of 22 *Enterococcus* strains of marine origin were predicted using antiSMASH5 and Bagel4 bioinformatic software. At least one gene cluster encoding a putative bioactive compound precursor was identified in each genome. Collectively, 73 putative antimicrobial compounds were identified, including 61 bacteriocins (83.56%), 10 terpenes (13.70%), and 2 (2.74%) related to putative nonribosomal peptides (NRPs). Two of the species studied, *Enterococcus avium* and *Enterococcus mundtii*, are rare causes of human disease and were found to lack any known pathogenic determinants but yet possessed bacteriocin biosynthetic genes, suggesting possible additional utility as probiotics. Wild marine animal-associated enterococci from human-remote ecosystems provide a potentially rich source for new antimicrobial compounds of therapeutic and industrial value and potential probiotic application.

Keywords: enterococci; genome-wide analysis; bacteriocins; probiotics; wild marine species

1. Introduction

Drug-resistant bacteria kill an estimated 700,000 people worldwide each year, and the discovery of new antimicrobial drugs is urgently needed [1–3]. This is motivating the search for new ecologies for novel natural products of potential therapeutic value. Human-proximal terrestrial life has been screened for diverse natural products to a much greater extent than larger but less accessible marine ecosystems. Blue biotechnology (or marine biotechnology) is an emerging field that investigates the rich diversity of bioactive molecules produced by marine organisms with potential industrial and therapeutic applications [4–9]. Early successes include compounds derived from a gastropod (e.g., ziconotide, commercial name Prialt [10]), sponge (e.g., eribulin mesylate, commercial name Halaven [11]), cyanobacteria (e.g., dolastatin 10 [12], apratoxin A [13], and barbamide [14]), fungi (e.g., penicillipyrone A and B [15], and aszonapyrone A [16]), algae (e.g., neolaurene [17] and diphlorethohydroxycarmalol (DPHC) [18]), and bacteria (e.g., salinosporamide A [19], abyssomicin C [20], forazoline A [21], and farnesylquinone [22].

Recently, host-associated microbes also have drawn attention as a potential source for low toxicity agents compatible with host health but active against pathogenic microbes [23,24]. It was, therefore, of interest to us to explore marine animals from remote habitats for host-associated microbes that encode novel natural product biosynthetic pathways. Further, we focused on host-associated enterococci, a genus of gut microbes associated with all classes of land animals studied [25], and with animals that have returned to the marine environment [26]. Although most enterococci exist as harmless commensals, some lineages of the species *Enterococcus faecalis* and *Enterococcus faecium* have emerged as leading causes of multidrug-resistant hospital infection [25,27–30].

Enterococci are known to produce bacteriocins with narrow to broad antimicrobial activity [31–33]. Bacteriocins have found use as natural antimicrobial agents so far, mainly in the food industry but could complement traditional antibiotics in controlling important human and animal pathogens [34,35]. Different classification schemes have been proposed for bacteriocins produced by Lactic Acid Bacteria (LAB), although still a subject of debate [33,36,37]. Class I bacteriocins are posttranslationally modified peptides with less than 10 kDa that require enzymatic modification during biosynthesis, and thereby, the molecules have uncommon amino acids and structures that impact their properties [36]. Class II bacteriocins are also less than 10 kDa, although they are heat stable and unmodified peptides [36] with the exception of disulfide bridging, circularization, and methionine formylation [33]. This class has been subclassified: IIa—pediocin-like bacteriocins; IIb—two-peptide bacteriocins; circular bacteriocins; leaderless; and other bacteriocins that do not fall into any of the recognized subclasses [33]. On the other hand, Class III bacteriocins are large-molecular-weight (more than 10 kDa) and heat-labile antimicrobial proteins usually composed of different domains [36]. Divergently, some authors have been classified circular bacteriocins as class IV [38] or as Class Ib [36] since these head-to-tail cyclized peptides whose N- and C-termini are linked by a peptide bond, thereby rendering a circular molecule [36].

The bacteriocins synthetized by enterococci, enterocins, are generally small molecular weight (20–60 amino acids), often post-translationally modified peptides with cationic, hydrophobic, and heat-stable properties [32,33,36]. They vary in their mode of action, activity spectrum (restricted or broad), molecular mass, biochemical properties, and genetic origin [33,39,40]. Most known enterocins are produced by *E. faecium* and *E. faecalis*, but a few peptides have also been isolated from *Enterococcus mundtii*, *Enterococcus avium*, *Enterococcus durans*, *Enterococcus hirae*, and *Enterococcus lactis* [33,38]. Most characterized enterocins derive from enterococci associated with food, waste, feces, and gastrointestinal tract of humans and other animals [32,33,41]. Few have been described from enterococci from wild ecologies [8,26,42–44].

Traditionally, new bioactive compounds have been identified by screening microorganism extracts for biological activity or by amplification of new genes using polymerase chain reaction (PCR) [45–48]. These screening strategies are limited by time-consuming and laborious test methods [24,49]. Advances in molecular biology, bioinformatics, and genomics have been providing important new tools for exploration and development [50–52]. Genome screening has identified a large pool of potential compounds encoded by biosynthetic gene clusters (BGCs) in DNA databases [1,53–56]. The identification of new BGCs may be performed by applying algorithms based on indicators (e.g., evolutionary hallmarks, signature protein domains, and distant paralogs of primary metabolic enzymes) and using bioinformatic tools, such as antiSMASH5 [57] and BAGEL4 [58]. High throughput computational technologies are being used for screening, presumptive chemical elucidation, and understanding of activities and biological aspects of new compounds [7,24].

Therefore, genome mining may represent a fertile strategy for identifying new biomolecules for future therapeutic and industrial applications. In this sense, the aim of the present study was to examine 22 genomes of *Enterococcus* species isolated from fecal samples of 17 wild marine animals from remote ecologies for potential antimicrobial compounds and/or probiotics strains.

2. Results

2.1. Diversity of Wild Marine Animals Associated-Enterococci

The genomes of 22 *Enterococcus* spp. isolated from wild sea turtles, seabirds, and marine mammals were sequenced (Table 1). A summary of the sequencing statistics is presented in Supplementary Table S1. The genomes sizes were between 2.6–4.5 Mb, with GC contents ranging from 36.3% to 42.4%. All genomes share average nucleotide identities (ANI) above 95% with known species [59], confirming designation as *Enterococcus avium* (4.54%); *Enterococcus casseliflavus* (13.64%); *Enterococcus faecalis* (45.45%); *Enterococcus hirae* (27.27%); *Enterococcus lactis* (4.54%); *Enterococcus mundtii* (4.54%) species (Table 1; Supplementary Table S2).

2.2. Marine Enterococcal Genomes Harbor Diverse Biosynthetic Gene Clusters (BGCs) Coding for Antimicrobial Compounds

Two informatic packages, antiSMASH5 [57] and Bagel4 [58], accurately predict all known enterococcal bacteriocins whose properties have been well studied [32,33], including bacteriocin 31, bacteriocin T8, durancin Q, enterocin 96, enterocin1071A and 1071B, enterocin_A, enterocin B, enterocin CRL35, enterocin EJ97, enterocin SE-K4, enterocin P, enterocin Xα and Xβ, enterolysin A, hiracin JM79, mundticin KS, and others. This also includes the *E. faecalis* cytolysin, a highly divergent two-component lantipeptide-type bacteriocin active against nearly all Gram positives [60], which also possesses lytic activity for some eukaryotic cells [61]. Therefore, antiSMASH5 [57] and Bagel4 [58] were used to mine the genomes of all 22 genomes for putative bacteriocin biosynthesis operons (Supplementary Table S3). This analysis identified one or more gene clusters encoding a bioactive compound precursor in each genome. In total, 73 antimicrobial compound BGCs were predicted, including 61 (83.56%) bacteriocins, 10 (13.70%) related to terpene synthesis, and 2 (2.74%) related to putative nonribosomal peptides (NRPs). The NRPs biosynthetic gene clusters were found only in *E. lactis* genome (MP10-1), whereas terpene BGCs were found among *E. casseliflavus* (HT1-1, J2, J4), *E. hirae* (C7, DMW1-1, MP1-1, MP1-2, MP1-4, MP1-5), and *E. mundtii* (MP7-18) species (Supplementary Table S3). NRP and terpene BGCs were predicted only by antiSMASH5 [57], whereas bacteriocins were identified by both tools.

Table 1. The description of the origin of enterococci genomes associated with wild marine animals.

Animal	Common Name	Scientific Name	Age [1]	Code [2]	Collection Date	Location	Enterococci Genomes [3]	Species Identification (ANI [5])	Collection from
Sea turtles	green turtle	*Chelonia mydas*	Y	2	29-May-13	Cidreira	GT3-2	*E. faecalis* (98.38)	Prichula et al. (2016) Prichula et al. (2020)
	green turtle	*Chelonia mydas*	Y	1	25-Apr-14	Tramandaií	GT6-1	*E. faecalis* (98.53)	
	hawksbill turtle	*Eretmochelys imbricata*	Y	1	23-Dec-12	Tramandaií	HT1-3	*E. casseliflavus* (98.56)	
Seabirds	Magellanic penguin	*Spheniscus magellanicus*	Y	1	2-Nov-12	Cidreira	MP1-1	*E. hirae* (98.36)	
							MP1-2	*E. hirae* (98.37)	
							MP1-4	*E. hirae* (99.34)	
							MP1-5	*E. hirae* (98.68)	
	Magellanic penguin	*Spheniscus magellanicus*	Y	1	13-Nov-12	Xangri-laí	MP2-6 [4]	*E. faecalis* (98.55)	
	Magellanic penguin	*Spheniscus magellanicus*	Y	2	27-Jul-13	Cidreira	MP5-1 [4]	*E. faecalis* (98.54)	
	Magellanic penguin	*Spheniscus magellanicus*	Y	1	19-Sep-13	Imbeí	MP7-18	*E. mundtii* (97.04)	
	Magellanic penguin	*Spheniscus magellanicus*	Y	1	14-Oct-13	Cidreira	MP8-1 [4]	*E. faecalis* (98.52)	
							MP8-17 [4]	*E. faecalis* (98.67)	
	Magellanic penguin	*Spheniscus magellanicus*	Y	1	16-Oct-13	Cidreira	MP9-10 [4]	*E. faecalis* (98.52)	
	Magellanic penguin	*Spheniscus magellanicus*	Y	1	23-Dec-13	Torres	MP10-1	*E. lactis* (98.92)	
	snowy-crowned tern	*Sterna trudeaui*	A	2	4-Dec-13	Arroio do Sal	ST1-20	*E. faecalis* (98.63)	
Marine Mammals	dwarf minke whale	*Balaenoptera acutorostrata*	Y	2	21-Jun-13	Tramandaií	DMW1-1	*E. hirae* (98.09)	
	Risso's dolphin	*Grampus griseus*	A	2	4-Jul-13	Balneaírio Pinhal	RD1-1	*E. faecalis* (98.71)	
	South American fur seal	*Arctocephalus australis*	-	2	2-Aug-12	Torres	B9	*E. faecalis* (98.81)	Santestevan et al. (2015)
	South American fur seal	*Arctocephalus australis*	A	2	2-Aug-12	Xangri-laí	C7	*E. hirae* (98.67)	
	South American fur seal	*Arctocephalus australis*	A	2	12-Jul-12	Palmares do Sul	J2	*E. casseliflavus* (98.56)	
							J4	*E. casseliflavus* (98.57)	
	South American fur seal	*Arctocephalus australis*	-	2	21-Jul-12	Tramandaií	L8	*E. avium* (98.06)	

[1] Age of the animals: A: adult; Y: young. [2] Code based on Geraci and Lounsbury (2005). [3] Strains were sequenced in this study. GT—green turtle; HT—hawksbill turtle; MP—Magellanic penguin; ST—snowy-crowned tern; DMW—dwarf minke whale; RD—Risso's dolphin, and B, C, J or L—South American fur seal. [4] Genomes sequenced in a previous study (Prichula et al., 2020). [5] The enterococci species were confirmed by pairwise comparison of their average nucleotide identity (ANI) using as reference the following genomes: *Enterococcus avium* ATCC14025; *Enterococcus casseliflavus* ATCC12755; *Enterococcus faecalis* ATCC19433; *Enterococcus hirae* ATCC 9790; *Enterococcus lactis* KCTC 21015; *Enterococcus mundtii* ATCC 882.

2.3. Diversity of Bacteriocins Genes among Wild Marine Animals-Associated Enterococci

A total of 30 unique bacteriocin species were identified, including 8 belonging to class I, 19 to class II, and 3 to class III (Figure 1). Although class II bacteriocins showed the greatest diversity, class III bacteriocins were most common and widely distributed. Interestingly, eight new putative bacteriocins with no significant identity to known peptides were found amongst marine enterococci genomes, including two new putative lanthipeptides (I and II) identified as class I, five unknown bacteriocins (I, II, III, IV, and V) identified as class II, and one unknown class III bacteriocin (VI) (Figure 1; Supplementary Table S4).

The most frequent class I bacteriocins were putative sactipeptides (n = 9), followed by unknown lanthipeptide 1 (n = 5), lasso peptides (n = 4), and thiopeptides (n = 4). Enterocin SE-K4 (n = 5) and enterocin P (n = 3) were the most frequent class II bacteriocins. In turn, the class III bacteriocin enterolysin A (n = 17) was the most frequent bacteriocin found in the 22 sequenced genomes (Figure 1).

Eight enterococcal genomes belonging to *E. hirae* (C7, DMW1-1, MP1-5), *E. avium* (L8), and *E. faecalis* (GT3-2, GT6-1, MP8-1, and ST1-20) species showed four or more bacteriocin biosynthetic genes (Figure 1). Four of these genomes (C7, DMW1-1, MP1-5, and MP8-1) encode bacteriocins belonging to three different classes (I, II, and III). Moreover, four enterococci genomes (C7, L8, ST1-20, and MP1-2) exhibited evidence of bacteriocin gene duplication (Figure 1; Supplementary Table S3). Because of their potentially new bacteriocins and/or amenability large-scale synthesis, putative class II and III bacteriocins were of special interest for further analysis.

2.4. Phylogenetic Relationship among Class II and III Bacteriocins Predicted from Wild Marine Animal-Associated Enterococcal Genomes

To gain insights into the phylogeny of the 30 class II and 19 class III bacteriocins genes identified, phylogenetic analysis was performed (Figure 2) to determine their relationship (Supplementary Table S5) to 16 reference sequences in Bagel4 and Uniprot databases (Supplementary Table S6). This identified two groups with significant branch support (Figure 2). Group 1 included bacteriocins of both classes II and III. Class II bacteriocin gene clusters in Group 1 could be divided into subclasses a, b, and others. Included within each are: *IIa*) mundticin AT06, enterocin P, bacteriocin T8, bacteriocin 31, and enterocin SE-K4; *IIb*) enterocin X chain alpha, enterocin X chain beta; *II leaderless*) enterocin EJ97; *II circular bacteriocin*) carnocyclin A; *II other subclasses*) sakacin Q, enterocin 96, uviB, and enterocin NKR-5-3D; and unknown bacteriocins I, II, III, IV, and V. Class III bacteriocins in Group 1 included: enterolysin A, propionicin SM1, and unknown bacteriocin VI. In contrast, phylogenetic Group 2 included only the class II bacteriocin, lactococcin 972.

Interestingly, the 17 Class III enterolysin A-related sequences occurring in Group 1 could be grouped into three subclades. The first and second branches included sequences derived from *E. hirae* strains C7, MP1-1, MP1-2, MP1-4, MP1-5, DMW1-1, while the third branch included enterolysins A from *E. faecalis* strains GT3-2, ST1-20, MP8-1, RD1-1, MP5-1, MP9-10, and B9. The alignment of enterolysin A sequences within each branch (Supplementary Figures S1–S3) shows high similarity among them, although they have few conserved amino acids compared to the enterolysin A reference sequences (Supplementary Figure S4).

The alignment of the other bacteriocin sequences with reference sequences was performed (Supplementary Figures S5–S10). Among identities found were conserved motifs such as YGN and cysteine residues (all class IIa bacteriocins can be found in Supplementary Figure S6), and GxxxG or AxxxA motifs among class IIb and circular bacteriocin members (Supplementary Figures S7 and S8).

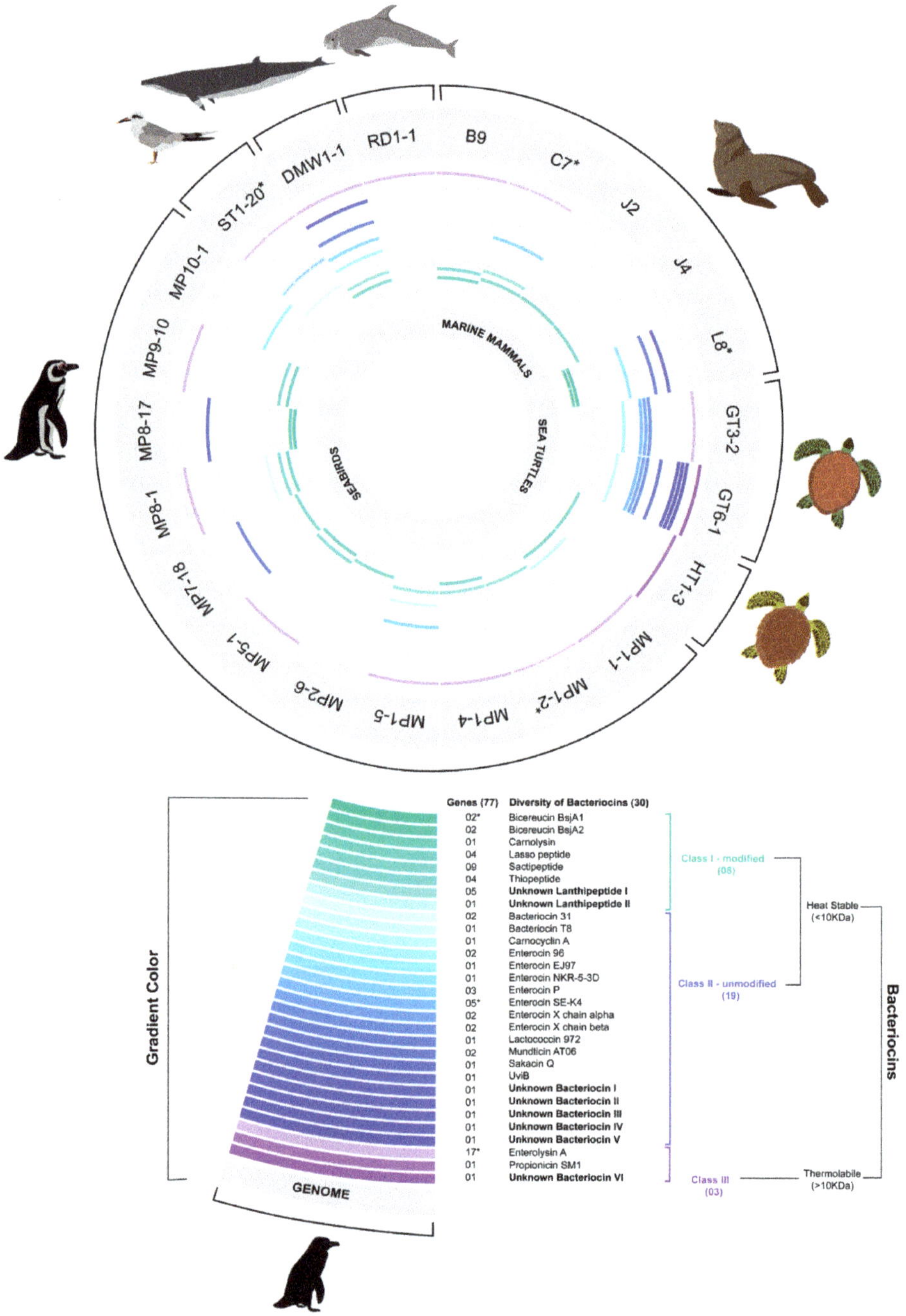

Figure 1. Biosynthetic bacteriocins genes were found within 22 *Enterococcus* spp. genomes from wild marine animals. The *Enterococcus* genomes are represented in the external circle (grey). Diversity of bacteriocin genes within 22 *Enterococcus* spp. genomes are represented by color gradients: Class I (green gradient) and Class II (blue gradient), and Class III (purple). * Genomes showing duplicated bacteriocin genes (rectangles indicate the number of these genes). The illustration was designed using a D3 and Adobe Illustrator.

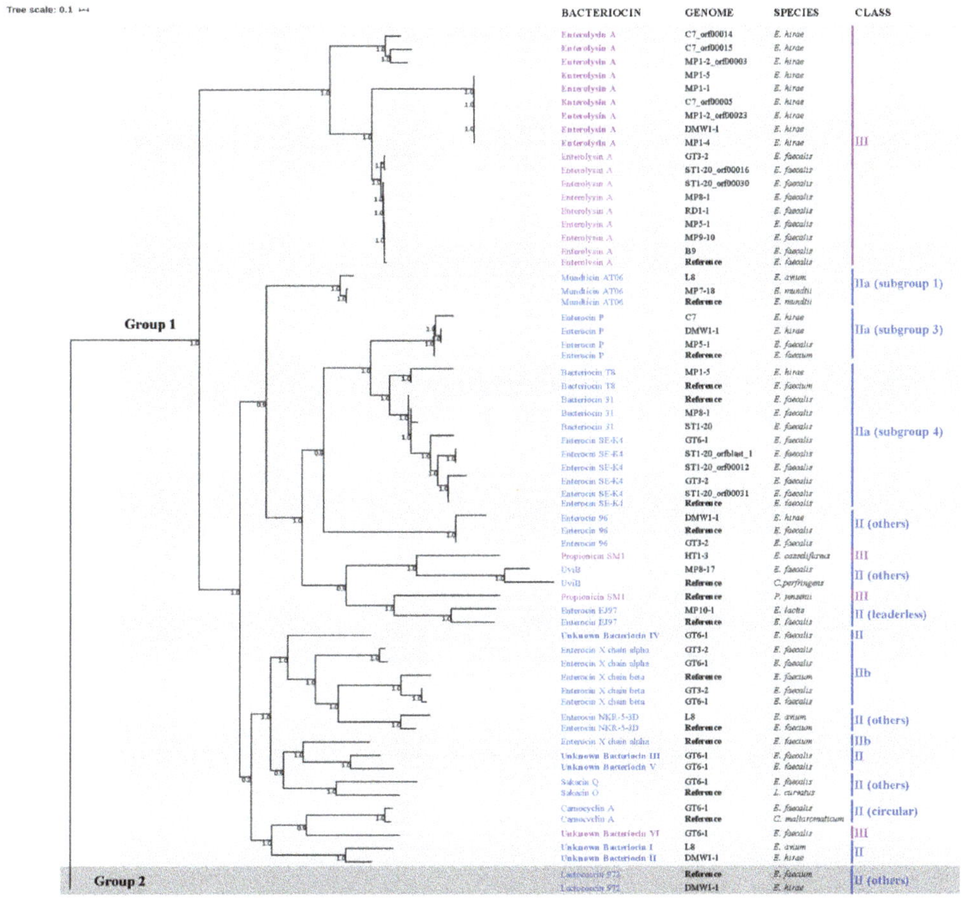
Tree scale: 0.1
BACTERIOCIN
GENOME
SPECIES
CLASS
Enterolysin A C7_orf00014 E. hirae
Enterolysin A C7_orf00015 E. hirae
Enterolysin A MP1-2_orf00003 E. hirae
Enterolysin A MP1-5 E. hirae
Enterolysin A MP1-1 E. hirae
Enterolysin A C7_orf00005 E. hirae
Enterolysin A MP1-2_orf00023 E. hirae
Enterolysin A DMW1-1 E. hirae
Enterolysin A MP1-4 E. hirae
Enterolysin A GT3-2 E. faecalis
Enterolysin A ST1-20_orf00016 E. faecalis
Enterolysin A ST1-20_orf00030 E. faecalis
Enterolysin A MP8-1 E. faecalis
Enterolysin A RD1-1 E. faecalis
Enterolysin A MP5-1 E. faecalis
Enterolysin A MP9-10 E. faecalis
Enterolysin A B9 E. faecalis
Enterolysin A Reference E. faecalis
III
Mundticin AT06 L8 E. avium
Mundticin AT06 MP7-18 E. mundtii
Mundticin AT06 Reference E. mundtii
IIa (subgroup 1)
Enterocin P C7 E. hirae
Enterocin P DMW1-1 E. hirae
Enterocin P MP5-1 E. faecalis
Enterocin P Reference E. faecium
IIa (subgroup 3)
Bacteriocin T8 MP1-5 E. hirae
Bacteriocin T8 Reference E. faecium
Bacteriocin 31 Reference E. faecalis
Bacteriocin 31 MP8-1 E. faecalis
Bacteriocin 31 ST1-20 E. faecalis
Enterocin SE-K4 GT6-1 E. faecalis
Enterocin SE-K4 ST1-20_orfblast_1 E. faecalis
Enterocin SE-K4 ST1-20_orf00012 E. faecalis
Enterocin SE-K4 GT3-2 E. faecalis
Enterocin SE-K4 ST1-20_orf00031 E. faecalis
Enterocin SE-K4 Reference E. faecalis
IIa (subgroup 4)
Enterocin 96 DMW1-1 E. hirae
Enterocin 96 Reference E. faecalis
Enterocin 96 GT3-2 E. faecalis
II (others)
Propionicin SM1 HT1-3 E. casseliflavus
III
UviB MP8-17 E. faecalis
UviB Reference C.perfringens
II (others)
Propionicin SM1 Reference P. jensenii
III
Enterocin EJ97 MP10-1 E. lactis
Enterocin EJ97 Reference E. faecalis
II (leaderless)
Unknown Bacteriocin IV GT6-1 E. faecalis
II
Enterocin X chain alpha GT3-2 E. faecalis
Enterocin X chain alpha GT6-1 E. faecalis
Enterocin X chain beta Reference E. faecium
Enterocin X chain beta GT3-2 E. faecalis
Enterocin X chain beta GT6-1 E. faecalis
IIb
Enterocin NKR-5-3D L8 E. avium
Enterocin NKR-5-3D Reference E. faecium
II (others)
Enterocin X chain alpha Reference E. faecium
IIb
Unknown Bacteriocin III GT6-1 E. faecalis
Unknown Bacteriocin V GT6-1 E. faecalis
II
Sakacin Q GT6-1 E. faecalis
Sakacin Q Reference L. curvatus
II (others)
Carnocyclin A GT6-1 E. faecalis
Carnocyclin A Reference C. maltaromaticum
II (circular)
Unknown Bacteriocin VI GT6-1 E. faecalis
III
Unknown Bacteriocin I L8 E. avium
Unknown Bacteriocin II DMW1-1 E. hirae
II
Lactococcin 972 Reference E. faecium
Lactococcin 972 DMW1-1 E. hirae
II (others)
Group 1
Group 2

Figure 2. The phylogenetic relationships among bacteriocins (Class II and III) predicted for wild marine animals-associated enterococci genomes. The different groups are represented by grey colors (light grey: Group 1 and dark grey: Group 2). Class II is represented in blue and class III in purple (bold purple are enterolysins A from *E. hirae*, and regular purple are enterolysins A from *E. faecalis*). Unknown bacteriocins are highlighted in bold blue (I, II, III, IV, and V) and bold purple (VI).

New putative bacteriocins I, II, and VI showed greater similarity to carnocyclin A, while the unknown bacteriocins III, IV and V were more closely related to enterocin X chain alpha (Xα) (Figure 2). Alignment of unknown bacteriocins with carnocyclin A and Enterocin Xα reference sequences allowed detection of conserved amino acid residues and motifs such as GxxxG or AxxxA (Figure 3). Putative novel bacteriocins I, II, VI and carnocyclin A showed only 1.3% overall amino acid sequence identity (Figure 3A), whereas bacteriocins I and II share 55.22% identity between them (Figure 3B). Putative bacteriocins III, IV, and V, which were closely related to enterocin Xα, have 9.2% overall amino acid sequence identity (Figure 3C); and bacteriocins III and V share 43.4% identity between them (Figure 3D). Structural modeling of these putative class II and III bacteriocins using the I-TASSER [62] package to build models using a combination of fragment and ab initio model building [63] is shown in Figure 4. Insights into structural features are important for the biosynthesis, mode of action, and biological activity of bacteriocins. The molecular models are in agreement with the expected protein folds (mostly alpha-helices with coil regions). Likewise, the most divergent model (Bacteriocin VI) is also isolated in its group in the phylogenetic reconstruction, supporting its uniqueness among other unknown bacteriocins.

A)

GENOME	BACTERIOCIN	AA SEQUENCE	
Reference (Bagel: 148.1)	**Carnocyclin A**	--	0
E. faecalis GT6-1	Unknow Bacteriocin VI	MVPNIRKKAGDFMELQVSRKSKFFCLAMALLIALGMFISAGTSVYAAEVNNDISEEDKVI	60
E. avium L8	Unknow Bacteriocin I	------------------------MIKKDV------------------------------	6
E. hirae DMW1-1	Unknow Bacteriocin II	---------------------------MKK------------------------------	3
	Consensus	--	
Reference (Bagel: 148.1)	**Carnocyclin A**	---------------------------------------MLYELVAYGIAQGT-------	14
E. faecalis GT6-1	Unknow Bacteriocin VI	LDNIDVNSFYSDANKGLNEFFSKAVSANPINGKLALNEIGAKDMFGEGIEYEAVVSFIEF	120
E. avium L8	Unknow Bacteriocin I	-----------------------------------LKKVDLKKVIGGGGASGT-------	24
E. hirae DMW1-1	Unknow Bacteriocin II	-----------------------------------LTAEEMKQVVGG----RV-------	17
		.:.. .	
	Consensus	--	
Reference (Bagel: 148.1)	**Carnocyclin A**	-------------A--EKVVSL------IN---AGLTVGSII----SILGGVTVGLS-GV	45
E. faecalis GT6-1	Unknow Bacteriocin VI	FNSDNNFNELGRFEFRDSLKTLAQGNLPIQTRAGGALAKCAVEWAK---NTFGVGISVAA	177
E. avium L8	Unknow Bacteriocin I	-------------WLDSKTKAC------INGQAGGMLAGSPGGLGGIIIGGIGGAIAGGC	65
E. hirae DMW1-1	Unknow Bacteriocin II	-------------HLSNNTKAC------INGQLGGMLTGSVGGIGGIILGGIAGAIAGGC	58
		.. : *: .* . . . . .:: .	
	Consensus	----------------------------**I**-----**G**-------------------------	
Reference (Bagel: 148.1)	**Carnocyclin A**	**F**TAVKAAIAKQGIKKAIQL--------------------------------	64
E. faecalis GT6-1	Unknow Bacteriocin VI	**F**KSV---LNTYGYAKAAAWLAGKVASSTGRKAAAVLTLVWTAMTCAPIEAE	225
E. avium L8	Unknow Bacteriocin I	**F**G---	67
E. hirae DMW1-1	Unknow Bacteriocin II	**F**N---	60
		*	
	Consensus	**F**--	

Figure 3. *Cont.*

B)

GENOME	BACTERIOCIN	AA SEQUENCE	
E. avium L8	Unknow Bacteriocin I	MIKKDVLKKVDLKKVIGGGGASGTWLDSKTKACINGQAGGMLAGSPGGLGGIIIGGIGGAIAGGCFG	67
E. hirae DMW1-1	Unknow Bacteriocin II	---MKKLTAEEMKQVVGG----RVHLSNNTKACINGQLGGMLTGSVGGIGGIILGGIAGAIAGGCFN	60
		. *. ::*:*:** . *..:******** ****:** **:****:***.********.	
	Consensus	------L-----K-V-GG-------L---TKACINGQ-GGML-GS-GG-GGII-GGI-GAIAGGCF-	

C)

GENOME	BACTERIOCIN	AA SEQUENCE	
Reference (Bagel: 96.2)	**Enterocin X chain alpha**	MQNVKEVSVKEMKQIIGGSNDSL--------WYGVGQFMGKQANCITNHPVKHMIIPGYCLSKILG--------------	58
E. faecalis GT6-1	Unknow Bacteriocin III	MENFKELTVKEMQKISGGGWQTMSFTPNMECWNGIL----KTGNCRVKWDVVANQAVNNVTSAMIGGFGRGR--------	68
E. faecalis GT6-1	Unknow Bacteriocin IV	MTKFKELTVQEMKQISGGKHGKPIYFKDLP-WA--------QQKCILSVA--GGALIGTTTGGPLGALLGAGSQAWGCL-	68
E. faecalis GT6-1	Unknow Bacteriocin V	MQNMKELTAKDTQQINGGGWSTPPGLSNIECKNGHL----AVGNCRAKWGDISNGLVNQLVSCAVNGMYGGRCKQPGKFY	76
		* :.**::.:: ::* ** . :* . . . :.	
	Consensus	M---KE--------I-GG------------------------C-------------------------------------	

D)

GENOME	BACTERIOCIN	AA SEQUENCE	
E. faecalis GT6-1	Unknow Bacteriocin III	MENFKELTVKEMQKISGGGWQTMSFTPNMECWNGILKTGNCRVKWDVVANQAVNNVTSAMIGGFGRGR--------	68
E. faecalis GT6-1	Unknow Bacteriocin V	MQNMKELTAKDTQQINGGGWSTPPGLSNIECKNGHLAVGNCRAKWGDISNGLVNQLVSCAVNGMYGGRCKQPGKFY	76
		::****.*: *:*.****.* *:** ** * .****.**. ::* **::.*. :.*: **	
	Consensus	M-N-KELT-K--Q-I-GGGW-T-----N-EC-NG-L--GNCR-KW----N--VN---S----G---GR--------	

Figure 3. The alignment of putative unknown Class II bacteriocins and reference sequences using Clustal Omega software. (**A**) Alignment among I, II, VI, and carnocyclin A (reference) (Identity (*): 1.3%; Strongly similar (:): 2.2%; Weakly similar (.): 4.4%]. (**B**) The alignment between I and II [Identity (*): 55.22%; Strongly similar (:): 11.94%; Weakly similar (.) 10.45%]. (**C**) Alignment among III, VI, V, and enterocin Xα (reference) [Identity (*): 9.2%; Strongly similar (:): 11.8%; Weakly similar (.): 9.2%]. (**D**) Alignment between I and II [Identity (*): 43.4%; Strongly similar (:): 14.5%; Weakly similar (.) 11.8%). Identical residues are shaded in grey, and GxxxG or AxxxA motives are represented in red color. (-) Gaps introduced to optimize alignments. (*) Positions with a single conserved residue. (:) Conservation between groups with strongly similar properties. (.) Conservation between groups with weakly similar properties.

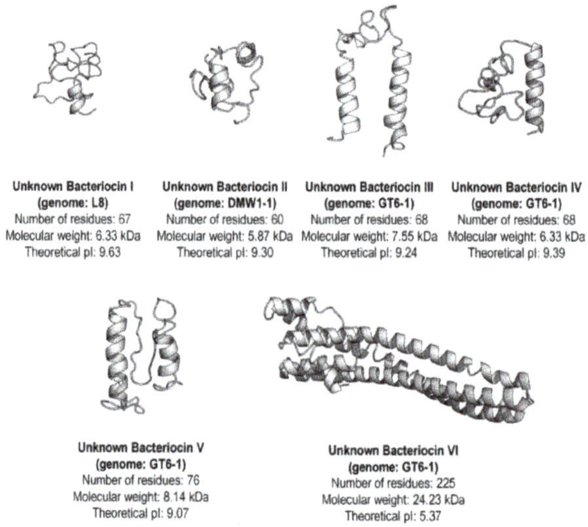

Figure 4. The structural modeling of unknown Class II enterococcal bacteriocins from wild marine animals.

2.5. Detection of Genes Associated with Enhanced Enterococcal Virulence

Among the 22 genomes evaluated, *E. avium* (L8) and *E. mundtii* (MP7-18) were found to be devoid of determinants that have mainly been identified in *E. faecalis* and *E. faecium* strains associated with enhanced virulence (Figure 5A,B). All other enterococci strains possessed at least one potential virulence-associated trait (Figure 5B). As expected, these were most common in *E. faecalis*, where they have been most thoroughly studied. Some of these traits are encoded within the core genomes [25,26]. The unique *E. lactis* harbored *efa*Afm and *acm* genes, while all *E. faecalis* contained several genes associated with adhesion (*ace*, *efa*Afs), biofilm production (*ebp*A, *ebp*B and *ebp*C), proteases (*gel*E and *srt*A), protection against oxidative stress (*tpx*), and quorum sensing and sex pheromone (*cad*, *cam*E, *c*CF10, *c*OB1, and *fsr*B). *Enterococcus faecalis* genomes varied in the presence of hyaluronidase genes (*hyl*A and *hyl*B) and adhesion-associated gene (*Elr*A).

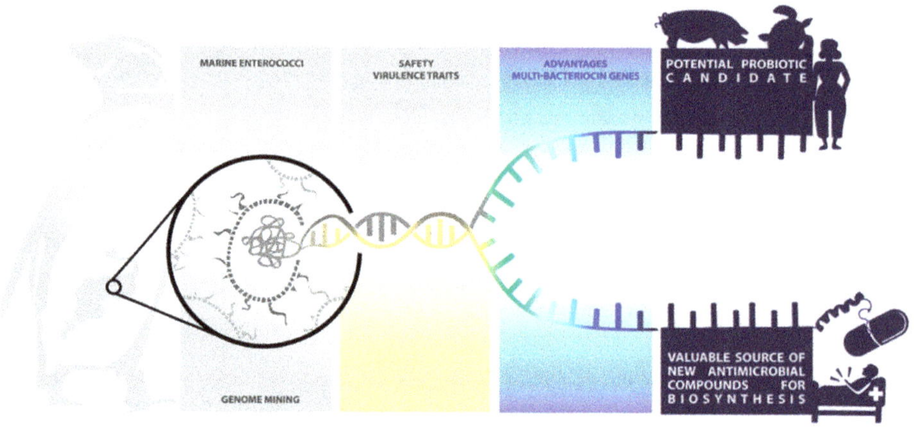

(A)

Figure 5. *Cont.*

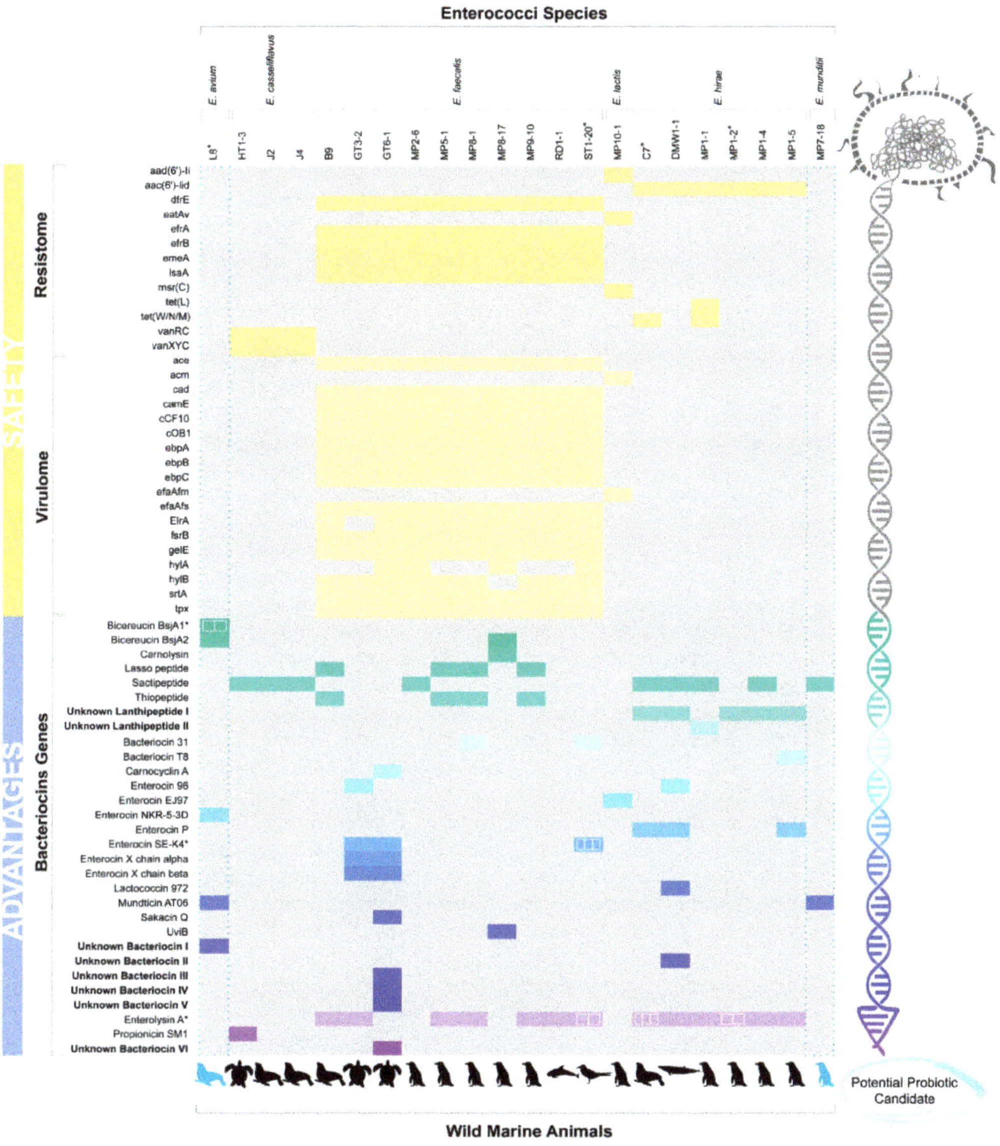

(B)

Figure 5. Wild marine animals-associated enterococci might represent a potentially valuable source of new compounds for biotechnological application and generation of new drug leads and potential probiotic application. (**A**) Scheme showing the main marine enterococci biotechnological applications suggested in this study. (**B**) Virulence markers analysis revealed potential probiotic enterococci from wild marine animals. Determinants of resistance (light yellow) and virulence (dark yellow) were associated with the results of in silico screening by bacteriocins (green, blue, and purple colors). * Genomes showing duplicated bacteriocin genes (rectangles are representing the number of these genes). Blue dash representing the potential probiotic candidate strains (L8 and MP7-18). The illustration was designed using D3, R software, and Adobe Illustrator.

Resistome analysis (Figure 5B) revealed that all *E. casseliflavus* genomes (n = 3) possessed genes related to low-level vancomycin resistance (*van*RC and *van*XYC), as expected since these are part of the core genome for that species [64]. All *E. faecalis* genomes (n = 10) contained genes within the core genomes [26] conferring resistance to trimethoprim (*dfr*E); to macrolide, fluoroquinolone, and rifamycin (*efr*A and *efr*B); to pleuromutilin, lincosamide, and streptogramin (*lsa*A); and have a multidrug and toxic compound extrusion transporter (*eme*A). On the other hand, the unique *E. lactis* genome possessed genes related to the resistance to aminoglycosides (*aac*(6′)-Ii); to macrolide, lincosamide, streptogramin, tetracycline, oxazolidinone, phenicol, pleuromutilin (*eat*Av); and to macrolide, lincosamide, streptogramin (*msr*C). In addition, *E. hirae* genomes harbored genes related to aminoglycoside (*acc*(6′)-Iid; n = 6), and tetracycline [*tet*(W/N/M), n = 2; *tet*(L); n = 1] resistance.

3. Discussion

Microbes associated with marine animals from remote ecologies may be important sources for new tools to manage human and/or microbial interactions. In this study, we explored *Enterococcus* strains from the microbiota of wild sea birds, sea turtles, and marine mammals that range from the Antarctic to the coast of Brazil to identify potentially novel BGCs. These prospective BCGs were found in generalist species *E. faecalis*, as well as less common and less studied species, including *E. avium*, *E. casseliflavus*, *E. hirae*, *E. lactis*, and *E. mundtii*.

Putative bacteriocin genes were present in all enterococcal strains investigated, highlighting the competitive nature of the gut niche. Bacteriocin-encoding genes are known to be widely disseminated among enterococci species of different origins [33,54,55]. However, likely because of the novel environmental source of these strains, we found considerable diversity and novelty (Figure 1), with eight genomes possessing four or more bacteriocin gene clusters. This may be driven by variation in wild marine animal diets along migratory routes, combined with selection pressure for factors to control population structure and niche control in the host gut.

Enterococcal bacteriocins are of interest because of their antimicrobial activities, with activity against different Gram-positive and Gram-negative bacteria, including species of *Listeria*, *Clostridium*, *Staphylococcus*, *Streptococcus*, *Cutibacterium*, *Pseudomonas*, and *Salmonella* [6,33,34,65]. Enterocins have also been described as effective agents against antibiotic-resistant bacteria such as vancomycin-resistant enterococci (VRE) and methicillin-resistant *Staphylococcus aureus* (MRSA) [35,46]. Furthermore, antiviral activities have been reported against herpes simplex viruses (HSV-1 and HSV-2), polio virus (PV3), measles virus, and influenza virus [41,66]. Immunomodulatory and anticancer properties of enterocins have not been widely explored but may also be of potential interest [67–69].

In this study, we identified known bacteriocins, natural variants of known bacteriocins, and potentially new bacteriocins distributed among different enterococcal species. The potency and spectrum of bacteriocins against important pathogens vary according to the peptide subclass [34,35,66,70]. Class I bacteriocins were identified in our in silico screening, with sactipeptides, new lanthipeptides I, lasso peptides, and thiopeptides being found in high numbers (Figure 1). Sactipeptides are produced mainly by Gram-positive organisms, and according to previous studies, the sactipeptides from *Bacillus subtilis* (subtilisin A) and *Bacillus thuringiensis* (Thuricin CD) have broad and narrow antimicrobial activity spectra, respectively [34,71]. A previous study also identified sactipeptide BGC in *Enterococcus mudtii* QU25 [36], similar to one found in this study. Lantibiotics and thiopeptides are most active against Gram-positive pathogens, including MRSA, VRE, and *Clostridium difficile* [23,34]. In contrast, most lasso peptides show activity against Gram-negative pathogens, e.g., bacteriocin MccJ25, which is active against some strains of *Escherichia coli* and *Salmonella* spp. [34].

The present study provides further evidence of the significant biodiversity of BGCs for class II, 19 bacteriocins, including five new putative bacteriocins (Figures 1 and 2; Supplementary Table S4). Class II bacteriocins are of special interest as potential therapeutic agents and have been proposed on a larger scale production, whether in the food industry or in human health and veterinary medicine [72–74]. Because they consist of unmodified peptides, they do not require enzymes for their maturation and are small structures, less than 10 kDa [36,73], that may subject to low-cost production than other classes by chemical synthesis [73]. Complementing the recombinant technologies, chemical synthesis of bacteriocins may allow further molecular engineering for enhanced potency, improved pharmacological properties, increased stability and modified spectra of activity [73]. Class II bacteriocins and analogs thereof have been successfully prepared by chemical syntheses, such as aureocin A53 (AucA), durancin A5-11, enterocin CRL35, lactococcin MMFII, leucocin A, pediocin PA-1, curvacin A, lacticin Q (LnqQ), mesentericin Y105, and sakacin P [72–74].

In general, the class II bacteriocins are most active against Gram-positive pathogens, especially the class IIa bacteriocins, which are active against *L. monocytogenes* and other Gram-positive pathogens [33,34,72,75]. Enterocin SE-K4 and enterocin P were the most frequent class II bacteriocins in this study (Figure 1). Enterocin SE-K4 has been reported to exhibit antimicrobial activity against Gram-positive bacteria, *B. subtilis*, *Clostridium beijerinckii*, *E. faecium*, *E. faecalis*, and *L. monocytogenes* [40]. In contrast, enterocin P has a broad antimicrobial spectrum that includes activity against food-borne pathogens, *C. botulinum*, *C. perfringens*, *L. monocytogenes*, and *S. aureus* [64], as well as clinical strains, *L. monocytogenes*, *Salmonella* (S.) *typhi*, *Salmonella paratyphi* C, *Shigella dysenteriae*, vancomycin-resistant enterococci (VRE), and carbapenem-resistant *Pseudomonas aeruginosa* [75,76].

It is also important to highlight that class III bacteriocins were most common and widely distributed from wild marine animals and also included the unknown bacteriocin VI (Figure 1). Furthermore, three different enterolysin A sequences were verified among enterococci species, with two of them from *E. hirae* genomes that are reported for the first time in this species. Enterolysin A is a cell wall-degrading bacteriocin first reported to be produced by *E. faecalis* isolated from fish in Iceland [77]. Despite class III bacteriocins are large proteins (more than 10 kDa) and complex produced by chemical approaches [61], enterolysin A have been reported as broad-spectrum activity against pathogenic and nonpathogenic bacteria; acting on cleave the peptide bonds within the stem peptide as well as in the interpeptide bridge of Gram-positive bacterial cell walls [33,78].

In addition to bacteriocins, a wide variety of novel gene clusters encoding putative terpenes, NRPs, polyketides, and other active compounds have been uncovered by in silico analysis, creating new opportunities for drug development [23,24,49,79]. NRPs and terpenes have been reported with activity against several antibiotic-resistant strains [80–85]. A small library of predicted NRP peptides was chemically synthesized, based on the primary sequence of NRP clusters in the human microbiome, and a potent anti-MRSA (methicillin-resistant *Staphylococcus aureus*) peptide with a new mechanism of action, named humimycin, was identified [80]. The antitubercular agent levesquamide is a new polyketide-nonribosomal peptide (PK-NRP) hybrid of a marine natural product (BGC) identified and isolated from *Streptomyces* sp. [84]. Furthermore, the antibacterial activity of 33 free terpenes commonly found in essential oils was evaluated, with 16 compounds showing antimicrobial activity, including eugenol, which exhibited rapid bactericidal action against *Salmonella enterica* serovar *Typhimurium*. Further, terpineol showed excellent bactericidal activity against *S. aureus* strains, and carveol, citronellol, and geraniol were rapidly bactericidal for *E. coli* [81]. In this study, we also found terpene biosynthesis-related clusters in *E. casseliflavus*, *E. hirae*, and *E. mundtii* species. Terpenes are secondary metabolites found in plants, bacteria, and fungi and have been shown to act as antibiotics, hormones, flavor or odor constituents, and pigments [86–88]. Beukers and collaborators [89] also identified putative genes or operons involved in terpene synthesis in *E. hirae*, *E. villorum*, *E. gallinarum*, *E. durans*, and *E. casseliflavus* strains isolated from bovine feces. The role of terpenes in enterococcal biology, including their possible involvement as bacteriocins, remains unclear [89].

Previous studies have examined the probiotic potential of enterococci from the marine environment [43,90,91]. Marine probiont strains have been used in finfish aquaculture due to their health beneficial effect and low potential to transfer antibiotic resistance genes to pathogens through horizontal gene transfer [92]. The potential of 13 enterococci isolated from wild seals was evaluated in a previous study from our group, and five (36.46%) showed activity against *L. monocytogenes* ATCC 35152 in the double-agar layer test, and one of them should be a good candidate for probiotic application [43]. In the present study, genome screening for bacteriocins highlighted potential probiotic enterococcal strains lacking known virulence or resistance traits (Figure 5A, B). In particular, the *E. avium* (L8) genome contained gene clusters for bicereucin BsjA1 and BsjA2, enterocin NKR-5-3D, mundticin AT06, and unknown bacteriocin I; and the *E. mundtii* genome (MP7-18) encoded sacpeptide and mundticin AT06 variants. Members of the genus *Enterococcus* have not yet obtained the status of generally recognized as safe (GRAS), although some are already being used as probiotics and in the production of animal food additives to prevent diseases or to improve growth [93,94]. New regulations for probiotics that distinguish between safe and potentially harmful strains are needed [35]. The application of genomic approaches in probiotic research would improve the understanding of the molecular mechanisms that endow the genera with safe and favorable traits [95].

Host-associated microbes are a rich source of factors that regulate community structure in a manner compatible with host health [96,97]. Our findings show a considerable novelty of biosynthetic pathways to be found by exploring the genomes of wild marine-animals-associated microbes in remote ecologies with the potential to shape host-associated microbial population structures. The novel compounds and natural bacteriocin variants were discovered to provide the first leads for deriving new approaches for managing human-microbe interactions in health and disease. Besides, this data will inform and broaden the limits of known structural variation, knowledge of how structure relates to activity, and synthetic biology. In this context, as a perspective for further studies, the data generated here may be associated with recombinant technologies, chemical synthesis, molecular engineering, and other strategies to increase the biological potency, stability, and pharmacological properties in order to guarantee or modify the antimicrobial activity. Therefore, our results may contribute to promote the future development of bacteriocin-based drugs for potential use in managing animal and human health and as food preservatives.

4. Materials and Methods

4.1. Bacterial Strains

Twenty-two enterococci strains previously described [26,98,99] were evaluated in the present study. Briefly, the collection includes *Enterococcus* species isolated from fecal samples (cloacal/anal swabs or intestinal content) collected from 17 wild marine animals. These animals, including sea turtles (n = 3), seabirds (n = 8), and marine mammals (n = 6), were found along the North Coast of Rio Grande do Sul, Southern Brazil, from Torres Beach (29°21′32.2″ S; 49°44′10.3″ W) to Dunas Altas Beach, Palmares do Sul (30°23′58.75″ S; 50°17′24.73″ W), between July 2012 and April 2014 (Table 1). The enterococci collection was stored frozen at −20 °C in skim milk supplemented with 20% glycerol, and cultures were routinely grown in brain heart infusion (BHI) at 37 °C for 18 h.

4.2. Genomic DNA Preparation, High-Throughput Sequencing, Assembly, and Annotation

The *Enterococcus* spp. strains were grown in BHI at 37 °C for 18 h. Genomic DNA was extracted using a commercial kit (QIAGEN DNeasy Blood & Tissue Kit, San Luis, MO, USA). Manufacturer instructions were followed with minor modification, namely, the addition of 50 µL of lysozyme (50 mg/mL) and 10 µL mutanolysin (2500 U/mL, Sigma-Aldrich, Germantown, MD, USA) for 30 min at 37 °C before the addition of 20 µL proteinase K (20 mg/mL). Extracted DNA was quantified using the Qubit double-stranded DNA (dsDNA) high-sensitivity (HS) assay kit (Life Technologies, Carlsbad, CA, USA). Libraries for genome sequencing were prepared using the Nextera XT DNA kit and index primers

(Illumina), and reads were generated by HiSeq/MiSeq reagent kit version 2 with 250 cycles on an Illumina HiSeq/Miseq platforms. Reads were subjected to de novo assembly using the CLC genomics workbench v8.0.3, and open reading frames (ORFs) were predicted using the NCBI Prokaryotic Annotation Pipeline—PGAP [100]. The enterococci species assignment was confirmed by pairwise comparison of their average nucleotide identity (ANI) using JSpeciesWS [101] and the following reference genomes available from GenBank (https://www.ncbi.nlm.nih.gov (accessed on 15 December 2020): *Enterococcus avium* ATCC 14025; *Enterococcus casseliflavus* ATCC 12755; *Enterococcus faecalis* ATCC 19433; *Enterococcus faecium* Aus0004 (Clade A1); *Enterococcus faecium* EnGen0007 (Clade A2); *Enterococcus faecium* Com12 (Clade B); *Enterococcus hirae* ATCC 9790; *Enterococcus lactis* KCTC 21015; *Enterococcus mundtii* ATCC 882. The GenBank accession number of reference strains is presented in Supplementary Table S2.

4.3. Genome Mining for Antimicrobial Compounds

Putative biosynthetic gene clusters (BGCs) were predicted using *anti*SMASH (antibiotics and Secondary Metabolite Analysis Shell 5.0) [57] and Bagel4 (bacteriocins and RiPP—Ribosomally synthesized and Post-translationally modified Peptides) [58] using the default parameters. The bacteriocin classification is in accordance with previous proposals for enterococci [33] and lactic acid bacteria [36] that accommodate the novel subclasses that are appearing over the last years, based on the biosynthesis mechanism and biological activity.

4.4. Phylogenetic Analysis

Amino acid sequences corresponding to bacteriocin genes (class II and class III) found in this work, along with reference sequences identified by AntiSMASH 5.0 [57] and Bagel4 [58], and Uniprot databases were aligned using MAFFT [102]. Guidance2 [103] was used to filter unreliable positions and generate a mega alignment encompassing 5 alternative alignments for the sequences. The mega alignment was used to infer the evolutionary history of these proteins by using the Maximum Likelihood method, based on the VT model [104]. A discrete Gamma distribution was used to model evolutionary rate differences among sites, and the rate variation model allowed for some sites to be evolutionarily invariable [105]. Significance was assessed via aLRT [106]. All evolutionary analyses were conducted in PhyML 3.0 [107]. Tree visualization and annotation were performed on Interactive Tree Of Life (iTOL) v [108].

4.5. Molecular Modeling

The structural modeling of unknown bacteriocins (I, II, III, IV, and VI) was performed using the I-TASSER package [62,63] since they were not suitable for traditional comparative modeling, requiring a combination of fragment and ab initio model building. UCSF Chimera [109] was used to visualize and edit the new bacteriocin structural models. Physico-chemical parameters were calculated with ProtParam [110].

4.6. Potential Virulence Markers

The comprehensive antibiotic resistance database (CARD/RGI-2017) [111] and Resfinder 3.2 [112] were used to identify antimicrobial resistance genes with default parameters and identification threshold of 60% identity over a length of 60% coverage, respectively. Virulence genes were predicted using VirulenceFinder [113], with a threshold of 85% identity over a length of 60%.

4.7. Figures Design

Figures were designed using D3 (or D3.js, a JavaScript library for visualizing data using web standards) [114], R software (R Development Core Team, 2019) [115], and Adobe Illustrator.

5. Conclusions

Our findings show that there is a considerable novelty to be found through exploring the genomes of host-associated microbes from animals in remote ecologies for biosynthetic pathways with the potential to shape host-associated microbial population structures. The novel compounds and natural bacteriocin variants discovered provide first leads for the derivation of new approaches for managing human-microbe interactions in health and disease.

Supplementary Materials: The following are available online at https://www.mdpi.com/article/10.3390/md19060328/s1, Table S1: Sequencing statistics, genome sizes, fold coverage, G+C content, of the *Enterococcus* spp. sequenced. Table S2: Reference genomes used to confirm the enterococci species. Table S3: Putative antimicrobial compounds biosynthesis gene clusters (BGCs) data predicted with antiSMASH5 and Bagel4 software. Table S4: Class I, class II, and class III unknown bacteriocins BGCs data that were not previously identified in antiSMASH5 and Bagel4 databases. Table S5: Class II and class III bacteriocin sequences predicted with antiSMASH5 and Bagel4 software. Table S6: Reference sequences from Bagel4 and Uniprot databases. Figure S1: The alignment of putative enterolysin A (class III) sequences (first branch) from *E. hirae* genomes using Clustal Omega software. Figure S2: The alignment of putative enterolysin A (class III) sequences (second branch) from *E. hirae* genomes using Clustal Omega software. Figure S3: The alignment of putative enterolysin A (class III) sequences (third branch) from *E. faecalis* genomes using Clustal Omega software. Figure S4: The alignment of four different enterolysin A (class III) and three different references (Bagel 62.3: *E. faecalis* LMG 2333; Bagel 63.3: *E. faecalis*; and Bagel 64.3: *Lactobacillus acidophilus*) using Clustal Omega software. Figure S5: The alignment of putative propionicin SM1 (class III) and reference sequence using Clustal Omega software. Figure S6: The alignment of putative Class IIa bacteriocins and reference sequences using Clustal Omega software. Figure S7: The alignment of putative class IIb bacteriocins and reference sequences using Clustal Omega software. Figure S8: The alignment of putative class II circular bacteriocin carnocyclin A and reference sequence using Clustal Omega software. Figure S9: The alignment of putative class II leaderless bacteriocin enterocin EJ97 and reference sequence using Clustal Omega software. Figure S10: The alignment of putative class II other bacteriocins and reference sequences using Clustal Omega software.

Author Contributions: J.P., A.S., M.P.-B. and M.S.G. designed the study. Samples were collected by M.T. The bacteria isolation, extraction, and genome sequencing were performed by J.P. and T.G.S.P. Bioinformatics approaches, analyze of data, and figures were designed by J.P., M.P.-B., R.C.Z.L., Í.M.S.C. and R.L.-B. The original draft manuscript was written by J.P., M.P.-B., A.S. and M.S.G. This study was funded and/or supervised by A.S., J.F., P.A.d., A.P.G.F. and M.S.G. All authors have read and agreed to the published version of the manuscript.

Funding: This research was funded by the NIH grant AI083214—*Harvard-wide program on antibiotic resistance*–, Conselho Nacional de Desenvolvimento Científico e Tecnológico do Brasil, and Coordenação e Aperfeiçoamento de Pessoal de Nível Superior (CAPES) of the Brazilian government (CNPq; 40788/2018-4).

Data Availability Statement: The novel genome sequences were deposited at DDBJ/ENA/GenBank as whole-genome shotgun projects under the accession numbers according to Table S1.

Acknowledgments: The authors would like to thank the Center for Coastal Studies, Limnology and Marine (CECLIMAR) for assistance in collecting samples and to members of the *Enteromar* Research Group for critical feedback on the manuscript.

Conflicts of Interest: The authors declare no conflict of interest.

References

1. Wohlleben, W.; Mast, Y.; Stegmann, E.; Ziemert, N. Antibiotic Drug Discovery. *Microb. Biotechnol.* **2016**, *9*, 541–548. [CrossRef]
2. Willyard, C. The Drug-Resistant Bacteria that Pose the Greatest Health Threats. *Nature* **2017**, *543*, 15. [CrossRef]
3. Tacconelli, E.; Carrara, E.; Savoldi, A.; Harbarth, S.; Mendelson, M.; Monnet, D.L.; Pulcini, C.; Kahlmeter, G.; Kluytmans, J.; Carmeli, Y.; et al. Discovery, Research, and Development of New Antibiotics: The WHO Priority List of Antibiotic-Resistant Bacteria and Tuberculosis. *Lancet Infect. Dis.* **2018**, *18*, 318–327. [CrossRef]
4. Buonocore, F. Marine Biotechnology: Developments and Perspectives. *J. Aquac. Res. Dev.* **2013**, *4*, 9546. [CrossRef]

5. Reen, F.J. Emerging Concepts Cromising New Horizons for Marine Biodiscovery and Synthetic Biology. *Mar. Drugs* **2015**, *31*, 2924–2954. [CrossRef] [PubMed]
6. Calle, F. Marine Microbiome as Source of Natural Products. *Microb. Biotechnol.* **2017**, *10*, 1293–1296. [CrossRef] [PubMed]
7. Smith, D. Discovery Pipelines for Marine Resources: An Ocean of Opportunity for Biotechnology? *World J. Microbiol. Biotechnol.* **2019**, *8*, 1293–1296. [CrossRef] [PubMed]
8. Desriac, F. Bacteriocin as Weapons in the Marine Animal-Associated Bacteria Warfare: Inventory and Potential Applications as an Aquaculture Probiotic. *Mar. Drugs* **2010**, *25*, 1153–1177. [CrossRef] [PubMed]
9. Debbab, A.; Aly, A.H.; Lin, W.H.; Proksch, P. Bioactive Compounds from Marine Bacteria and Fungi. *Microb. Biotechnol.* **2010**, *20*, 544–563. [CrossRef] [PubMed]
10. Deer, T.R.; Pope, J.E.; Hanes, M.C.; McDowell, G.C. Intrathecal Therapy for Chronic Pain: A Review of Morphine and Ziconotide as Firstline Options. *Pain Med.* **2019**, *20*, 784–798. [CrossRef] [PubMed]
11. Fujisawa, Y.; Fujimura, T.; Matsushita, S.; Yamamoto, Y.; Uchi, H.; Otsuka, A.; Funakoshi, T.; Miyagi, T.; Hata, H.; Gosho, M.; et al. The Efficacy of Eribulin Mesylate for Patients with Cutaneous Angiosarcoma Previously Treated with Taxane: A Multicentre Prospective Observational Study. *Br. J. Dermatol.* **2020**, *183*, 831–839. [CrossRef] [PubMed]
12. Luesch, H.; Moore, R.E.; Paul, V.J.; Mooberry, S.L.; Corbett, T.H. Isolation of Dolastatin 10 from the Marine Cyanobacterium *Symploca* Species VP642 and Total Stereochemistry and Biological Evaluation of Its Analogue Symplostatin 1. *J. Nat. Prod.* **2001**, *64*, 907–910. [CrossRef]
13. Luesch, H.; Chanda, S.K.; Raya, R.M.; DeJesus, P.D.; Orth, A.P.; Walker, J.R.; Izpisúa Belmonte, J.C.; Schultz, P.G. A Functional Genomics Approach to the Mode of Action of Apratoxin A. *Nat. Chem. Biol.* **2006**, *2*, 158–167. [CrossRef]
14. Galonić, D.P.; Barr, E.W.; Walsh, C.T.; Bollinger, J.M.; Krebs, C. Two Interconverting Fe (IV) Intermediates in Aliphatic Chlorination by the Halogenase CytC3. *Nat. Chem. Biol.* **2007**, *3*, 113–116. [CrossRef]
15. Liao, L.; Lee, J.-H.; You, M.; Choi, T.J.; Park, W.; Lee, S.K.; Oh, D.-C.; Oh, K.-B.; Shin, J. Penicillipyrones A and B, Meroterpenoids from a Marine-Derived *Penicillium* Sp. Fungus. *J. Nat. Prod.* **2014**, *77*, 406–410. [CrossRef]
16. Mayer, A.M.S.; Guerrero, A.J.; Rodríguez, A.D.; Taglialatela-Scafati, O.; Nakamura, F.; Fusetani, N. Marine Pharmacology in 2014–2015: Marine Compounds with Antibacterial, Antidiabetic, Antifungal, Anti-Inflammatory, Antiprotozoal, Antituberculosis, Antiviral, and Anthelmintic Activities; Affecting the Immune and Nervous Systems, and Other Miscellaneous Mechanisms of Action. *Mar. Drugs* **2019**, *18*, 5.
17. Kamada, T.; Vairappan, C.S. New Laurene-Type Sesquiterpene from Bornean *Laurencia nangii*. *Nat. Prod. Commun.* **2015**, *10*, 843–844. [CrossRef]
18. Piao, M.; Hewage, S.; Han, X.; Kang, K.; Kang, H.; Lee, N.; Hyun, J. Protective Effect of Diphlorethohydroxycarmalol against Ultraviolet B Radiation-Induced DNA Damage by Inducing the Nucleotide Excision Repair System in HaCaT Human Keratinocytes. *Mar. Drugs* **2015**, *13*, 5629–5641. [CrossRef] [PubMed]
19. Tsueng, G.; Teisan, S.; Lam, K.S. Defined Salt Formulations for the Growth of *Salinispora tropica* Strain NPS21184 and the Production of Salinosporamide A (NPI-0052) and Related Analogs. *Appl. Microbiol. Biotechnol.* **2008**, *78*, 827–832. [CrossRef] [PubMed]
20. Freundlich, J.S.; Lalgondar, M.; Wei, J.-R.; Swanson, S.; Sorensen, E.J.; Rubin, E.J.; Sacchettini, J.C. The Abyssomicin C Family as in Vitro Inhibitors of *Mycobacterium tuberculosis*. *Tuberculosis* **2010**, *90*, 298–300. [CrossRef] [PubMed]
21. Wyche, T.P.; Piotrowski, J.S.; Hou, Y.; Braun, D.; Deshpande, R.; McIlwain, S.; Ong, I.M.; Myers, C.L.; Guzei, I.A.; Westler, W.M.; et al. Forazoline A: Marine-Derived Polyketide with Antifungal In Vivo Efficacy. *Angew. Chem. Int. Ed.* **2014**, *53*, 11583–11586. [CrossRef] [PubMed]
22. Liu, D.; Yang, A.; Wu, C.; Guo, P.; Proksch, P.; Lin, W. Lipid-Lowering Effects of Farnesylquinone and Related Analogues from the Marine-Derived *Streptomyces nitrosporeus*. *Bioorg. Med. Chem. Lett.* **2014**, *24*, 5288–5293. [CrossRef]
23. Donia, M.S.; Cimermancic, P.; Schulze, C.J.; Wieland Brown, L.C.; Martin, J.; Mitreva, M.; Clardy, J.; Linington, R.G.; Fischbach, M.A. A Systematic Analysis of Biosynthetic Gene Clusters in the Human Microbiome Reveals a Common Family of Antibiotics. *Cell* **2014**, *158*, 1402–1414. [CrossRef] [PubMed]
24. Wang, L.; Ravichandran, V.; Yin, Y.; Yin, J.; Zhang, Y. Natural Products from Mammalian Gut Microbiota. *Trends Biotechnol.* **2019**, *37*, 492–504. [CrossRef] [PubMed]
25. Lebreton, F.; Manson, A.L.; Saavedra, J.T.; Straub, T.J.; Earl, A.M.; Gilmore, M.S. Tracing the Enterococci from Paleozoic Origins to the Hospital. *Cell* **2017**, *169*, 849–861. [CrossRef]
26. Prichula, J.; Van Tyne, D.; Schwartzman, J.; Sant'Anna, F.H.; Pereira, R.I.; da Cunha, G.R.; Tavares, M.; Lebreton, F.; Frazzon, J.; d'Azevedo, P.A.; et al. Enterococci from Wild Magellanic Penguins (*Spheniscus magellanicus*) as an Indicator of Marine Ecosystem Health and Human Impact. *Appl. Environ. Microbiol.* **2020**, *86*, e01662-20. [CrossRef]
27. Lebreton, F.; van Schaik, W.; Manson McGuire, A.; Godfrey, P.; Griggs, A.; Mazumdar, V.; Corander, J.; Cheng, L.; Saif, S.; Young, S.; et al. Emergence of Epidemic Multidrug-Resistant Enterococcus Faecium from Animal and Commensal Strains. *mBio* **2013**, *4*, e00534-13. [CrossRef] [PubMed]
28. Raven, K.E.; Reuter, S.; Reynolds, R.; Brodrick, H.J.; Russell, J.E.; Török, M.E.; Parkhill, J.; Peacock, S.J. A Decade of Genomic History for Healthcare-Associated *Enterococcus faecium* in the United Kingdom and Ireland. *Genome Res.* **2016**, *26*, 1388–1396. [CrossRef] [PubMed]

29. Raven, K.E.; Reuter, S.; Gouliouris, T.; Reynolds, R.; Russell, J.E.; Brown, N.M.; Török, M.E.; Parkhill, J.; Peacock, S.J. Genome-Based Characterization of Hospital-Adapted *Enterococcus faecalis* Lineages. *Nat. Microbiol.* **2016**, *1*, 15033. [CrossRef]
30. Fiore, E.; Van Tyne, D.; Gilmore, M.S. Pathogenicity of Enterococci. *Microbiol. Spect.* **2019**, *7*, 378–397.
31. Brock, T.D.; Peacher, B.; Pierson, D. Survey of the Bacteriocines of Enterococci. *J. Bacteriol.* **1963**, *86*, 702–707. [CrossRef]
32. Nes, I.F.; Diep, D.B.; Holo, H. Bacteriocin Diversity in *Streptococcus* and *Enterococcus*. *J. Bacteriol.* **2007**, *189*, 1189–1198. [CrossRef]
33. Ness, I.F.; Diep, D.B.; Ike, Y. Enterococcal Bacteriocins and Antimicrobial Proteins that Contribute to Niche Control. In *Enterococci: From Commensals to Leading Causes of Drug Resistant Infection*; Gilmore, M.S., Clewell, D.B., Ike, Y., Shankar, N., Eds.; Massachusetts Eye and Ear Infirmary: Boston, MA, USA, 2014.
34. Cotter, P.D.; Ross, R.P.; Hill, C. Bacteriocins—A Viable Alternative to Antibiotics? *Nat. Rev. Microbiol.* **2013**, *11*, 95–105. [CrossRef]
35. Hanchi, H.; Mottawea, W.; Sebei, K.; Hammami, R. The Genus Enterococcus: Between Probiotic Potential and Safety Concerns—An Update. *Front. Microbiol.* **2018**, *9*, 1–16. [CrossRef] [PubMed]
36. Alvarez-Sieiro, P.; Montalbán-López, M.; Mu, D.; Kuipers, O.P. Bacteriocins of Lactic Acid Bacteria: Extending the Family. *Appl. Microbiol. Biotechnol.* **2016**, *100*, 2939–2951. [CrossRef]
37. Zimina, M.; Babich, O.; Prosekov, A.; Sukhikh, S.; Ivanova, S.; Shevchenko, M.; Noskova, S. Overview of Global Trends in Classification, Methods of Preparation and Application of Bacteriocins. *Antibiotics* **2020**, *9*, 553. [CrossRef] [PubMed]
38. Maqueda, M.; Sánchez-Hidalgo, M.; Fernández, M.; Montalbán-López, M.; Valdivia, E.; Martínez-Bueno, M. Genetic Features of Circular Bacteriocins Produced by Gram-Positive Bacteria. *FEMS Microbiol. Rev.* **2008**, *32*, 2–22. [CrossRef]
39. Chen, H.; Hoover, D.G. Bacteriocins and Their Food Applications. *Compr. Rev. Food Sci. Food Saf.* **2003**, *2*, 82–100.
40. Franz, C.M.A.P.; Van Belkum, M.J.; Holzapfel, W.H.; Abriouel, H.; Gálvez, A. Diversity of Enterococcal Bacteriocins and Their Grouping in a New Classification Scheme. *FEMS Microbiol. Rev.* **2007**, *31*, 293–310. [CrossRef]
41. Todorov, S.D.; Wachsman, M.B.; Knoetze, H.; Meincken, M.; Dicks, L.M.T. An Antibacterial and Antiviral Peptide Produced by *Enterococcus mundtii* ST4V Isolated from Soya Beans. *Int. J. Antimicrob. Agents* **2005**, *25*, 508–513. [CrossRef]
42. Poeta, P.; Costa, D.; Rojo-Bezares, B.; Zarazaga, M.; Klibi, N.; Rodrigues, J.; Torres, C. Detection of Antimicrobial Activities and Bacteriocin Structural Genes in Faecal Enterococci of Wild Animals. *Microbiol. Res.* **2007**, *162*, 257–263. [CrossRef] [PubMed]
43. Comerlato, C.B.; Buboltz, J.R.; Santestevan, N.A. Antimicrobial compounds produced by *Enterococcus* spp. isolates from fecal samples of wild South American fur seals. *J. Microbiol. Antimicrob.* **2016**, *8*, 14–21.
44. Ghomrassi, H.; Hani, K.; Chobert, J.M.; Ghrairi, T. Evaluation of Marine Bacteriocinogenic *Enterococci* Strains with Inhibitory Activity against Fish-Pathogenic Gram-Negative Bacteria. *Dis. Aquat. Organ.* **2016**, *118*, 31–43. [CrossRef] [PubMed]
45. Ogaki, M.B.; Rocha, K.R.; Terra, M.R.; Furlaneto, M.C.; Furlaneto-Maia, L. Screening of the Enterocin-Encoding Genes and Antimicrobial Activity in *Enterococcus* Species. *J. Microbiol. Biotechnol.* **2016**, *26*, 9. [CrossRef]
46. Phumisantiphong, U.; Siripanichgon, K.; Reamtong, O.; Diraphat, P. A Novel Bacteriocin from Enterococcus faecalis 478 Exhibits a Potent Activity against Vancomycin-Resistant *Enterococci*. *PLoS ONE* **2017**, *12*, e0186415. [CrossRef]
47. Rahmeh, R. Characterization of Semipurified Enterocins Produced by *Enterococcus faecium* Strains Isolated from Raw Camel Milk. *J. Dairy Sci.* **2016**, *101*, 4944–4952. [CrossRef]
48. Vandera, E. Approaches for Enhancing in Situ Detection of Enterocin Genes in Thermized Milk, and Selective Isolation of Enterocin-Producing *Enterococcus faecium* from Baird-Parker Agar. *Int. J. Food Microbiol.* **2018**, *281*, 23–31. [CrossRef]
49. Zhao, X.-Q. Genome-Based Studies of Marine Microorganisms to Maximize the Diversity of Natural Products Discovery for Medical Treatments. *Evid.-Based Complementary Altern. Med.* **2011**, *2011*, 1–12. [CrossRef]
50. Zhang, M.M. Using Natural Products for Drug Discovery: The Impact of the Genomics Era. *Expert. Opin. Drug Discov.* **2017**, *12*, 475–487. [CrossRef]
51. Gregory, K.; Salvador, L.A.; Akbar, S.; Adaikpoh, B.I.; Stevens, D.C. Survey of Biosynthetic Gene Clusters from Sequenced Myxobacteria Reveals Unexplored Biosynthetic Potential. *Microorganisms* **2019**, *7*, 181. [CrossRef] [PubMed]
52. Sekurova, O.N.; Schneider, O.; Zotchev, S.B. Novel Bioactive Natural Products from Bacteria via Bioprospecting, Genome Mining and Metabolic Engineering. *Microb. Biotechnol.* **2019**, *12*, 828–844. [CrossRef] [PubMed]
53. Xin, B.; Liu, H.; Zheng, J.; Xie, C.; Gao, Y.; Dai, D.; Peng, D.; Ruan, L.; Chen, H.; Sun, M. In Silico Analysis Highlights the Diversity and Novelty of Circular Bacteriocins in Sequenced Microbial Genomes. *Msystems* **2020**, *5*, e00047-20. [CrossRef]
54. Bonacina, J.; Suárez, N.; Hormigo, R.; Fadda, S.; Lechner, M.; Saavedra, L. A Genomic View of Food-Related and Probiotic Enterococcus Strains. *DNA Res.* **2016**, *24*, 11–24. [CrossRef]
55. Suárez, N.E.; Bonacina, J.; Hebert, E.M.; Saavedra, M.L. Genome Mining and Transcriptional Analysis of Bacteriocin Genes in *Enterococcus faecium* CRL1879. *J. Data Min. Genom. Proteom.* **2015**, *6*, 1–8.
56. Vezina, B.; Rehm, B.H.A.; Smith, A.T. Bioinformatic Prospecting and Phylogenetic Analysis Reveals 94 Undescribed Circular Bacteriocins and Key Motifs. *BMC Microbiol.* **2020**, *20*, 1–16. [CrossRef]
57. Blin, K. AntiSMASH 5.0: Updates to the Secondary Metabolite Genome Mining Pipeline. *Nucleic Acids Res.* **2019**, *47*, W81–W87. [CrossRef]
58. van Heel, A.J.; de Jong, A.; Song, C.; Viel, J.H.; Kok, J.; Kuipers, O.P. BAGEL4: A User-Friendly Web Server to Thoroughly Mine RiPPs and Bacteriocins. *Nucleic Acids Res.* **2018**, *46*, W278–W281. [CrossRef] [PubMed]
59. Richter, M.; Rosselló-Móra, R. Shifting the Genomic Gold Standard for the Prokaryotic Species Definition. *Proc. Natl. Acad. Sci. USA* **2009**, *106*, 19126–19131. [CrossRef]

60. Coburn, P.S. *Enterococcus faecalis* Senses Target Cells and in Response Expresses Cytolysin. *Science* **2004**, *306*, 2270–2272. [CrossRef] [PubMed]
61. Van Tyne, D.; Martin, M.; Gilmore, M. Structure, Function, and Biology of the *Enterococcus faecalis* Cytolysin. *Toxins* **2013**, *5*, 895–911. [CrossRef]
62. Yang, J.; Yan, R.; Roy, A.; Xu, D.; Poisson, J.; Zhang, Y. The I-TASSER Suite: Protein Structure and Function Prediction. *Nat. Methods* **2015**, *12*, 7–8. [CrossRef]
63. Zhang, Y. I-TASSER Server for Protein 3D Structure Prediction. *BMC Bioinf.* **2008**, *9*, 1–8. [CrossRef]
64. Palmer, K.L.; Godfrey, P.; Griggs, A.; Kos, V.N.; Zucker, J.; Desjardins, C.; Cerqueira, G.; Gevers, D.; Walker, S.; Wortman, J.; et al. Comparative Genomics of Enterococci: Variation in *Enterococcus faecalis*, Clade Structure in *E. faecium*, and Defining Characteristics of *E. gallinarum* and *E. casseliflavus*. *mBio* **2012**, *3*, e00318-11. [CrossRef]
65. Jennes, W.; Dicks, L.M.T.; Verwoerd, D.J. Enterocin 012, a Bacteriocin Produced by *Enterococcus gallinarum* Isolated from the Intestinal Tract of Ostrich. *J. Appl. Microbiol. Biochem.* **2000**, *88*, 349–357. [CrossRef] [PubMed]
66. Ermolenko, E.I. Anti–Influenza Activity of Enterocin B In Vitro and Protective Effect of Bacteriocinogenic Enterococcal Probiotic Strain on Influenza Infection in Mouse Model. *Probiotics Antimicrob. Proteins* **2019**, *11*, 705–712. [CrossRef] [PubMed]
67. Al-Fakharany, O.M.; Aziz, A.A.A.; El-Banna, T.E.-S.; Sonbol, F.I. Immunomodulatory and Anticancer Activities of Enterocin Oe-342 Produced by *Enterococcus faecalis* Isolated from Stool. *J. Clin. Cell. Immunol.* **2018**, *9*, 1000558. [CrossRef]
68. Ankaiah, D.; Palanichamy, E.; Antonyraj, C.B.; Ayyanna, R.; Perumal, V.; Ahamed, S.I.B.; Arul, V. Cloning, Overexpression, Purification of Bacteriocin Enterocin-B and Structural Analysis, Interaction Determination of Enterocin-A, B against Pathogenic Bacteria and Human Cancer Cells. *Int. J. Biol. Macromol.* **2018**, *116*, 502–512. [CrossRef] [PubMed]
69. Pirkhezranian, Z.; Tanhaeian, A.; Mirzaii, M.; Sekhavati, M.H. Expression of Enterocin-P in HEK Platform: Evaluation of Its Cytotoxic Effects on Cancer Cell Lines and Its Potency to Interact with Cell-Surface Glycosaminoglycan by Molecular Modeling. *Int. J. Pept. Res. Ther.* **2020**, *26*, 1503–1512. [CrossRef]
70. Caly, D.L. The Safe Enterocin DD14 Is a Leaderless Two-Peptide Bacteriocin with Anti-*Clostridium perfringens* Activity. *J. Antimicrob. Agents* **2017**, *49*, 282–289. [CrossRef]
71. Mathur, H.; Rea, M.; Cotter, P.; Hill, C.; Ross, R. The Sactibiotic Subclass of Bacteriocins: An Update. *CPPS* **2015**, *16*, 549–558. [CrossRef]
72. Bédard, F.; Hammami, R.; Zirah, S.; Rebuffat, S.; Fliss, I.; Biron, E. Synthesis, Antimicrobial Activity and Conformational Analysis of the Class IIa Bacteriocin Pediocin PA-1 and Analogs Thereof. *Sci. Rep.* **2018**, *8*, 9029. [CrossRef]
73. Bédard, F.; Biron, E. Recent Progress in the Chemical Synthesis of Class II and S-Glycosylated Bacteriocins. *Front. Microbiol.* **2018**, *9*, 1048. [CrossRef] [PubMed]
74. Lander, A.J.; Li, X.; Jin, Y.; Luk, L.Y. Total Chemical Synthesis of Aureocin A53, Lacticin Q and Their Enantiomeric Counterparts. *ChemRxiv. Preprint.* **2020**. [CrossRef]
75. Tanhaeian, A.; Damavandi, M.S.; Mansury, D.; Ghaznini, K. Expression in Eukaryotic Cells and Purification of Synthetic Gene Encoding Enterocin P: A Bacteriocin with Broad Antimicrobial Spectrum. *AMB Expr.* **2019**, *9*, 1–9. [CrossRef] [PubMed]
76. Cintas, L.M.; Casaus, P.; Håvarstein, L.S.; Hernández, P.E.; Nes, I.F. Biochemical and Genetic Characterization of Enterocin P, a Novel Sec-Dependent Bacteriocin from *Enterococcus faecium* P13 with a Broad Antimicrobial Spectrum. *Appl. Environ. Microbiol.* **1997**, *63*, 4321–4330. [CrossRef]
77. Nilsen, T.; Nes, I.F.; Holo, H. Enterolysin A, a Cell Wall-Degrading Bacteriocin from *Enterococcus faecalis* LMG 2333. *AEM* **2003**, *69*, 2975–2984. [CrossRef] [PubMed]
78. Khan, H.; Flint, S.H.; Yu, P.-L. Determination of the Mode of Action of Enterolysin A, Produced by *Enterococcus faecalis* B9510. *J. Appl. Microbiol.* **2013**, *115*, 484–494. [CrossRef]
79. Tran, P.N.; Yen, M.-R.; Chiang, C.-Y.; Lin, H.-C.; Chen, P.-Y. Detecting and Prioritizing Biosynthetic Gene Clusters for Bioactive Compounds in Bacteria and Fungi. *Appl. Microbiol. Biotechnol.* **2019**, *103*, 3277–3287. [CrossRef]
80. Chu, J.; Vila-Farres, X.; Inoyama, D.; Ternei, M.; Cohen, L.J.; Gordon, E.A.; Reddy, B.V.B.; Charlop-Powers, Z.; Zebroski, H.A.; Gallardo-Macias, R.; et al. Discovery of MRSA Active Antibiotics Using Primary Sequence from the Human Microbiome. *Nat. Chem. Biol.* **2016**, *12*, 1004–1006. [CrossRef]
81. Guimarães, A.C.; Meireles, L.M.; Lemos, M.F.; Guimarães, M.C.C.; Endringer, D.C.; Fronza, M.; Scherer, R. Antibacterial Activity of Terpenes and Terpenoids Present in Essential Oils. *Molecules* **2019**, *24*, 2471. [CrossRef]
82. Basalla, J.; Chatterjee, P.; Burgess, E.; Khan, M.; Verbrugge, E.; Wiegmann, D.D.; LiPuma, J.J.; Wildschutte, H. Loci Encoding Compounds Potentially Active against Drug-Resistant Pathogens amidst a Decreasing Pool of Novel Antibiotics. *Appl. Environ. Microbiol.* **2019**, *85*, e01438-19. [CrossRef] [PubMed]
83. Cappiello, F.; Loffredo, M.R.; Del Plato, C.; Cammarone, S.; Casciaro, B.; Quaglio, D.; Mangoni, M.L.; Botta, B.; Ghirga, F. The Revaluation of Plant-Derived Terpenes to Fight Antibiotic-Resistant Infections. *Antibiotics* **2020**, *9*, 325. [CrossRef]
84. Liang, L.; Haltli, B.; Marchbank, D.H.; Fischer, M.; Kirby, C.W.; Correa, H.; Clark, T.N.; Gray, C.A.; Kerr, R.G. Discovery of an Isothiazolinone-Containing Antitubercular Natural Product Levesquamide. *J. Org. Chem.* **2020**, *85*, 6450–6462. [CrossRef]
85. Jiang, M.; Wu, Z.; Guo, H.; Liu, L.; Chen, S. A Review of Terpenes from Marine-Derived Fungi: 2015–2019. *Mar. Drugs* **2020**, *18*, 321. [CrossRef] [PubMed]
86. Brahmkshatriya, P.P.; Brahmkshatriya, P.S. Terpenes: Chemistry, Biological Role, and Therapeutic Applications. In *Natural Products*; Ramawat, K.G., Mérillon, J.M., Eds.; Springer: Berlin/Heidelberg, Germany, 2013; pp. 2665–2691.

87. Chen, R.; Wong, H.; Burns, B. New Approaches to Detect Biosynthetic Gene Clusters in the Environment. *Medicines* **2019**, *6*, 32. [CrossRef] [PubMed]
88. Ziko, L.; Adel, M.; Malash, M.N.; Siam, R. Insights into Red Sea Brine Pool Specialized Metabolism Gene Clusters Encoding Potential Metabolites for Biotechnological Applications and Extremophile Survival. *Mar. Drugs* **2019**, *17*, 273. [CrossRef]
89. Beukers, A.G. Comparative Genomics of *Enterococcus* Spp. Isolated from Bovine Feces. *BMC Microbiol.* **2017**, *17*, 1–18. [CrossRef]
90. Román, L.; Padilla, D.; Acosta, F.; Sorroza, L.; Fátima, E.; Déniz, S.; Grasso, V.; Bravo, J.; Real, F. The Effect of Probiotic *Enterococcus gallinarum* L-1 on the Innate Immune Parameters of Outstanding Species to Marine Aquaculture. *J. Appl. Anim. Res.* **2015**, *43*, 177–183. [CrossRef]
91. Safari, R.; Adel, M.; Lazado, C.C.; Caipang, C.M.A.; Dadar, M. Host-Derived Probiotics *Enterococcus casseliflavus* Improves Resistance against *Streptococcus iniae* Infection in Rainbow Trout (*Oncorhynchus mykiss*) via Immunomodulation. *Fish Shellfish Immunol.* **2016**, *52*, 198–205. [CrossRef]
92. Ringø, E.; Hoseinifar, S.H.; Ghosh, K.; Doan, H.V.; Beck, B.R.; Song, S.K. Lactic Acid Bacteria in Finfish—An Update. *Front. Microbiol.* **2018**, *9*, 1818. [CrossRef]
93. Rubner-Institute, M. Enterococci as Probiotics and Their Implications in Food Safety. *Int. J. Food Microbiol.* **2001**, *151*, 125–140.
94. Huys, G.; Botteldoorn, N.; Delvigne, F.; De Vuyst, L.; Heyndrickx, M.; Pot, B.; Dubois, J.; Daube, G. Microbial Characterization of Probiotics—Advisory Report of the Working Group "8651 Probiotics" of the Belgian Superior Health Council (SHC). *Mol. Nutr. Food Res.* **2013**, *57*, 1479–1504. [CrossRef] [PubMed]
95. Joseph, J.P. Probiotic genomes: Sequencing and annotation in the past decade. *Int. J. Pharm. Sci. Res.* **2018**, *9*, 1351–1362.
96. Donia, M.S.; Fischbach, M.A. Small Molecules from the Human Microbiota. *Science* **2016**, *349*, 1254766. [CrossRef] [PubMed]
97. Hashempour-Baltork, F.; Hosseini, H.; Shojaee-Aliabadi, S.; Torbati, M.; Alizadeh, A.M.; Alizadeh, M. Drug Resistance and the Prevention Strategies in Food Borne Bacteria: An Update Review. *Adv. Pharm. Bull.* **2019**, *9*, 335–347. [CrossRef]
98. Prichula, J.; Pereira, R.I.; Wachholz, G.R.; Cardoso, L.A.; Tolfo, N.C.C.; Santestevan, N.A.; Medeiros, A.W.; Tavares, M.; Frazzon, J.; d'Azevedo, P.A.; et al. Resistance to Antimicrobial Agents among Enterococci Isolated from Fecal Samples of Wild Marine Species in the Southern Coast of Brazil. *Mar. Pollut. Bull.* **2016**, *105*, 51–57. [CrossRef]
99. Santestevan, N.A. Antimicrobial Resistance and Virulence Factor Gene Profiles of *Enterococcus* Spp. Isolates from Wild *Arctocephalus australis* (South American Fur Seal) and *Arctocephalus tropicalis* (Subantarctic Fur Seal). *World J. Microbiol. Biotechnol.* **2015**, *31*, 1935–1946. [CrossRef]
100. Haft, D.H.; DiCuccio, M.; Badretdin, A.; Brover, V.; Chetvernin, V.; O'Neill, K.; Li, W.; Chitsaz, F.; Derbyshire, M.K.; Gonzales, N.R.; et al. RefSeq: An Update on Prokaryotic Genome Annotation and Curation. *Nucleic Acids Res.* **2018**, *46*, D851–D860. [CrossRef]
101. Richter, M.; Rossello, R.J. Species WS: A Web Server for Prokaryotic Species Circumscription Based on Pairwise Genome Comparison. *Bioinformatics* **2016**, *32*, 929–931. [CrossRef] [PubMed]
102. Katoh, K.; Kuma, K.; Toh, H.; Miyata, T. MAFFT Version 5: Improvement in Accuracy of Multiple Sequence Alignment. *Nucleic Acids Res.* **2005**, *33*, 511–518. [CrossRef] [PubMed]
103. Sela, I.; Ashkenazy, H.; Katoh, K.; Pupko, T. GUIDANCE 2: Accurate Detection of Unreliable Alignment Regions Accounting for the Uncertainty of Multiple Parameters. *Nucleic Acids Res.* **2015**, *43*, W7–W14. [CrossRef] [PubMed]
104. Müller, T.; Vingron, M. Modeling Amino Acid Replacement. *J. Comput. Biol.* **2000**, *7*, 761–776. [CrossRef]
105. Lefort, V.; Longueville, J.-E.; Gascuel, O. SMS: Smart Model Selection in PhyML. *Mol. Biol. Evol.* **2017**, *34*, 2422–2424. [CrossRef]
106. Anisimova, M.; Gascuel, O. Approximate Likelihood-Ratio Test for Branches: A Fast, Accurate, and Powerful Alternative. *Syst. Biol.* **2006**, *55*, 539–552. [CrossRef] [PubMed]
107. Hordijk, W.; Gascuel, O. New Algorithms and Methods to Estimate Maximum-Likelihood Phylogenies: Assessing the Performance of PhyML 3.0. *Syst. Biol.* **2010**, *59*, 307–321.
108. Letunic, I.; Bork, P. Interactive Tree Of Life (ITOL) v4: Recent Updates and New Developments. *Nucleic Acids Res.* **2019**, *47*, W256–W259. [CrossRef]
109. Pettersen, E.F.; Goddard, T.D.; Huang, C.C.; Couch, G.S.; Greenblatt, D.M.; Meng, E.C.; Ferrin, T.E. UCSF Chimera—A Visualization System for Exploratory Research and Analysis. *J. Comput. Chem.* **2004**, *25*, 1605–1612. [CrossRef]
110. Gasteiger, E.; Hoogland, C.; Gattiker, A.; Wilkins, M.R.; Appel, R.D.; Bairoch, A. Protein identification and analysis tools on the ExPASy server. In *The Proteomics Protocols Handbook*; Walker, J.M., Ed.; Humana Press: Totowa, NJ, USA, 2005; pp. 571–607.
111. Jia, B.; Raphenya, A.R.; Alcock, B.; Waglechner, N.; Guo, P.; Tsang, K.K.; Lago, B.A.; Dave, B.M.; Pereira, S.; Sharma, A.N.; et al. CARD 2017: Expansion and Model-Centric Curation of the Comprehensive Antibiotic Resistance Database. *Nucleic Acids Res.* **2017**, *45*, D566–D573. [CrossRef]
112. Zankari, E.; Hasman, H.; Cosentino, S.; Vestergaard, M.; Rasmussen, S.; Lund, O.; Aarestrup, F.M.; Larsen, M.V. Identification of Acquired Antimicrobial Resistance Genes. *J. Antimicrob. Chemoth.* **2012**, *67*, 2640–2644. [CrossRef]
113. Joensen, K.G.; Scheutz, F.; Lund, O.; Hasman, H.; Kaas, R.S.; Nielsen, E.M.; Aarestrup, F.M. Real-Time Whole-Genome Sequencing for Routine Typing, Surveillance, and Outbreak Detection of Verotoxigenic *Escherichia Coli*. *J. Clin. Microb.* **2014**, *52*, 1501–1510. [CrossRef]

114. Bostock, M.; Ogievetsky, V.; Heer, J. D3 Data-Driven Documents. *IEEE Trans. Visual. Comput. Graph.* **2011**, *17*, 2301–2309. [CrossRef] [PubMed]
115. R Core Team. *R: A Language and Environment for Statistical Computing*; R Foundation for Statistical Computing: Vienna, Austria. Available online: https://www.R-project.org/ (accessed on 18 December 2019).

marine drugs

MDPI

Article

Genome Reduction and Secondary Metabolism of the Marine Sponge-Associated Cyanobacterium *Leptothoe*

Despoina Konstantinou [1], Rafael V. Popin [2], David P. Fewer [2], Kaarina Sivonen [2] and Spyros Gkelis [1,*]

[1] Department of Botany, School of Biology, Aristotle University of Thessaloniki, GR-541 24 Thessaloniki, Greece; kidespoi@bio.auth.gr

[2] Department of Microbiology, University of Helsinki, Viikinkaari 9, FI-00014 Helsinki, Finland; rafael.popin@helsinki.fi (R.V.P.); david.fewer@helsinki.fi (D.P.F.); kaarina.sivonen@helsinki.fi (K.S.)

* Correspondence: sgkelis@bio.auth.gr; Tel.: +30-2310-998083

Abstract: Sponges form symbiotic relationships with diverse and abundant microbial communities. Cyanobacteria are among the most important members of the microbial communities that are associated with sponges. Here, we performed a genus-wide comparative genomic analysis of the newly described marine benthic cyanobacterial genus *Leptothoe* (Synechococcales). We obtained draft genomes from *Le. kymatousa* TAU-MAC 1615 and *Le. spongobia* TAU-MAC 1115, isolated from marine sponges. We identified five additional *Leptothoe* genomes, host-associated or free-living, using a phylogenomic approach, and the comparison of all genomes showed that the sponge-associated strains display features of a symbiotic lifestyle. *Le. kymatousa* and *Le. spongobia* have undergone genome reduction; they harbored considerably fewer genes encoding for (i) cofactors, vitamins, prosthetic groups, pigments, proteins, and amino acid biosynthesis; (ii) DNA repair; (iii) antioxidant enzymes; and (iv) biosynthesis of capsular and extracellular polysaccharides. They have also lost several genes related to chemotaxis and motility. Eukaryotic-like proteins, such as ankyrin repeats, playing important roles in sponge-symbiont interactions, were identified in sponge-associated *Leptothoe* genomes. The sponge-associated *Leptothoe* stains harbored biosynthetic gene clusters encoding novel natural products despite genome reduction. Comparisons of the biosynthetic capacities of *Leptothoe* with chemically rich cyanobacteria revealed that *Leptothoe* is another promising marine cyanobacterium for the biosynthesis of novel natural products.

Keywords: cyanobacteria; symbionts; marine sponges; comparative genomics; natural products; biosynthetic gene clusters

Citation: Konstantinou, D.; Popin, R.V.; Fewer, D.P.; Sivonen, K.; Gkelis, S. Genome Reduction and Secondary Metabolism of the Marine Sponge-Associated Cyanobacterium *Leptothoe*. *Mar. Drugs* **2021**, *19*, 298. https://doi.org/10.3390/md19060298

Academic Editor: Max Crüsemann

Received: 30 April 2021
Accepted: 21 May 2021
Published: 24 May 2021

1. Introduction

Sponges host abundant and remarkable diverse microbial communities [1] that exhibit biological complexity similar to the human microbiome [2,3]. Cyanobacteria are an ancient lineage of photosynthetic prokaryotes demonstrating ecological key roles (e.g., oxygen production, nitrogen fixation, carbon flux) in a broad range of habitats, including sponges [4,5], with which they are often found in symbiosis (cyanobionts). Several approaches including whole-genome sequencing of symbiotic microbes and metagenomic binning have provided insights into the functional potential of the symbionts [6,7]. For instance, it has been shown that across sponge-associated bacteria taxa there are pathways involved in carbon fixation, B-vitamin synthesis, taurine metabolism, sulfite oxidation, and most steps of nitrogen metabolism [7,8]. *Candidatus Synechococcus spongiarum*, a widespread (yet uncultivated) sponge symbiont, has specific adaptations to life inside sponges [9]. This obligate cyanobiont showed extreme genome reduction [9], similarly to other bacterial sponge symbionts such as *Candidatus Endohaliclona renieramycinifaciens* [10]. Genome reduction is the major genomic feature of bacterial symbionts [11] and is thought to be a process that reduces the cost of genome replication [12].

Cyanobacteria are a prolific source of natural products with complex chemical structures and interesting bioactivities [13]. Advances in genomics have greatly expanded our knowledge and understanding of cyanobacterial natural product biosynthesis [13] with known natural products linked to biosynthetic gene clusters and new natural products discovered through genome mining (e.g., [14–17]). However, the majority of natural products from cyanobacteria are described from a relative limited number of genera [13]. This phenomenon is attributed to problems with cyanobacterial taxonomy that obfuscates the true distribution of natural products in marine cyanobacteria.

Marine sponges are also prolific sources of natural products of great interest for drug development, contributing to nearly 30% (more than 4850 compounds) of all marine natural products discovered [18]. Sponge-associated bacteria are widely thought to be responsible for sponge natural product diversity [2,3,19], with cyanobacteria being among the major producers [20].

Sponge-associated members of the newly described marine cyanobacterium *Leptothoe* [21,22] were found to be highly cytotoxic against human breast, skin, and colon cancer epithelial cells [23]. Extracts of *Le. kymatousa* TAU-MAC 1615 were found to have antibacterial activity [23]. In this study, we sequenced two draft *Leptothoe* genomes, *Le. kymatousa* TAU-MAC 1615 and *Le. spongobia* TAU-MAC 1115, previously isolated form the marine sponges *Chondrilla nucula* and *Acanthella acuta*, respectively [21,24]. We performed comparative genomic analyses of sponge-associated, other host-associated and free-living members of *Leptothoe* genus, and other marine cyanobacterial genera, aiming to (a) identify symbiosis factors and (b) gain insight into their natural product biosynthetic potential.

2. Results and Discussion

Two new sponge-associated cyanobacterial draft genomes belonging to the newly described *Leptothoe* genus were recovered from the isolates TAU-MAC 1615 and 1115 (Figure S1, Table 1). To date, most microbial isolates derived from sponges have been mainly affiliated with Proteobacteria [7,25,26]. A limited number of cyanobacterial strains have been isolated from sponges [24]. Indeed, only one genome assembly from a sponge-associated cyanobacterial strain is available in public databases for a *Myxosarcina*-like cyanobacterium isolated from *Terpios hoshinota* [27]. Recently, a considerable number of novel genera and species of cyanobacteria were found to be associated with Aegean Sea sponges [21,22].

The size of the assembled sponge-associated *Leptothoe* genomes ranged between 4.06 Mb for *Le. kymatousa* TAU-MAC 1615 and 5.24 Mb for *Le. spongobia* TAU-MAC 1115, with G+C contents of 50.5% and 47.3%, respectively (Figure S1, Table 1). Table 1 summarizes the basic genome features of sponge-associated *Leptothoe* genomes, *Leptothoe* genomes associated with other macro-organisms (isolated from turfs), and free-living *Leptothoe* genomes used for comparative genomic analyses in this study after verification of genome-wide relatedness using phylogenomic approaches (Figure 1). The draft assemblies of sponge-associated strains showed the smallest genome sizes (Table 1). Although the genome coverage of sponge-associated strains was high (approximately $\times 450$ and $\times 90$ for TAU-MAC 1615 and TAU-MAC 1115, respectively), the genome completeness estimated by the marker sets used by CheckM (encode essential functions) was substantially complete ($\approx$70%) (Table 1). The GC% contents of the strains were quite similar, varying from 47.3% (TAU-MAC 1115, CCMR0081) to 50.5% (TAU-MAC 1615). Concerning the number of scaffolds, the SIO3F4 metagenome showed the highest number (1508) and the lowest N50 (7412). The number of coding sequences (CDSs) of sponge-associated strains was considerably lower (3638–4790) than the rest of the *Leptothoe* strains, while the amount of CDSs categorized in RAST subsystems (13–17%) was quite similar (Table 1). The remaining 84–87% of CDSs were not classified in any subsystem.

Table 1. Genome properties and quality metrics of *Leptothoe* strains used for comparative genomic analyses. Subsystem statistics were obtained using the RAST server [28] and SEED tool [29].

Genome Statistics	*Leptothoe kymatousa* TAU-MAC 1615	*Leptothoe spongobia* TAU-MAC 1115	*Leptolyngbya* sp. PCC 7375	*Leptolyngbya* sp. Heron Island J	Leptolyngbyaceae CCMR0081	Leptolyngbyaceae CCMR0082	*Leptolyngbya* sp. SIO3F4
Genome size (bp)	4,068,244	5,242,870	9,422,068	8,064,168	8,660,379	8,890,835	8,111,629
Genome coverage (x)	450	92	30	100	150	136	30
Genome completeness	71.92	70.38	99.73	98.64	99.18	99.46	97.64
Genome contamination	0.28	1.49	1.08	1.49	1.35	1.09	12.31
Scaffolds	18	92	5	119	17	21	1,508
Max scaffold length (bp)	1,235,479	2,951,16	-	-	-	-	-
Min scaffold length (bp)	5043	256	-	-	-	-	-
Mean scaffold size (bp)	226,014	56,988	-	-	-	-	-
Median scaffold size (bp)	161,613	42,147	-	-	-	-	-
Scaffold N50	300,414	99,444	5,859,380	103,122	51,381	147,025	7412
GC (%)	50.5	47.3	47.60	48	47.3	47.4	45.7
Pseudogenes	34	79	-	0	303	260	236
Mobile elements	**14**	**68**	**460**	**196**	**115**	**82**	**76**
Phages	0	6	8	4	2	5	3
Transposons	6	32	86	53	36	16	26
Insertion sequences	8	30	366	139	77	61	47
Subsystem annotation statistics							
Number of subsystems	185	183	298	285	303	303	300
Number of coding sequences	3638	4790	9182	7785	8186	8350	8779
Coding sequences in subsystems	526 (15%)	616 (13%)	1251 (14%)	1175 (16%)	1204 (15%)	1196 (15%)	1470 (17%)
Coding sequences not in subsystems	3112 (85%)	4174 (87%)	7931 (86%)	6610 (84%)	6982 (85%)	71154 (85%)	7390 (83%)
Lifestyle	Sponge-associated	Sponge-associated	Free-living	Free-living	Associated with macroalgae and corals *	Associated with macroalgae and corals *	Associated with macroalgae and other microbes †
GenBank Accession numbers	This study	This study	NZ_ALVN00000000	NZ_AWNH00000000	NZ_QXHD00000000	NZ_QZCE00000000	JAAHHO000000000

* Isolated from turf samples growing over corals; † isolated from turf samples.

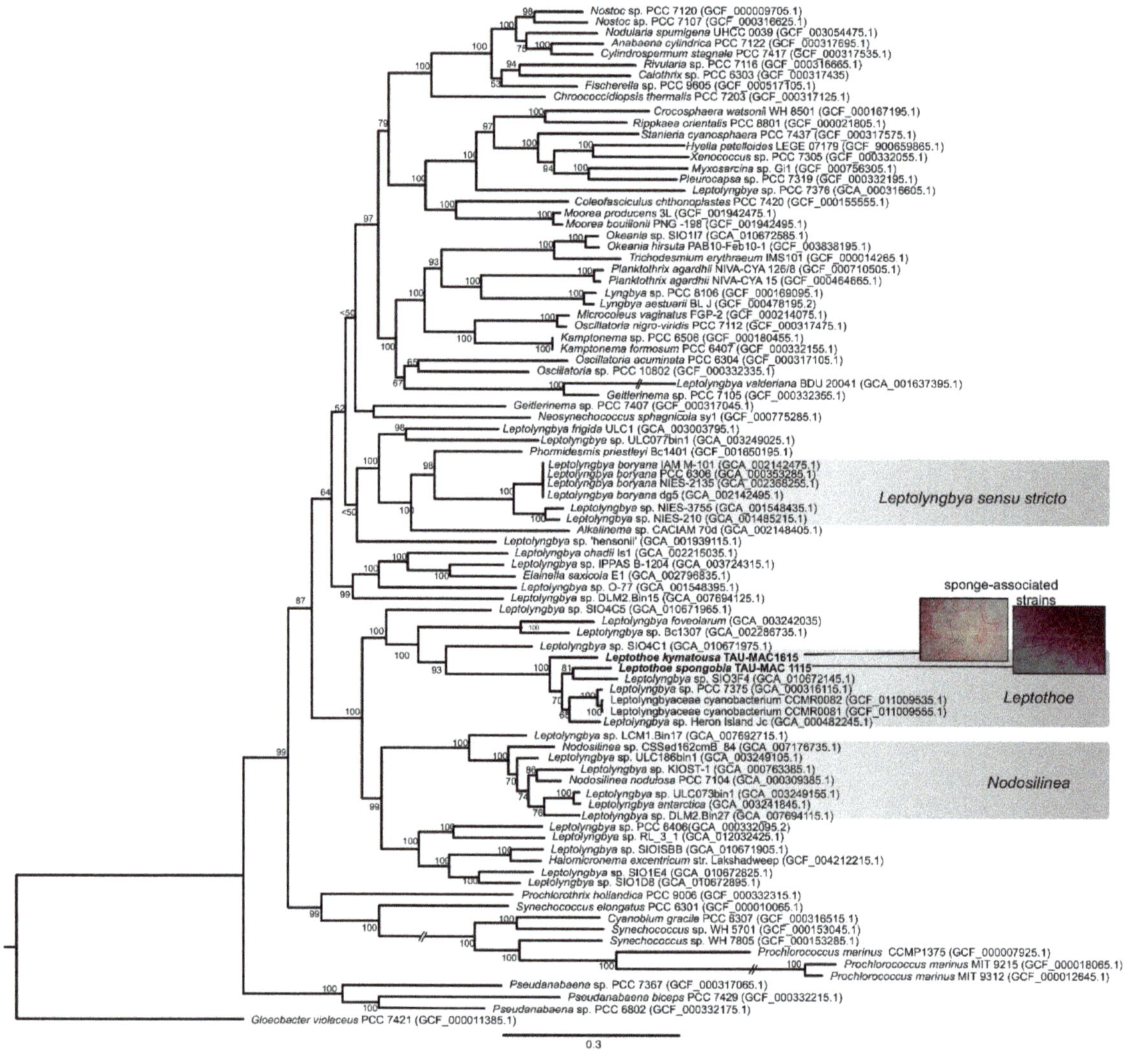

Figure 1. Maximum likelihood phylogenomic tree based on 120 conserved proteins in cyanobacterial genomes. The sponge-associated *Leptothoe* strains sequenced in the present study are shown in bold. Accession numbers of the sequences are presented in parentheses.

The phylogenomic reconstruction based on 120 bacterial single-copy conserved marker genes indicated that our two sponge-associated strains were placed inside *Leptothoe* clade and grouped together with 5 of the 35 public cyanobacterial genomes identified as *Leptolyngbya* or Leptolyngbyaceae (Figure 1). *Leptothoe* is a thin marine filamentous cyanobacterium with benthic lifestyle being epilithic, epizoic, or epiphytic, recently separated from the polyphyletic filamentous genus *Leptolynbya* by a taxonomic re-evaluation [21].

The remaining 30 cyanobacteria, identified as *Leptolyngbya* or Leptolyngbyaceae, were grouped in different clades spread across a variety of cyanobacteria orders (Figure 1). This analysis further supported the evolutionary divergence of *Leptothoe* from *Leptolyngbya* sensu stricto and other thin filamentous genera separated from *Leptolyngbya* such as *Nodosilinea* and *Elainella* (Figure 1). The analysis also supported the evolutionary distinction of the two sponge-associated strains, TAU-MAC 1115 and TAU-MAC 1615, which belong to different species *Le. spongobia* and *Le. kymatousa* (Figure 1). The free-living strains PCC 7375 and Heron Island J were placed separately within a subclade along with two strains (CCMR0081 and CCMR0081) isolated from turf samples growing over corals, while the metagenome-assembled genome SIO3F4 isolated from turfs assembles in Panama was placed in the same subclade with *Le. spongobia* TAU-MAC 1115 (Figure 1). Further, our phylogenomic analysis showed that the members of genus *Leptothoe* (seven in total) were not grouped on the basis of the isolation source (host-associated or free-living), indicating the lack of host-specific clustering. Other marine bacterial genera, including free-living and host-associated members such as *Pseudovibrio*, have shown a lack of host-specific clustering [30]. However, the sponge-associated *Le. kymatousa* TAU-MAC 1615 was placed separately in the phylogenomic tree, likely suggesting its independent evolution from other host-associated strains of the genus. These results might indicate distinct patterns of evolution among members of genus *Leptothoe*.

2.1. Genomic Hallmarks of a Symbiotic Lifestyle

2.1.1. Genome Reduction of Sponge-Associate Strains

Leptothoe kymatousa TAU-MAC 1615 and *Leptothoe spongobia* TAU-MAC 1115 are not obligate sponge symbionts and can sustain growth in pure cultures. However, these two strains showed considerable smaller genome size (Figure 2a). This pattern of genome reduction was also observed for the obligate sponge cyanobiont *Candidatus Synechococcus spongiarum* [9,31]. Genome reduction is widely observed mainly in obligate bacterial symbionts [11], although signs of genome reduction have been identified in facultative symbionts too [32]. Both cyanobionts are slow growing in culture conditions, and thus they could be considered as facultative symbionts that are generally not essential for the host's survival, although they may contribute to host fitness. Recently evolved symbionts, which have undergone genome reduction, are generally characterized by a proliferation of pseudogenes and mobile elements [11]. The two *Leptothoe* sponge-associated genomes reported here showed lower numbers of those traits compared to the other members of the genus (Table 1); on the basis of these data, we hypothesized that sponges did not recently acquire the *Leptothoe* symbionts.

The number of coding sequences of the sponge-associated strains were also half compared to the remaining strains (Figure 2b). An overview of different subsystems obtained using the RAST and SEED annotation showed that the sponge-associated *Leptothoe* strains harbored considerably fewer genes related to several essential functions (Figure 2c, Table S1). Remarkably, *Le. kymatousa* TAU-MAC 1615 and *Le. spongobia* TAU-MAC 1115 have undergone extreme reduction of the number of genes encoding for cofactors, vitamins, prosthetic groups, pigments, proteins, and amino acid biosynthesis (Figure 2c, Table S1). Sponge-associated strains may be dependent on co-occurring microbes for lost metabolic capacities [33]. A complete loss of genes involved in DNA recombination and fewer genes involved in DNA repair were observed in their genomes, while they retained approximately the same number of genes for DNA replication as the rest of the *Leptothoe* genomes. The sponge-associated strains have lost several genes involved in potassium, sulfur, and phosphorus metabolism (Table S1). They were also found to have fewer genes related to stress response, mainly genes coding for antioxidant enzymes, as well as fewer genes responsible for the biosynthesis of capsular polysaccharide (CPS) and extracellular polysaccharides (Table S1). Our *Leptothoe* genomes were characterized by a complete or near complete lack of chemotaxis and motility traits, which are among the most depleted functions in sponge-associated bacteria genomes [34].

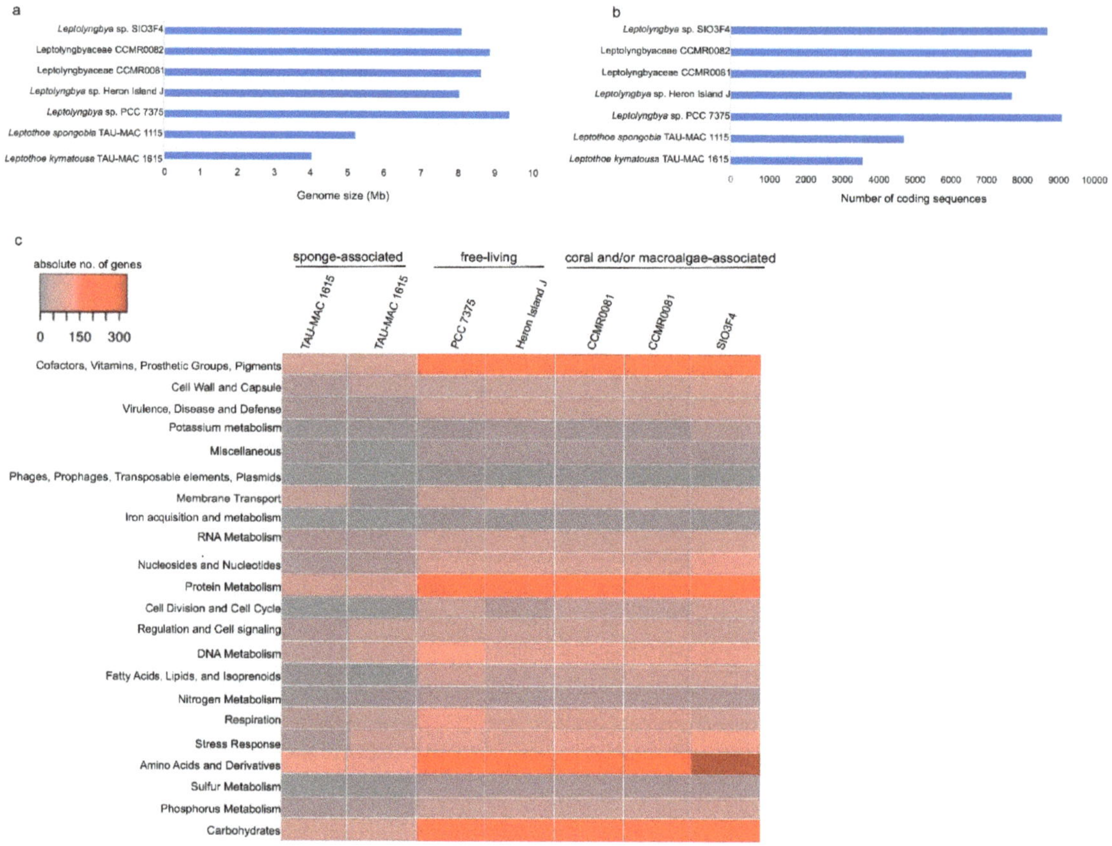

Figure 2. Comparison of genome size (**a**), number of coding sequences (**b**), and number of genes in each RAST subsystem [28] (**c**) of the analyzed *Leptothoe* genomes.

The number of COGs (clusters of orthologous groups of proteins) per genome ranged from 6594 in free-living PCC 7375 strain to 2925 in the sponge-associated TAU-MAC 1615 strain. *Leptothoe* strains shared > 80% average amino acid identity (AAI) (Figure S2), while only 1602 COG entries that account for approximately half (for sponge-associated strains) or even lower (≈25% for the rest of the strains) of the total number of COG entries were common in all genomes (Figure 3), likely suggesting specific adaptations for different lifestyles and for different symbiont types. Genome streamlining process forces adaptations of cyanobacterial genomes to specific niches that are also reflected in their different functional capacities [12]. Previously, sponge-associated and free-living *Synechococcus* genomes have also been found to share half of their total number of COGs, suggesting variability and specific adaptations of each member of the genus [9]. Comparisons based on COG categories among the sponge-associated, coral, and/or macroalgae-associated and free-living *Leptothoe* revealed a relative lower abundance of genes belonging to the different functional categories in the sponge-associated strains. This analysis identified an overrepresentation of functional categories 'J' (translation, ribosomal structure, and biogenesis), 'L' (replication, recombination, and repair), 'O' (posttranslational modification, protein turnover, chaperones), and 'P' (inorganic ion transport and metabolism) and was observed in the genomes of the coral and/or macroalgae-associated strains (Figure S3). A uniform distribution of genes belonging to COG functional categories between the two sponge-associated strains was detected.

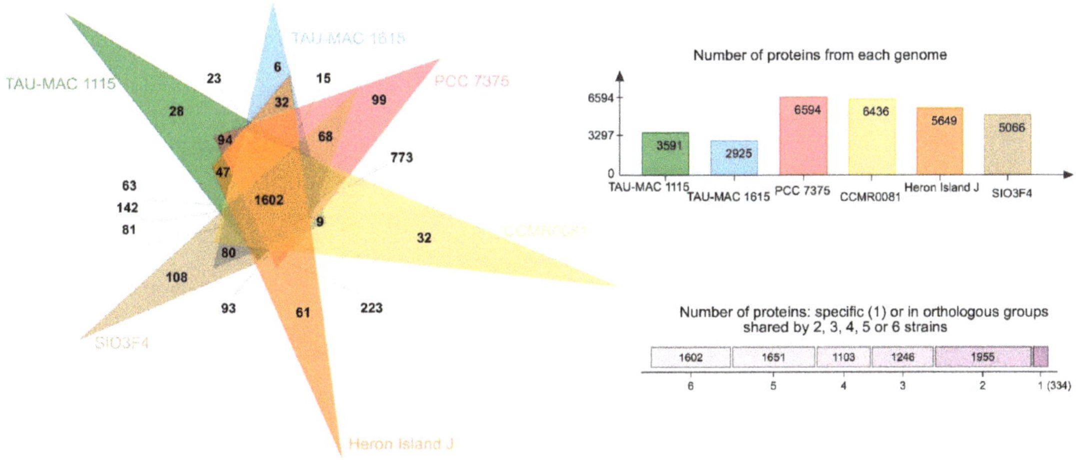

Figure 3. Analysis of homologous protein clusters in the genomes of *Le. kymatousa* TAU-MAC 1615, *Le. spongobia* TAU-MAC 1115, Leptolyngbyaceae sp. CCMR0081, Leptolyngbyaceae sp. CCMR0082, *Leptolyngbya* sp. SIO3F4 *Leptolyngbya* sp. PCC 7375, and *Leptolyngbya* sp. Hero Island J.

The sponge-associated strains possess biosynthetic gene clusters (BGCs) encoding for natural products despite undergoing genome reduction (Figure 4a,b). It has been proposed that maintenance of such clusters sustains the symbiotic interaction [35]. Natural product BGCs were previously detected in another cyanobacterial sponge symbiont, *Hormoscilla spongilae*, suggesting that these biosynthetic capacities to produce metabolically expensive natural products may contribute to host fitness [36].

2.1.2. Eukaryotic-Like Protein (ELP)-Encoding Genes

Genes encoding eukaryotic-like proteins (ELPs) such as ankyrin-like domains (ANKs), tetratricopeptide repeats (TPRs), Leucine-rich repeat (LRR) protein, and pyrroloquinoline quinone (PQQ) were detected in the two sponge-associated *Leptothoe* strains (Table 2); ELPs are often detected in facultative or obligate symbionts and play a key role in the modulation of cellular protein–protein interactions [37,38]. In particular, abundance of ANKs seems to be a major genomic feature of sponge symbionts [6,26] as they have been thought to be involved in preventing phagocytosis by the sponge host. Indeed, the role of ANKs in modulating the amoebal phagocytosis in sponge symbionts was experimentally validated [39]. Genome analyses of sponge-associated Alphaproteobacteria [7,26,30], Deltaproteobacteria [40], and Poribacteria [41] have revealed the presence of ELPs, as well as the particular abundance of ANKs. The obligate sponge symbionts *Hormoscilla spongeliae* and *Candidatus Synechococcus spongiarum* had a great number of ELP repeats, while different free-living cyanobacteria taxa such as *Nodosilinea*, *Leptolyngbya*, *Synechococcus*, *Prochlorococcus*, and *Cyanobium gracile* almost lacked ANK domains, the typical genomic signature of sponge symbionts (Table 2). We also detected the different ELP types in varying proportions in other host-associated and free-living members of the genus *Leptothoe*. Similarly, ELPs have been previously detected in host-associated and free-living members of Alphaproteobacteria, likely suggesting the ability of strains to infect a different range of marine hosts and attach to various marine niches [26,30].

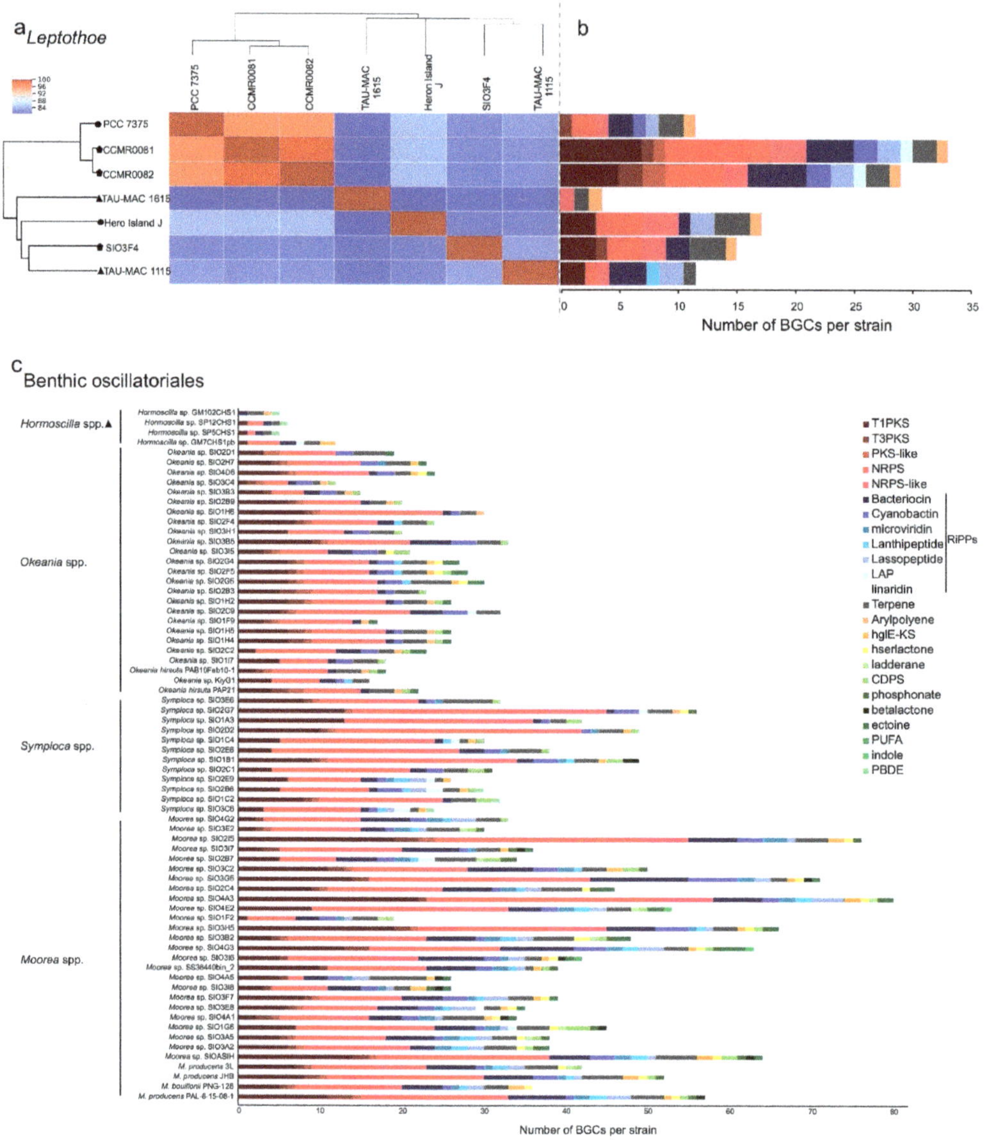

Figure 4. Average nucleotide identity heatmap (**a**) and composition of BGCs identified in *Leptothoe* genomes (**b**) and composition of BGCs identified in marine benthic filamentous Oscillatoriales (**c**). The absolute number of BGCs per strain assigned to each BGC class is shown. Triangle, sponge associated strains; polygon, coral and/or macroalgae-associated strains; circle, free-living strains.

2.2. Biosynthetic Potential of *Leptothoe*

The genomic repertoire for secondary metabolism of seven *Leptothoe* genomes was predicted using antiSMASH (Figure 4a,b). *Leptothoe* genomes were found to harbor a considerable number of BGCs (121), the majority of which have no known end product. BGCs with unknown end products are present in almost all cyanobacterial genomes [42], and on the other hand, there are still natural products for which a biosynthetic origin is unknown [43]. The vast majority of BGCs in *Leptothoe* genomes were predicted to encode non-ribosomal peptide synthetases (NRPS) (24 BGCs), followed by type I polyketide synthase (T1PKS) (20 BGCs) and bacteriocin (17 BGCs) (Figure 4, Table S2). Previously, genome-mining efforts have revealed that a major fraction of cyanobacterial natural products is produced using NRPS or PKS enzymes systems [43,44]. Bacteriocin BGCs, which are widespread in cyanobacterial genomes [45], were detected in almost all *Leptothoe* genomes (except for *Le. kymatousa* TAU-MAC 1615). Bacteriocins have been mainly reported to exhibit antimicrobial activity [46], but are also promising as antivirals, plant protection agents, and anticancer agents [47]. Further, it is suggested that bacteriocins may be involved in shaping bacterial communities through inter- and intra-specific interactions [47]. In addition, lassopeptide and terpene synthase BGCs were detected with high relative abundance in almost all the *Leptothoe* genomes, while cyanobactin and arylpolyene BGCs were rarely found in some of the genomes. Terpene BGCs, reported in a wide variety of bacteria including cyanobacteria [48], were also present in all *Leptothoe* genomes. The considerably similar *Leptothoe* strains CCMR0081 and CCMR0081 (96% average nucleotide identity) associated with corals and macroalgae (isolated from turfs) showed the highest number of natural product BGCs (Figure 4a,b, Table S2). In contrast, the two sponge-associated *Leptothoe* species (sharing ≈84% average nucleotide identity) showed the lowest number of natural product BGCs. Interestingly *Le. spongobia* strain harbored a BGC encoding for a lanthipeptide (Figure 4b). Lanthipeptides are ribosomally synthesized and post-translationally modified peptides (RiPPs) that display a wide variety of biological activities [49], while their detection and isolation are restricted to bacteria [43]. Lanthipeptide BGCs are particularly found in the genomes of many genera of Firmicutes, Actinobacteria, Proteobacteria, Bacteroidetes, and Cyanobacteria [50].

Table 2. Eukaryotic-like protein repeats across symbiotic and free-living cyanobacterial genomes.

		Strains	Eukaryotic-Like Domain			
			Tetratricopeptide Repeats	**Ankyrin Repeats**	**Leucine-Rich Repeats**	**Pyrroloquinoline Quinone**
***Leptothoe* clade**	*Sponge symbionts*	***Le. kymatousa*TAU-MAC 1615**	41	7	6	0
		***Le. spongobia*TAU-MAC 1115**	60	3	5	1
	Host associated	Leptolyngbyaceae CCMR0081	99	10	10	0
		Leptolyngbyaceae CCMR0082	83	9	9	0
	Free-living	*Leptolyngbya* sp. SIO3F4	93	5	22	0
		Leptolyngbya sp. PCC 7375	102	4	5	0
		Leptolyngbya sp. Heron Island J	70	5	8	0
Other cyanobacterial taxa	**Sponge symbionts**	*Hormoscilla spongeliae GM7CHS1pb*	70	4	56	0
		Candidatus Synechococcus spongiarum SH4	3	17	9	0
	Free-living	*Nodosilinea nodulosa PCC 7104*	73	1	3	0
		Leptolyngbya boryana PCC 6306	70	1	0	1
		Synechococcus sp. WH 5701	17	0	0	0
		Prochlorococcus marinus CCMP137	6	0	2	0
		Cyanobium gracile PCC 6307	12	0	0	0

We assigned producers of known natural products to the *Leptothoe* lineage by combining 16S rRNA phylogenetic analysis with the "Comprehensive database of secondary metabolites from cyanobacteria 'CyanoMetDB'" [51]. We searched the database for entries attributed to *Leptolyngbya*, *Pseudanabaena* (*Pseudanabaena persicina* = *Leptolyngbya ectocarpi*), *Phormidium* (*Phormidium ectocarpi* = *Leptolyngbya ectocarpi*), or thin filamentous strains of pinkish color, and where a sequence was available, it was included in our phylogenetic analysis (Table S3, Figure 5). This analysis demonstrated that two strains previously assigned to *Leptolyngbya*, *Leptolyngbya ectocarpi* SAG 60.90, and *Leptolyngbya* sp. RS03, reported to produce compounds such as hierridin B, grassypeptolides D and E, a lyngbyastatin analogue, and dolastatin 12, belong to the *Leptothoe* genus (Table S3, Figure 5). However, the natural product BGCs involved in the biosynthesis of the abovementioned compounds have not been studied as the genomes of these *Leptothoe* strains have not been sequenced yet. Our phylogenetic analysis revealed that *Leptothoe* was closely affiliated with three other marine benthic cyanobacteria, *Salileptolyngbya* and two strains with unknown taxonomic status (Cyanobacterium csf1 and Filamentous cyanobacterium FLK9); csf1 was found to produce two new cyclic depsipeptides, companeramides A and B (Figure 5; CyanoMetDB). Further, in our analysis, other genera of marine origin with benthic lifestyle and often with a reddish to pinkish thallus color, known for the production of natural products such as linear and cyclic peptides, linear and cyclic non-peptides, and linear and cyclic depsipeptides, were extracted from the CyanoMetDB database. These chemically rich genera—*Moorea*, *Caldora*, *Symploca*, *Okeania*, and *Hormoscilla*—were placed in separate clades inside Oscillatoriales and were found to be distantly related to *Leptothoe* (Figure 5).

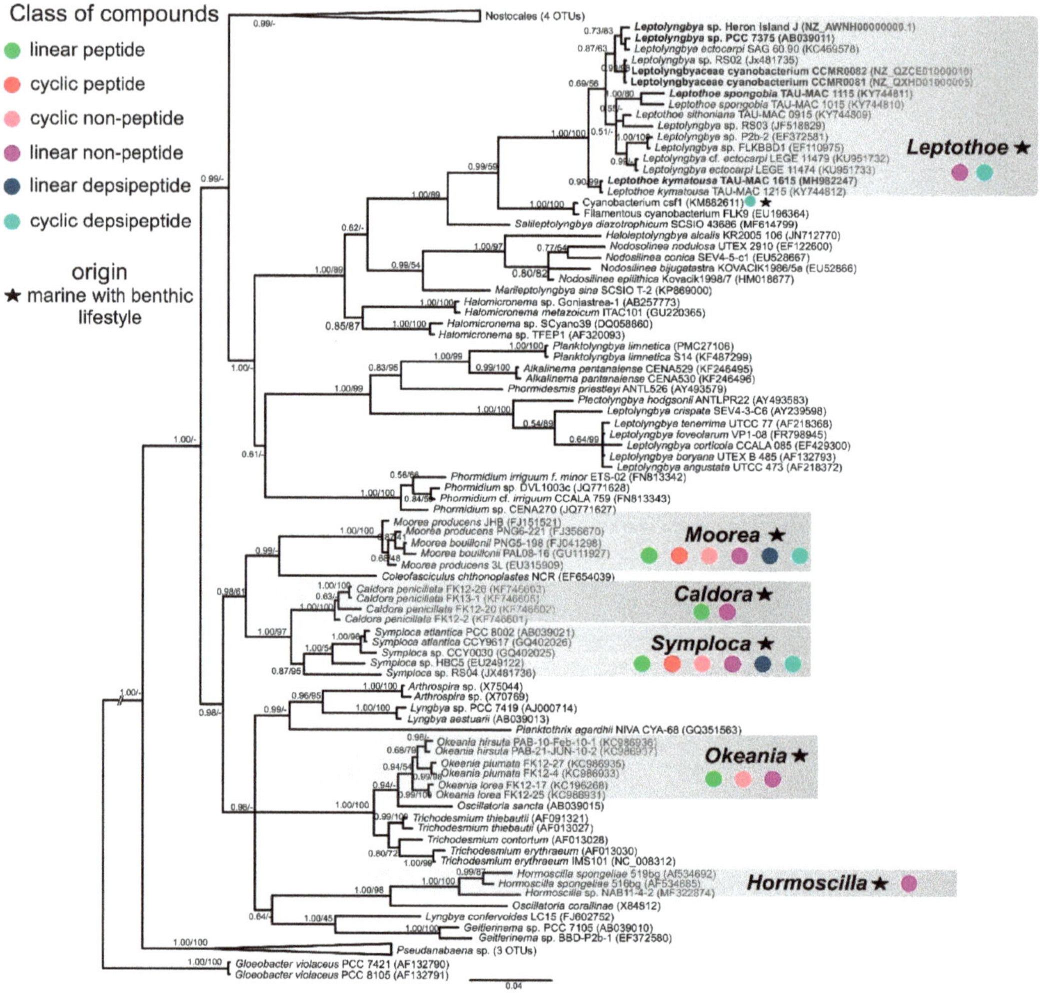

Figure 5. Phylogenetic relationships of *Leptothoe* strains based on the 16S rRNA gene sequence, in relationship to representative strains of other marine filamentous cyanobacteria with benthic lifestyle, with *Gloeobacter* violaceus as outgroup. The tree was constructed with the Bayesian inference (BI) method and the maximum-likelihood (ML) method; BI topology is demonstrated. Support values are indicated as posterior probability for Bayesian inference and bootstrap support for maximum likelihood analysis. The bar represents 0.04 nucleotide substitutions per site.

Most of the natural products from marine cyanobacteria have been isolated from *Moorea* [52], which occur in high densities in marine environments of tropical and subtropical regions, making the harvest of biomass easily accessible [52]. Similarly, *Symploca, Caldora,* and *Okeania* form large populations attached to hard substrates in marine habitats [53,54] and yield a great number of natural products. Novel compounds with strong anticancer properties such as apratoxins, grassypeptolides, wewakazole B, odoamide, and caldoramide are isolated from these marine genera [55–59]. Interestingly, cyclic depsipeptides are the main peptides with cytotoxic effects isolated from marine cyanobacteria, including 76 compounds [60]. Genome-mining analysis conducted in the present study for >70 marine cyanobacteria also highlighted the high metabolic potential of the well-studied Oscillatoriales; numerous BGCs were identified in their genomes (Figure 4c). On the other hand, other marine filamentous cyanobacteria with smaller trichomes and a slower growth rate, such as *Leptolyngbya*-like or *Pseudanabaena*-like, have been overlooked [52], as well as the members of *Leptothoe* genus according to our analysis. Herein, we revealed another promising benthic marine cyanobacterium for novel natural products biosynthesis, *Leptothoe*, that warrants further exploration.

3. Materials and Methods

3.1. Sponge-Associated Strains and Growth Conditions

Leptothoe kymatousa TAU-MAC 1615 and *Le. spongobia* TAU-MAC 1115 were previously isolated from the marine sponges *Chondrilla nucula* and *Acanthella acuta*, accordingly, from a rocky sublittoral zone of the North Aegean Sea [21,24]. The strains were purified, and an axenic culture was obtained only for *Le. kymatousa* TAU-MAC 1615 due to difficulties in producing pure cultures stemming from tightly associated heterotrophic bacteria. Axenic and mono-clonal cultures were grown in MN medium [61] for 20–25 days at 20–25 °C, at a photo irradiance of 8–15 μmol photons m^{-2} s^{-1}. These strains are maintained in the Microalgae and Cyanobacteria Collection (TAU-MAC) of the Aristotle University of Thessaloniki [62].

3.2. Total Genomic DNA Extraction

The genomic DNA of *Leptothoe kymatousa* TAU-MAC 1615 was extracted using a DNA extraction kit (E.Z.N.A.® SP Plant DNA Mini Kit Protocol—Fresh/Frozen Samples, Omega Bio-Tek, Norcross, GA, USA). We harvested 50 mL cultures by centrifugation at 7000× *g* for 10 min, and the pellets were transferred to microcentrifuge tubes. A total of 200 μL of glass beads (two different sizes: 425 to 600 μm and 710 to 1180 μm; Sigma-Aldrich, St. Louis, MO, USA) and SP buffer were added, and the cells were disrupted mechanically with a FastPrep-24 homogenizer (MP Biomedicals, Irvine, CA, USA) at 6.5 m/s for 30 s (2 cycles). The sample of lysed cells was extracted as described in the manufacturers' protocol.

A total of 50 mL cultures of *Le. spongobia* TAU-MAC 1115 were harvested by centrifugation at 7000× *g* for 10 min, washed twice with washing buffer (50 mM Tris-HCl, 100 mM EDTA, 100 mM NaCl), and transferred to microcentrifuge tubes. After centrifugation (at 7000× *g* for 4 min), the supernatant was discarded, glass beads (two different sizes: 425 to 600 μm and 710 to 1180 μm; Sigma-Aldrich, St. Louis, MO, USA) were added, and the cells were frozen at −80 °C. The sample was thawed at 64 °C and 800 μL of GOS buffer (100 mM TrisHCl (pH 8), 1.5% SDS, 10 mM EDTA, 1% deoxycholate, 1% Igepal-CA630, 5 mM thiourea, 10 mM dithiothreitol) [63] was added. Disruption of the cells was performed using FastPrep at 5 m s^{-1} for 30 s (2 cycles). The rest of the extraction procedure was performed as previously described in detail [63].

The purity, concentration, and quality of the DNA were determined using a Nanodrop ND-1000 Spectrophotometer (Nanodrop Technologies, Wilmington, DE USA), gel electrophoresis, and an Agilent TapeStation (Agilent Technologies, Lexington, MA, USA).

3.3. Genome Sequencing and Assembly of Sponge-Associated Cyanobacteria

High-molecular-weight DNA was subjected to library construction (Illumina TruSeq PCR-free 150 bp) and sequenced by the Illumina HiSeq 2500 platform, with a paired-end 100-cycle run (Macrogen Europe, Amsterdam, the Netherlands). The quality of the raw data was initially assessed using FastQC v0.10.1 [64]. Prinseq [65] was used to perform quality filtering, and genome assembly was performed with SPAdes 3.5.0 [66], followed by scaffolding and gap-closing performed with Platanus 1.2.1 [67]. Scaffolds from culture contaminants were identified by Kraken 1.0 [68] and removed using ZEUSS 1.0.2 [69]. Genome assembly statistics were obtained using Assemblathon 2 [70]. Completeness and contamination of the genomes were accessed using CheckM v1.1.3 [71].

3.4. Phylogenomic and Phylogenetic Analysis

An alignment of 120 bacterial single-copy conserved marker genes was generated with the Genome Taxonomy Database GTDB-Tk [72] from 90 cyanobacterial genomes, including the two newly sequenced sponge-associated *Leptothoe* genomes as well as 35 genomes registered in GenBank as *Leptolyngbya* or Leptolyngbyaceae and representative taxa of Nostocales, Oscillatoriales, and Chroococcales. A maximum-likelihood phylogenomic tree was constructed by RAxML [73] that was based on the nucleotide substitution model LG +I +G assigned by a BIC calculation in ProtTest [74], with 1000 rapid bootstrap searches.

For 16S rRNA phylogenetic analysis, a dataset consisting of gene sequences belonging to *Leptothoe* genus (>94.5% sequence similarity via BLASTn searches) along with sequences of closely affiliated genera (such as *Salileptolyngbya*, *Nodosilinea*, *Halomicronema*), as well as sequences of other filamentous cyanobacteria was generated. Multiple sequence alignment was performed in MEGA v. 7.0 [75] using ClustalW [76]. The phylogenetic tree was constructed using maximum likelihood (ML) and Bayesian inference (BI). Two 16S rRNA gene sequences of the cyanobacterium *Gloeobacter violaceus* were used as outgroups (GenBank acc. no. AF132790, AF132791). The GTR+I+G model was determined by a BIC calculation in jModelTest 0.1.1 [77] as the most appropriate. The ML analysis was performed in MEGA v. 7 [75]. Bootstrap resampling was performed on 1000 replicates. Bayesian analysis was conducted using MrBayes 3.2.6 [78]. Four Metropolis-coupled MCMC chains (three heated chains and one cold) were run for 10,000,000 generations, the first 2,500,000 generations were discarded as burn-in, and the following datasets were sampled every 1000th generation. Phylogenomic and phylogenetic tree were visualized using the FigTree (V1.4.3) software (http://tree.bio.ed.ac.uk/software/figtree/, accessed on 12 March 2021).

3.5. Annotation and Comparative Analyses of Genomes

Open reading frames (ORFs) prediction and annotation were performed using the draft genomes of the two sponge-associated *Leptothoe* strains in the RAST (Rapid Annotation using Subsystem Technology) prokaryotic genome annotation server (version 2.0) [28] with standard procedures. For comparative analysis, five genomes of strains belonging to genus *Leptothoe* were identified in NCBI's GenBank [79] and selected. Prior to the comparative genomic analyses, all genome datasets were re-annotated using RAST [28] and PROKKA [80]. Subsystems annotation of all seven genomes was performed with the RAST server [28] and SEED tool [29]. CDSs (predicted using RAST) of all seven genomes were subjected to annotation on the basis of clusters of orthologous groups (COGs) of proteins using the on-line server WebMGA (e-value = 0.001) [81]. Pseudogenes were calculated using NCBI's annotation pipeline. The different classes of mobile elements were analyzed separately. PHASTER [82] was used for phage detection, TransposonPSI (http://transposonpsi.sourceforge.net/, accessed on 12 March 2021) for transposon identification, and ISEScan [83] for identification of insertion sequence elements. In order to detect eukaryotic-like proteins (ELPs) such as ankyrin repeats (ANKs), tetratricopeptide repeat (TPRs), leucine-rich repeats, WD40 proteins, and pyrroloquinoline quinone (PQQ), we searched the annotation files manually using the key words 'repeats', 'Ankyrin', 'Tetratricopeptide', 'leucine', and 'PQQ' (similar to Karimi et al. [7,34]).

Heatmaps for average nucleotide and amino acid identities were estimated using the program GET_HOMOLOGUES [84]. All seven genomes were searched for in terms of the presence of natural product biosynthetic gene clusters (BGCs) using antiSMASH 5.1.1 [85], which was done in order to gain further insight to their metabolic potential.

3.6. Data Availability

The *Leptothoe kymatousa* TAU-MAC 1615 Whole Genome project was deposited at DDBJ/ENA/GenBank under the accession number JADOER000000000. The *Leptothoe spongobia* TAU-MAC 1115 Whole Genome Shotgun project was deposited at DDBJ/ENA/GenBank under the accession number JADOES000000000.

4. Conclusions

Here, we report the first two draft genomes of sponge-associated filamentous Synechococcales. Our comparative genomic analyses revealed symbiosis signatures of sponge-associated *Leptothoe* such as reduction of their gene content, functional dissimilarities to other host-associated and free-living members of *Leptothoe*, and presence of ELP repeats. Moreover, genome-mining analysis revealed the unique biosynthetic potential of *Leptothoe* with more than 100 natural product BGCs, emerging as an unexplored source of potent marine natural products. Additional studies are needed to identify and characterize these produced compounds. Future research to address the actual functioning of sponge-associated cyanobacteria should include metagenomics, metabolomics, and metatranscriptomics.

Supplementary Materials: The following are available online at https://www.mdpi.com/article/10.3390/md19060298/s1, Table S1. Number of genes in subsystems (obtained by RAST server and SEED tool) per *Leptothoe* strain. Table S2. Biosynthetic gene clusters per *Leptothoe* genome (antiSMASH results). Table S3. Compounds produced by *Leptothoe* cyanobacteria extracted from the CyanoMetDB (Jones et al., 2020). Figure S1. Circular view of the genomes of two sponge-associated *Leptothoe* species, generated with CGview (Stothard and Wishart, 2005). Circles from interior to exterior represent GC content and GC skew. Blue circles denote the coding sequences on forward and reverse strands. Figure S2. Average amino acid identity heatmap of *Leptothoe* genomes. Figure S3. Distribution of the categories of functional genes present in seven *Leptothoe* strains on the basis of the cluster of orthologous groups (COGs) of proteins. The alphabetic code for the COG categories is as follows: C, energy production and conversion; D, cell cycle control, cell division, chromosome partitioning; E, amino acid transport and metabolism; F, nucleotide transport and metabolism; G, carbohydrate transport and metabolism; H, coenzyme transport and metabolism; I, lipid transport and metabolism; J, translation, ribosomal structure, and biogenesis; K, transcription; L, replication, recombination, and repair; M, cell wall/membrane/envelope biogenesis; N, cell motility; O, posttranslational modification, protein turnover, chaperones; P, inorganic ion transport and metabolism; Q, secondary metabolite biosynthesis, transport, and catabolism; R, general function prediction only; S, function unknown; T, signal transduction mechanisms; U, intracellular trafficking, secretion, and vesicular transport; V, defense mechanisms.

Author Contributions: Conceptualization, D.K. and S.G.; methodology, D.K., R.V.P., and D.P.F.; validation, D.K., D.P.F., and S.G.; formal analysis, D.K. and R.V.P.; investigation, D.K.; resources, S.G., D.P.F., and K.S.; data curation, D.K.; writing—original draft preparation, D.K.; writing—review and editing, all authors.; visualization, D.K.; supervision, S.G. and D.P.F.; project administration, S.G.; funding acquisition, S.G. All authors have read and agreed to the published version of the manuscript.

Funding: This study was supported by the General Secretariat for Research and Technology (GSRT) and the Hellenic Foundation for Research and Innovation (HFRI), grant number 938 (http://www.elidek.gr/en/homepage/, accessed on 12 March 2021) to D.K. S.G. would like to acknowledge co-funding of this work by the European Union and Greek national funds through the Operational Program Competitiveness, Entrepreneurship and Innovation, under the call RESEARCH—CREATE—INNOVATE (project code: T1EDK-02681). R.V.P. received funding from the Doctoral Program in Microbiology and Biotechnology from the University of Helsinki.

Data Availability Statement: The *Leptothoe kymatousa* TAU-MAC 1615 Whole Genome project was deposited at DDBJ/ENA/GenBank under the accession number JADOER000000000. The *Leptothoe spongobia* TAU-MAC 1115 Whole Genome Shotgun project was deposited at DDBJ/ENA/GenBank under the accession number JADOES000000000.

Acknowledgments: We thank Lyudmila Saari for her kind assistance in purifying the sponge-associated strains.

Conflicts of Interest: The authors declare no conflict of interest. The funders had no role in the design of the study; in the collection, analyses, or interpretation of data; in the writing of the manuscript; or in the decision to publish the results.

References

1. Thomas, T.; Moitinho-Silva, L.; Lurgi, M.; Björk, J.R.; Easson, C.; Astudillo-García, C.; Olson, J.B.; Erwin, P.M.; López-Legentil, S.; Luter, H.; et al. Diversity, structure and convergent evolution of the global sponge microbiome. *Nat. Commun.* **2016**, *7*, 11870. [CrossRef] [PubMed]
2. Taylor, M.W.; Radax, R.; Steger, D.; Wagner, M. Sponge-Associated Microorganisms: Evolution, Ecology, and Biotechnological Potential. *Microbiol. Mol. Biol. Rev.* **2007**, *71*, 295–347. [CrossRef]
3. Hentschel, U.; Piel, J.; Degnan, S.M.; Taylor, M.W. Genomic insights into the marine sponge microbiome. *Nat. Rev. Microbiol.* **2012**. [CrossRef]
4. Adams, D.G.; Duggan, P.S.; Owen, J. Cyanobacterial Symbioses. In *Ecology of Cyanobacteria II: Their Diversity in Space and Time*; Whitton, B.A., Ed.; Spriger: Dordrecht, The Netherlands, 2012; pp. 593–636.
5. Whitton, B.A.; Potts, M. Introduction to the Cyanobacteria. In *Ecology of Cyanobacteria II: Their Diversity in Space and Time*; Whitton, B.A., Ed.; Springer: Dordrecht, The Netherlands, 2012; pp. 1–14.
6. Fan, L.; Reynolds, D.; Liu, M.; Stark, M.; Kjelleberg, S.; Webster, N.S.; Thomas, T. Functional equivalence and evolutionary convergence in complex communities of microbial sponge symbionts. *Proc. Natl. Acad. Sci. USA* **2012**, *109*, E1878–E1887. [CrossRef]
7. Karimi, E.; Keller-Costa, T.; Slaby, B.M.; Cox, C.J.; da Rocha, U.N.; Hentschel, U.; Costa, R. Genomic blueprints of sponge-prokaryote symbiosis are shared by low abundant and cultivatable Alphaproteobacteria. *Sci. Rep.* **2019**, *9*, 1999. [CrossRef]
8. Engelberts, J.P.; Robbins, S.J.; de Goeij, J.M.; Aranda, M.; Bell, S.C.; Webster, N.S. Characterization of a sponge microbiome using an integrative genome-centric approach. *ISME J.* **2020**, *14*, 1100–1110. [CrossRef] [PubMed]
9. Burgsdorf, I.; Slaby, B.M.; Handley, K.M.; Haber, M.; Blom, J.; Marshall, C.W.; Gilbert, J.A.; Hentschel, U.; Steindler, L. Lifestyle evolution in cyanobacterial symbionts of sponges. *mBio* **2015**, *6*, e00391-15. [CrossRef] [PubMed]
10. Tianero, M.D.; Balaich, J.N.; Donia, M.S. Localized production of defence chemicals by intracellular symbionts of Haliclona sponges. *Nat. Microbiol.* **2019**, *4*, 1149–1159. [CrossRef] [PubMed]
11. McCutcheon, J.P.; Moran, N.A. Extreme genome reduction in symbiotic bacteria. *Nat. Rev. Microbiol.* **2012**, *10*, 13–26. [CrossRef]
12. Larsson, J.; Nylander, J.A.A.; Bergman, B. Genome fluctuations in cyanobacteria reflect evolutionary, developmental and adaptive traits. *BMC Evol. Biol.* **2011**, *11*. [CrossRef]
13. Dittmann, E.; Gugger, M.; Sivonen, K.; Fewer, D.P. Natural Product Biosynthetic Diversity and Comparative Genomics of the Cyanobacteria. *Trends Microbiol.* **2015**, *23*, 642–652. [CrossRef] [PubMed]
14. Costa, M.; Sampaio-Dias, I.E.; Castelo-Branco, R.; Scharfenstein, H.; Rezende De Castro, R.; Silva, A.; Schneider, M.P.C.; Araújo, M.J.; Martins, R.; Domingues, V.F.; et al. Structure of hierridin c, synthesis of hierridins b and c, and evidence for prevalent alkylresorcinol biosynthesis in picocyanobacteria. *J. Nat. Prod.* **2019**, *82*, 393–402. [CrossRef]
15. Mattila, A.; Andsten, R.M.; Jumppanen, M.; Assante, M.; Jokela, J.; Wahlsten, M.; Mikula, K.M.; Sigindere, C.; Kwak, D.H.; Gugger, M.; et al. Biosynthesis of the Bis-Prenylated Alkaloids Muscoride A and B. *ACS Chem. Biol.* **2019**, *14*, 2683–2690. [CrossRef] [PubMed]
16. Pancrace, C.; Ishida, K.; Briand, E.; Pichi, D.G.; Weiz, A.R.; Guljamow, A.; Scalvenzi, T.; Sassoon, N.; Hertweck, C.; Dittmann, E.; et al. Unique Biosynthetic Pathway in Bloom-Forming Cyanobacterial Genus Microcystis Jointly Assembles Cytotoxic Aeruginoguanidines and Microguanidines. *ACS Chem. Biol.* **2019**, *14*, 67–75. [CrossRef] [PubMed]
17. Heinilä, L.M.P.; Fewer, D.P.; Jokela, J.K.; Wahlsten, M.; Jortikka, A.; Sivonen, K. Shared PKS Module in Biosynthesis of Synergistic Laxaphycins. *Front. Microbiol.* **2020**, *11*, 578878. [CrossRef]
18. Mehbub, M.F.; Lei, J.; Franco, C.; Zhang, W. Marine sponge derived natural products between 2001 and 2010: Trends and opportunities for discovery of bioactives. *Mar. Drugs* **2014**, *12*, 4539–4577. [CrossRef] [PubMed]
19. Lackner, G.; Peters, E.E.; Helfrich, E.J.N.; Piel, J. Insights into the lifestyle of uncultured bacterial natural product factories associated with marine sponges. *Proc. Natl. Acad. Sci. USA* **2017**, *114*, E347–E356. [CrossRef]
20. Thomas, T.R.A.; Kavlekar, D.P.; LokaBharathi, P.A. Marine drugs from sponge-microbe association—A review. *Mar. Drugs* **2010**, *8*, 1417–1468. [CrossRef]
21. Konstantinou, D.; Voultsiadou, E.; Panteris, E.; Zervou, S.-K.; Hiskia, A.; Gkelis, S. *Leptothoe*, a new genus of marine cyanobacteria (Synechococcales) and three new species associated with sponges from the Aegean Sea. *J. Phycol.* **2019**, *55*. [CrossRef]

22. Konstantinou, D.; Voultsiadou, E.; Panteris, E.; Gkelis, S. Revealing new sponge-associated cyanobacterial diversity: Novel genera and species. *Mol. Phylogenet. Evol.* **2021**, *155*, 106991. [CrossRef] [PubMed]
23. Konstantinou, D.; Mavrogonatou, E.; Zervou, S.K.; Giannogonas, P.; Gkelis, S. Bioprospecting Sponge-Associated Marine Cyanobacteria to Produce Bioactive Compounds. *Toxins* **2020**, *12*, 73. [CrossRef] [PubMed]
24. Konstantinou, D.; Gerovasileiou, V.; Voultsiadou, E.; Gkelis, S. Sponges-Cyanobacteria associations: Global diversity overview and new data from the Eastern Mediterranean. *PLoS ONE* **2018**. [CrossRef]
25. Esteves, A.I.S.; Hardoim, C.C.P.; Xavier, J.R.; Gonçalves, J.M.S.; Costa, R. Molecular richness and biotechnological potential of bacteria cultured from Irciniidae sponges in the north-east Atlantic. *FEMS Microbiol. Ecol.* **2013**, *85*, 519–536. [CrossRef] [PubMed]
26. Alex, A.; Antunes, A. Whole-genome comparisons among the genus shewanella reveal the enrichment of genes encoding ankyrin-repeats containing proteins in sponge-associated bacteria. *Front. Microbiol.* **2019**, *10*, 5. [CrossRef] [PubMed]
27. Yu, C.H.; Lu, C.K.; Su, H.M.; Chiang, T.Y.; Hwang, C.C.; Liu, T.; Chen, Y.M. Draft genome of myxosarcina sp. Strain Gi1, a baeocytous cyanobacterium associated with the marine sponge terpios hoshinota. *Stand. Genom. Sci.* **2015**, *10*, 28. [CrossRef] [PubMed]
28. Aziz, R.K.; Bartels, D.; Best, A.; DeJongh, M.; Disz, T.; Edwards, R.A.; Formsma, K.; Gerdes, S.; Glass, E.M.; Kubal, M.; et al. The RAST Server: Rapid annotations using subsystems technology. *BMC Genomics* **2008**, *9*, 75. [CrossRef]
29. Overbeek, R.; Olson, R.; Pusch, G.D.; Olsen, G.J.; Davis, J.J.; Disz, T.; Edwards, R.A.; Gerdes, S.; Parrello, B.; Shukla, M.; et al. The SEED and the Rapid Annotation of microbial genomes using Subsystems Technology (RAST). *Nucleic Acids Res.* **2014**, *42*, D206–D214. [CrossRef]
30. Alex, A.; Antunes, A. Genus-wide comparison of *Pseudovibrio* bacterial genomes reveal diverse adaptations to different marine invertebrate hosts. *PLoS ONE* **2018**, *13*, e0194368. [CrossRef] [PubMed]
31. Gao, Z.M.; Wang, Y.; Tian, R.M.; Wong, Y.H.; Batang, Z.B.; Al-Suwailem, A.M.; Bajic, V.B.; Qian, P.Y. Symbiotic Adaptation Drives Genome Streamlining of the Cyanobacterial Sponge Symbiont "Candidatus Synechococcus spongiarum". *mBio* **2014**, *5*, e00079-14. [CrossRef]
32. Sloan, D.B.; Moran, N.A. Genome reduction and co-evolution between the primary and secondary bacterial symbionts of psyllids. *Mol. Biol. Evol.* **2012**, *29*, 3781–3792. [CrossRef]
33. Morris, J.; Lenski, R.E.; Zinser, E.R. The Black Queen Hypothesis: Evolution of Dependencies through Adaptive Gene Loss. *mBio* **2012**, *3*, e00036-12. [CrossRef] [PubMed]
34. Karimi, E.; Slaby, B.M.; Soares, A.R.; Blom, J.; Hentschel, U.; Costa, R. Metagenomic binning reveals versatile nutrient cycling and distinct adaptive features in alphaproteobacterial symbionts of marine sponges. *FEMS Microbiol. Ecol.* **2018**, *94*, fiy074. [CrossRef] [PubMed]
35. Moya, A.; Peretó, J.; Gil, R.; Latorre, A. Learning how to live together: Genomic insights into prokaryote-animal symbioses. *Nat. Rev. Genet.* **2008**, *9*, 218–229. [CrossRef] [PubMed]
36. Schorn, M.A.; Jordan, P.A.; Podell, S.; Blanton, J.M.; Agarwal, V.; Biggs, J.S.; Allen, E.E.; Moore, B.S. Comparative Genomics of Cyanobacterial Symbionts Reveals Distinct, Specialized Metabolism in Tropical Dysideidae Sponges. *mBio* **2019**, *10*, 1–15. [CrossRef]
37. Díez-Vives, C.; Moitinho-Silva, L.; Nielsen, S.; Reynolds, D.; Thomas, T. Expression of eukaryotic-like protein in the microbiome of sponges. *Mol. Ecol.* **2017**, *26*, 1432–1451. [CrossRef]
38. Reynolds, D.; Thomas, T. Evolution and function of eukaryotic-like proteins from sponge symbionts. *Mol. Ecol.* **2016**, *25*, 5242–5253. [CrossRef]
39. Nguyen, M.T.H.D.; Liu, M.; Thomas, T. Ankyrin-repeat proteins from sponge symbionts modulate amoebal phagocytosis. *Mol. Ecol.* **2014**, *23*, 1635–1645. [CrossRef]
40. Liu, M.; Fan, L.; Zhong, L.; Kjelleberg, S.; Thomas, T. Metaproteogenomic analysis of a community of sponge symbionts. *ISME J.* **2012**, *6*, 1515–1525. [CrossRef]
41. Siegl, A.; Kamke, J.; Hochmuth, T.; Piel, J.; Richter, M.; Liang, C.; Dandekar, T.; Hentschel, U. Single-cell genomics reveals the lifestyle of Poribacteria, a candidate phylum symbiotically associated with marine sponges. *ISME J.* **2011**, *5*, 61–70. [CrossRef]
42. Wang, H.; Fewer, D.P.; Holm, L.; Rouhiainen, L.; Sivonen, K. Atlas of nonribosomal peptide and polyketide biosynthetic pathways reveals common occurrence of nonmodular enzymes. *Proc. Natl. Acad. Sci. USA* **2014**, *111*, 9259–9264. [CrossRef]
43. Welker, M.; Von Döhren, H. Cyanobacterial peptides—Nature's own combinatorial biosynthesis. *FEMS Microbiol. Rev.* **2006**, *30*, 530–563. [CrossRef] [PubMed]
44. Jones, A.C.; Monroe, E.A.; Eisman, E.B.; Gerwick, L.; Sherman, D.H.; Gerwick, W.H. The unique mechanistic transformations involved in the biosynthesis of modular natural products from marine cyanobacteria. *Nat. Prod. Rep.* **2010**, *27*, 1048–1065. [CrossRef]
45. Wang, H.; Fewer, D.P.; Sivonen, K. Genome mining demonstrates the widespread occurrence of gene clusters encoding bacteriocins in cyanobacteria. *PLoS ONE* **2011**, *6*, e22384. [CrossRef] [PubMed]
46. Piper, C.; Cotter, P.; Ross, R.; Hill, C. Discovery of Medically Significant Lantibiotics. *Curr. Drug Discov. Technol.* **2009**, *6*, 1–18. [CrossRef]
47. Drider, D.; Bendali, F.; Naghmouchi, K.; Chikindas, M.L. Bacteriocins: Not Only Antibacterial Agents. *Probiotics Antimicrob. Proteins* **2016**, *8*, 177–182. [CrossRef] [PubMed]

48. Yamada, Y.; Kuzuyama, T.; Komatsu, M.; Shin-ya, K.; Omura, S.; Cane, D.E.; Ikeda, H. Terpene synthases are widely distributed in bacteria. *Proc. Natl. Acad. Sci. USA* **2015**, *112*, 857–862. [CrossRef]
49. Zhang, Q.; Yu, Y.; Vélasquez, J.E.; Van Der Donk, W.A. Evolution of lanthipeptide synthetases. *Proc. Natl. Acad. Sci. USA* **2012**, *109*, 18361–18366. [CrossRef]
50. Repka, L.M.; Chekan, J.R.; Nair, S.K.; Van Der Donk, W.A. Mechanistic Understanding of Lanthipeptide Biosynthetic Enzymes. *Chem. Rev.* **2017**, *117*, 5457–5520. [CrossRef]
51. Jones, M.; Pinto, E.; Torres, M.; Dörr, F.; Mazur-Marzec, H.; Szubert, K.; Tartaglione, L.; Dell'Aversano, C.; Miles, C.; Beach, D.; et al. Comprehensive database of secondary metabolites from cyanobacteria. *Water Res.* **2021**, *196*, 117017. [CrossRef]
52. Martins, M.D.R.; Costa, M. Marine cyanobacteria compounds with anticancer properties: Implication of apoptosis. In *Handbook of Anticancer Drugs from Marine Origin*; Kim, S.-K., Ed.; Springer International Publishing: Cham, Switzerland, 2015; pp. 621–647, ISBN 9783319071459.
53. Engene, N.; Tronholm, A.; Salvador-Reyes, L.A.; Luesch, H.; Paul, V.J. Caldora penicillata gen. nov., comb. nov. (Cyanobacteria), a pantropical marine species with biomedical relevance. *J. Phycol.* **2015**, *51*, 670–681. [CrossRef]
54. Engene, N.; Paul, V.J.; Byrum, T.; Gerwick, W.H.; Thor, A.; Ellisman, M.H. Five chemically rich species of tropical marine cyanobacteria of the genus *Okeania* gen. nov. (Oscillatoriales, Cyanoprokaryota). *J. Phycol.* **2013**, *49*, 1095–1106. [CrossRef] [PubMed]
55. Thornburg, C.C.; Cowley, E.S.; Sikorska, J.; Shaala, L.A.; Ishmael, J.E.; Youssef, D.T.A.; McPhail, K.L. Apratoxin H and apratoxin A sulfoxide from the red sea cyanobacterium *Moorea producens*. *J. Nat. Prod.* **2013**, *76*, 1781–1788. [CrossRef]
56. Kwan, J.C.; Eksioglu, E.A.; Liu, C.; Paul, V.J.; Luesch, H. Grassystatins A-C from marine cyanobacteria, potent cathepsin E inhibitors that reduce antigen presentation. *J. Med. Chem.* **2009**, *52*, 5732–5747. [CrossRef]
57. Gunasekera, S.P.; Imperial, L.; Garst, C.; Ratnayake, R.; Dang, L.H.; Paul, V.J.; Luesch, H. Caldoramide, a Modified Pentapeptide from the Marine Cyanobacterium *Caldora penicillata*. *J. Nat. Prod.* **2016**, *79*, 1867–1871. [CrossRef]
58. Sueyoshi, K.; Kaneda, M.; Sumimoto, S.; Oishi, S.; Fujii, N.; Suenaga, K.; Teruya, T. Odoamide, a cytotoxic cyclodepsipeptide from the marine cyanobacterium *Okeania* sp. *Tetrahedron* **2016**, *72*, 5472–5478. [CrossRef]
59. Lopez, J.A.V.; Al-Lihaibi, S.S.; Alarif, W.M.; Abdel-Lateff, A.; Nogata, Y.; Washio, K.; Morikawa, M.; Okino, T. Wewakazole B, a Cytotoxic Cyanobactin from the Cyanobacterium *Moorea producens* Collected in the Red Sea. *J. Nat. Prod.* **2016**, *79*, 1213–1218. [CrossRef] [PubMed]
60. Mi, Y.; Zhang, J.; He, S.; Yan, X. New peptides isolated from marine cyanobacteria, an overview over the past decade. *Mar. Drugs* **2017**, *15*, 132. [CrossRef] [PubMed]
61. Rippka, R. Isolation and Purification of Cyanobacteria. *Methods Enzymol.* **1988**, *167*, 1–26.
62. Gkelis, S.; Panou, M. Capturing biodiversity: Linking a cyanobacteria culture collection to the "scratchpads" virtual research environment enhances biodiversity knowledge. *Biodivers. Data J.* **2016**, *4*, e7965-1. [CrossRef] [PubMed]
63. Jokela, J.; Heinilä, L.M.P.; Shishido, T.K.; Wahlsten, M.; Fewer, D.P.; Fiore, M.F.; Wang, H.; Haapaniemi, E.; Permi, P.; Sivonen, K. Production of high amounts of hepatotoxin nodularin and new protease inhibitors pseudospumigins by the brazilian benthic nostoc sp. CENA543. *Front. Microbiol.* **2017**, *8*, 1963. [CrossRef] [PubMed]
64. Brown, J.; Pirrung, M.; Mccue, L.A. FQC Dashboard: Integrates FastQC results into a web-based, interactive, and extensible FASTQ quality control tool. *Bioinformatics* **2017**, *33*, 3137–3139. [CrossRef] [PubMed]
65. Schmieder, R.; Edwards, R. Quality control and preprocessing of metagenomic datasets. *Bioinformatics* **2011**, *27*, 863–864. [CrossRef]
66. Bankevich, A.; Nurk, S.; Antipov, D.; Gurevich, A.A.; Dvorkin, M.; Kulikov, A.S.; Lesin, V.M.; Nikolenko, S.I.; Pham, S.; Prjibelski, A.D.; et al. SPAdes: A new genome assembly algorithm and its applications to single-cell sequencing. *J. Comput. Biol.* **2012**, *19*, 455–477. [CrossRef] [PubMed]
67. Kajitani, R.; Toshimoto, K.; Noguchi, H.; Toyoda, A.; Ogura, Y.; Okuno, M.; Yabana, M.; Harada, M.; Nagayasu, E.; Maruyama, H.; et al. Efficient de novo assembly of highly heterozygous genomes from whole-genome shotgun short reads. *Genome Res.* **2014**, *24*, 1384–1395. [CrossRef] [PubMed]
68. Wood, D.E.; Salzberg, S.L. *Kraken: Ultrafast Metagenomic Sequence Classification Using Exact Alignments*; BMC: Berlin/Heidelberg, Germany, 2014.
69. Alvarenga, D.O.; Fiore, M.F.; Varani, A.M. A metagenomic approach to cyanobacterial genomics. *Front. Microbiol.* **2017**, *8*, 809. [CrossRef] [PubMed]
70. Bradnam, K.R.; Fass, J.N.; Alexandrov, A.; Baranay, P.; Bechner, M.; Birol, I.; Boisvert, S.; Chapman, J.A.; Chapuis, G.; Chikhi, R.; et al. Assemblathon 2: Evaluating de novo methods of genome assembly in three vertebrate species. *Gigascience* **2013**, *2*, 10. [CrossRef]
71. Parks, D.H.; Imelfort, M.; Skennerton, C.T.; Hugenholtz, P.; Tyson, G.W. CheckM: Assessing the quality of microbial genomes recovered from isolates, single cells, and metagenomes. *Genome Res.* **2015**, *25*, 1043–1055. [CrossRef]
72. Chaumeil, P.A.; Mussig, A.J.; Hugenholtz, P.; Parks, D.H. GTDB-Tk: A toolkit to classify genomes with the genome taxonomy database. *Bioinformatics* **2020**, *36*, 1925–1927. [CrossRef]
73. Stamatakis, A. RAxML version 8: A tool for phylogenetic analysis and post-analysis of large phylogenies. *Bioinformatics* **2014**, *30*, 1312–1313. [CrossRef]

74. Darriba, D.; Taboada, G.L.; Doallo, R.; Posada, D. ProtTest 3: Fast selection of best-fit models of protein evolution. *Bioinformatics* **2011**, *27*, 1164–1165. [CrossRef]
75. Kumar, S.; Stecher, G.; Tamura, K. MEGA7: Molecular Evolutionary Genetics Analysis Version 7.0 for Bigger Datasets. *Mol. Biol. Evol.* **2016**, *33*, 1870–1874. [CrossRef] [PubMed]
76. Larkin, M.A.; Blackshields, G.; Brown, N.P.; Chenna, R.; Mcgettigan, P.A.; McWilliam, H.; Valentin, F.; Wallace, I.M.; Wilm, A.; Lopez, R.; et al. Clustal W and Clustal X version 2.0. *Bioinformatics* **2007**, *23*, 2947–2948. [CrossRef] [PubMed]
77. Posada, D. jModelTest: Phylogenetic model averaging. *Mol. Biol. Evol.* **2008**, *25*, 1253–1256. [CrossRef] [PubMed]
78. Ronquist, F.; Huelsenbeck, J.P. MrBayes 3: Bayesian phylogenetic inference under mixed models. *Bioinformatics* **2003**, *19*, 1572–1574. [CrossRef] [PubMed]
79. Clark, K.; Karsch-Mizrachi, I.; Lipman, D.J.; Ostell, J.; Sayers, E.W. GenBank. *Nucleic Acids Res.* **2016**, *44*, D67–D72. [CrossRef]
80. Seemann, T. Prokka: Rapid prokaryotic genome annotation. *Bioinformatics* **2014**, *30*, 2068–2069. [CrossRef] [PubMed]
81. Wu, S.; Zhu, Z.; Fu, L.; Niu, B.; Li, W. WebMGA: A customizable web server for fast metagenomic sequence analysis. *BMC Genom.* **2011**, *12*, 444. [CrossRef]
82. Arndt, D.; Grant, J.R.; Marcu, A.; Sajed, T.; Pon, A.; Liang, Y.; Wishart, D.S. PHASTER: A better, faster version of the PHAST phage search tool. *Nucleic Acids Res.* **2016**, *44*, W16–W21. [CrossRef]
83. Xie, Z.; Tang, H. ISEScan: Automated identification of insertion sequence elements in prokaryotic genomes. *Bioinformatics* **2017**, *33*, 3340–3347. [CrossRef]
84. Contreras-Moreira, B.; Vinuesa, P. GET_HOMOLOGUES, a versatile software package for scalable and robust microbial pangenome analysis. *Appl. Environ. Microbiol.* **2013**, *79*, 7696–7701. [CrossRef]
85. Blin, K.; Shaw, S.; Steinke, K.; Villebro, R.; Ziemert, N.; Lee, S.Y.; Medema, M.H.; Weber, T. AntiSMASH 5.0: Updates to the secondary metabolite genome mining pipeline. *Nucleic Acids Res.* **2019**, *47*, W81–W87. [CrossRef] [PubMed]

marine drugs

MDPI

Article

Metabolomic Characterization of a cf. *Neolyngbya* Cyanobacterium from the South China Sea Reveals Wenchangamide A, a Lipopeptide with In Vitro Apoptotic Potential in Colon Cancer Cells

Lijian Ding [1,2,†], Rinat Bar-Shalom [3,†], Dikla Aharonovich [2], Naoaki Kurisawa [4], Gaurav Patial [1], Shuang Li [1], Shan He [1], Xiaojun Yan [1], Arihiro Iwasaki [4,5], Kiyotake Suenaga [4,5], Chengcong Zhu [5], Haixi Luo [5], Fuli Tian [5], Fuad Fares [3], C. Benjamin Naman [1,5,*] and Tal Luzzatto-Knaan [2,*]

1. Li Dak Sum Yip Yio Chin Kenneth Li Marine Biopharmaceutical Research Center, Department of Marine Pharmacy, College of Food and Pharmaceutical Sciences, Ningbo University, Ningbo 315800, China; dinglijian@nbu.edu.cn (L.D.); gaurav.patial945@gmail.com (G.P.); lishuang9892@163.com (S.L.); heshan@nbu.edu.cn (S.H.); yanxiaojun@nbu.edu.cn (X.Y.)
2. Department of Marine Biology, Leon H. Charney School of Marine Sciences, University of Haifa, Haifa 31905, Israel; daharon1@univ.haifa.ac.il
3. Department of Human Biology, Faculty of Life Sciences, University of Haifa, Haifa 31905, Israel; rbar-shal@univ.haifa.ac.il (R.B.-S.); ffares@univ.haifa.ac.il (F.F.)
4. Department of Chemistry, Keio University, 3-14-1, Hiyoshi, Kohoku-ku, Yokohama, Kanagawa 223-8522, Japan; b8213011@gmail.com (N.K.); a.iwasaki@chem.keio.ac.jp (A.I.); suenaga@chem.keio.ac.jp (K.S.)
5. Key Laboratory of Medicinal and Edible Plant Resources of Hainan Province, Hainan Vocational University of Science and Technology, Haikou 571126, China; zhu1447262684@163.com (C.Z.); hluo@hvust.edu.cn (H.L.); ftian@imu.edu.cn (F.T.)

* Correspondence: bnaman@nbu.edu.cn (C.B.N.); tluzzatto@univ.haifa.ac.il (T.L.-K.)

† These authors contributed equally to the work.

Citation: Ding, L.; Bar-Shalom, R.; Aharonovich, D.; Kurisawa, N.; Patial, G.; Li, S.; He, S.; Yan, X.; Iwasaki, A.; Suenaga, K.; et al. Metabolomic Characterization of a cf. *Neolyngbya* Cyanobacterium from the South China Sea Reveals Wenchangamide A, a Lipopeptide with In Vitro Apoptotic Potential in Colon Cancer Cells. *Mar. Drugs* **2021**, *19*, 397. https://doi.org/10.3390/md19070397

Academic Editor: Max Crüsemann

Received: 2 May 2021
Accepted: 13 July 2021
Published: 16 July 2021

Abstract: Metabolomics can be used to study complex mixtures of natural products, or secondary metabolites, for many different purposes. One productive application of metabolomics that has emerged in recent years is the guiding direction for isolating molecules with structural novelty through analysis of untargeted LC-MS/MS data. The metabolomics-driven investigation and bioassay-guided fractionation of a biomass assemblage from the South China Sea dominated by a marine filamentous cyanobacteria, cf. *Neolyngbya* sp., has led to the discovery of a natural product in this study, wenchangamide A (**1**). Wenchangamide A was found to concentration-dependently cause fast-onset apoptosis in HCT116 human colon cancer cells in vitro (24 h IC_{50} = 38 μM). Untargeted metabolomics, by way of MS/MS molecular networking, was used further to generate a structural proposal for a new natural product analogue of **1**, here coined wenchangamide B, which was present in the organic extract and bioactive sub-fractions of the biomass examined. The wenchangamides are of interest for anticancer drug discovery, and the characterization of these molecules will facilitate the future discovery of related natural products and development of synthetic analogues.

Keywords: metabolomics; secondary metabolites; natural products; cyanobacteria; *Neolyngbya*; anticancer; drug discovery; South China Sea; wenchangamide

1. Introduction

Cyanobacteria have been shown to be prolific producers of structurally diverse natural products with a wide range of ecological and pharmacological activities [1–3]. Many discovered marine natural products have gone through clinical trials and even been accepted by regulatory agencies as drugs, and these include several antibody-drug conjugates that use a dolastatin/symplostatin marine cyanobacterium natural product derivative as an anti-cancer "warhead" [4]. Other cyanobacterial natural products have been advanced in anticancer drug discovery programs at the preclinical stage by means of total synthesis, medicinal chemistry analogue development, and pharmacological characterization of their mechanisms of action. Some notable lead molecules from cyanobacteria include the apratoxins, carmaphycins, coibamides, curacins, and largazoles, among others [1–3]. It is generally understood that the secondary metabolism of cyanobacteria, while energetically taxing, must serve some (often unknown) ecological function for the organisms. This has been demonstrated in a few specific cases, e.g., in the upregulation of microcystins production by some cyanobacteria in response to predation by grazers [5,6]. Filamentous cyanobacteria have also been reported to contain genetic information for biosynthesis of natural products comprising up to 20% of the genome, and even surpassing that in the example of some *Moorena* species, further supporting the importance to the organisms of this biosynthetic capacity on an evolutionary time scale [7]. However, it can be quite challenging to obtain or maintain filamentous cyanobacteria in axenic laboratory cultures, as well as perform molecular biology experiments with them [8]. A number of laboratory culture conditions is also understood to greatly impact not only the growth and survival of cyanobacteria, but also the associated natural product biosynthesis [9]. Accordingly, a majority of natural product chemicals reported historically from these organisms have come from larger environmental collections, or assemblages. A meta-analysis of all secondary metabolites reported from marine and microbial sources between 1941 and 2015 revealed that the chemistry of these samples is relatively source-specific, with the majority of cyanobacterial natural products being structurally dissimilar from those of all other producers examined [10].

The taxonomy of many documented filamentous cyanobacteria has come into question in the post-genomics era, and this is especially true for the *Lyngbya*-like and *Phormidium*-like morphotype [11–13]. For example, *Phormidium* is formally accepted as a part of the family *Oscillatoriaceae*, but it still appears in some literature reports and databases under *Phormidiaceae* (the *Phormidium*-like family) following previous taxonomic assignment and reclassification [14,15]. The genus *Phormidium* once comprised some 200 species; however, about 90% of these organisms have been redistributed into other genera, such as *Lyngbya*, and even different families in the order Oscillatoriales, including both *Oscillatoriaceae* and *Phormidiaceae*, after molecular characterization studies in recent years [16–18]. The members of genus *Lyngbya* have also been re-evaluated and revised several times [14]. After molecular characterization, several newly formed genera have emerged for organisms previously described as members of *Lyngbya*, notably including *Leptolyngbya*, *Moorena*, and *Okeania* [12,13,19,20]. More recently, the new genus *Neolyngbya* has also been created for several newly described *Lyngbya*-like organisms [21]. Despite having a reported biotechnological potential for drug discovery and development, only one new natural product has yet been reported from assemblages with *Neolyngbya*, namely the neurotoxic sesquiterpenoid eudesmacarbonate [22,23]. *Neolyngbya* organisms have not been previously reported in the South China Sea. Meanwhile, the South China Sea is home to a vastly understudied biodiversity of marine filamentous cyanobacteria [24,25]. This biodiversity resource has been largely under-examined, especially when compared to the vast chemical study of other types of microorganisms in China (actinomycetes, fungi, etc.) [26].

Metabolomics is useful for the large-scale analysis of molecules within a biological sample [27]. In recent years, this field has taken a central role in many natural product research programs, especially for studying the chemical space and diversity using both untargeted and targeted metabolomics [28]. Untargeted metabolomics allows for the generation of a broad overview of the chemical diversity in even a complex extract. This can also be used for the comparative analysis of multiple samples, or various treatment conditions, to identify potential characteristic and chemical markers. In contrast, targeted metabolomics is useful when the focus can be specified to a single compound of interest or a set of pre-determined molecules for further qualitative and quantitative analysis. Mass spectrometry-based metabolomics in the past decade has shown immense utility in the field of natural product discovery, and has yielded major impacts, mainly because of the accuracy, sensitivity, speed, and robustness of these methods, along with newly developed cutting-edge downstream platforms for data analysis [29–36]. These platforms have been made to provide structural information based on the fragmentation patterns of each molecule, allowing for the comparison of each with other known and unknown compounds in spectrometric libraries, natural product databases, and public or private collections of raw data. Altogether, this has facilitated the characterization of putative structures based on a similarity between the fragmentation of different compounds, minimized the rediscovery of known structures by virtual dereplication, and allowed for a more efficient discovery of new natural products and new chemical scaffolds prior to the isolation and characterization effort [29–36].

In this study, a metabolomics-based approach was used to explore the chemistry of a cf. *Neolyngbya* sp. environmental collection and characterize novel natural product chemistry. Moreover, the concurrent bioactivity-guided fractionation of this extract was expected to yield pure compounds produced with potential anti-cancer effects, as evaluated in vitro using an immortalized colorectal cancer cell line. Reported herein is the chemical and biological exploration of an environmental collection from the South China Sea that is dominated by a marine filamentous cyanobacteria, cf. *Neolyngbya* sp. This report details the characterization of the microbiome, metabolome, and associated pharmacology that allowed for the directed isolation of a new bioactive natural product, wenchangamide A (**1**; Figure 1). The structure elucidation and investigation of this molecule as a potential anticancer drug lead is also described, along with the expansion of this class of compound to include a new proposed bioactive analogue based on available metabolomics and bioassay testing data.

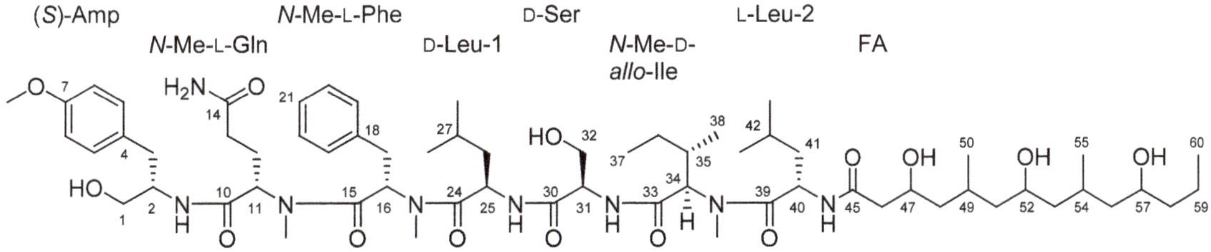

Figure 1. Structure and numbering scheme of wenchangamide A (**1**).

2. Results and Discussion

2.1. Sample Evaluation

An environmental sample of marine filamentous cyanobacteria, HAINAN-19SEP17-3, was collected near Wenchang, Hainan, China. Based on colonial morphology and light microscopy, the sample was initially classified as cf. *Neolyngbya* sp. (Figure 2). To validate this and determine the microbiome composition, a portion of the sample was analyzed by 16S rRNA gene sequencing using universal PCR primers, and this further supported the genetic identity of the predominant biomass as cyanobacteria categorized under *Phormidiaceae* (57%; certainly includes basionyms in *Oscillatoriaceae*) along with additional associated microbes from *Bacteroidetes* (22%), *Proteobacteria* (14%), and others at a lower abundance (Figure 2). The higher taxonomic order Oscillatoriales is presented for the majority of the cyanobacterial 16S gene sequence data in Figure 2 to avoid confounding basionyms that occur within its members, i.e., parts of the families *Oscillatoriaceae* and *Phormidiaceae*. The 16S gene sequence V3-V4 amplicon of the organism that dominates this consortium was found to clade with *Neolyngbya*. *Neolyngbya* is a recently described genus of the family *Oscillatoriaceae*, and was established from the *Lyngbya*-like morphotype that has historically also been a misclassification for some *Phormidium* organisms [16,17,21]. There is great difficulty in growing axenic cultures of cyanobacteria; therefore, it is important to refer to the collected consortia as a whole. While several studies demonstrated that the microbiome of cyanobacteria is relatively stable between environmental samples and non-axenic cultures (mainly *Proteobacteria* and *Bacteroidetes*) [37], little is known about the microbiome associated with *Lyngbya*-like and *Phormidium*-like organisms [38].

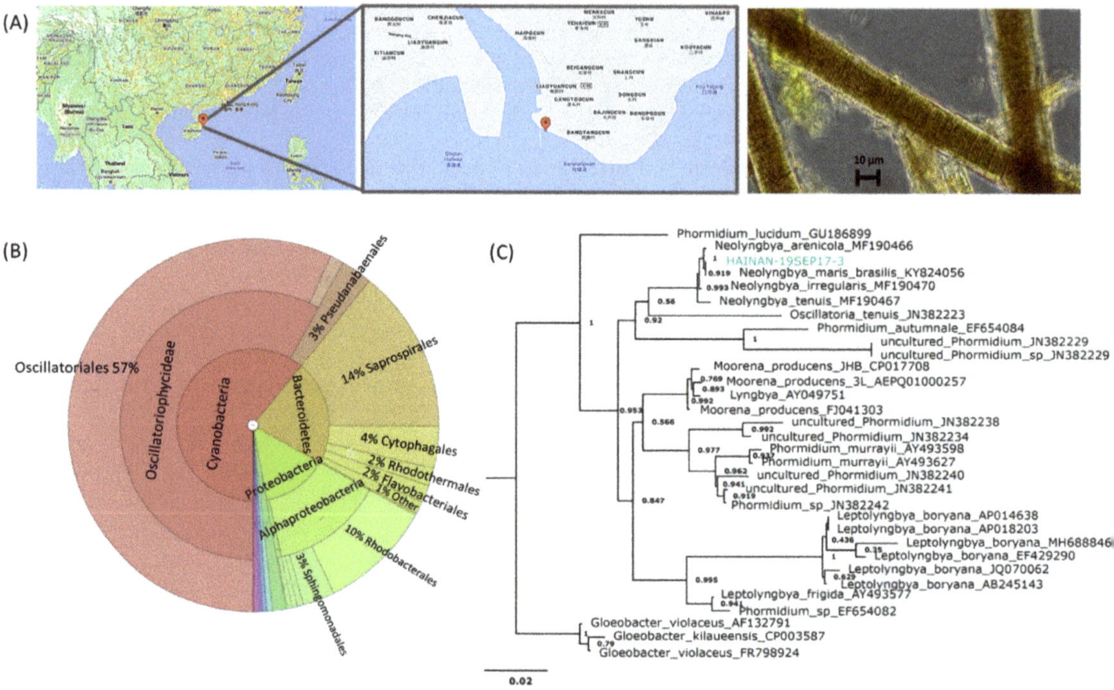

Figure 2. Sample information. (**A**) Collection site and morphology of HAINAN-19SEP17-3. (**B**) Microbiome analysis; the order Oscillatoriales contains the families *Oscillatoriaceae* and *Phormidiaceae*, and this higher taxonomy is presented here to avoid confounding basionyms within these two. (**C**) Phylogeny of the environmental assemblage dominated by cf. *Neolyngbya* sp. from the South China Sea that was evaluated in this study. Map generated with Google Earth. Taxonomy and phylogeny were evaluated using Silva and EMBL-EBI databases. *Gleobacter* was used as the outgroup.

An LC-MS/MS untargeted metabolomic approach [28] was utilized to overview the chemical potential of the prioritized South China Sea cf. *Neolyngbya* sp. sample. Feature detection and annotation analyses were done using the Global Natural Products Social (GNPS) Molecular Networking platform. This method aligns the fragmentation patterns obtained by MS/MS against various spectrometric databases and allows for the putative annotation of structural characteristics and chemical classifications [33,36]. Nearly 750 molecular features were present in the initial evaluation of this sample; however, reported cyanobacterial specialized metabolites were not able to be detected. Some common pigments (mainly chlorophylls and breakdown products thereof) were annotated in the dataset. Together, these data highlighted the potential for discovery of novel compounds and, at the same time, allowed ubiquitous pigment molecules to be avoided in the isolation procedure. Furthermore, most of the chemistry had no match to any known structure in the spectrometric libraries (84%), yet some had putative annotations to general chemical classes (5 super-classes; Figure 3A), based on the associated fragmentation patterns. The subset of classified molecules were further delineated into 19 putative chemical subclasses (Figure 3B) that highlight the chemical diversity and discovery potential of this complex extract. The main prevalent classes that were detected and annotated include peptides

(42%) and terpenoids (17%). Though databases on such molecules are largely incomplete, or hard to access, these molecular families are known to contain many types of bioactive natural products [39–41]. Nonribosomal peptides are a diverse group of natural products that have complex chemical structures and a vast array of bioactivity potentials as anti-cancer, anti-parasitic, anti-fungal, and cytotoxic agents, protease inhibitors and more [39]. The structures of natural products resulting from non-ribosomal peptide synthetase (NRPS) biosynthesis can be linear or cyclic, possess typical and/or unusual amino acids, and may even be hybridized with modules from polyketide synthase (PKS) genes. NRPS and PKS biosynthetic gene clusters are mostly common in bacteria, and many such hybridized biosynthetic mechanisms have been uniquely found in cyanobacteria or are rarely described from other organisms [39,42]. The metabolomic annotation of unknown peptides, depsipeptides and derivatives from the cyanobacteria sample here studied was accordingly encouraging for the potential to discover new bioactive molecules.

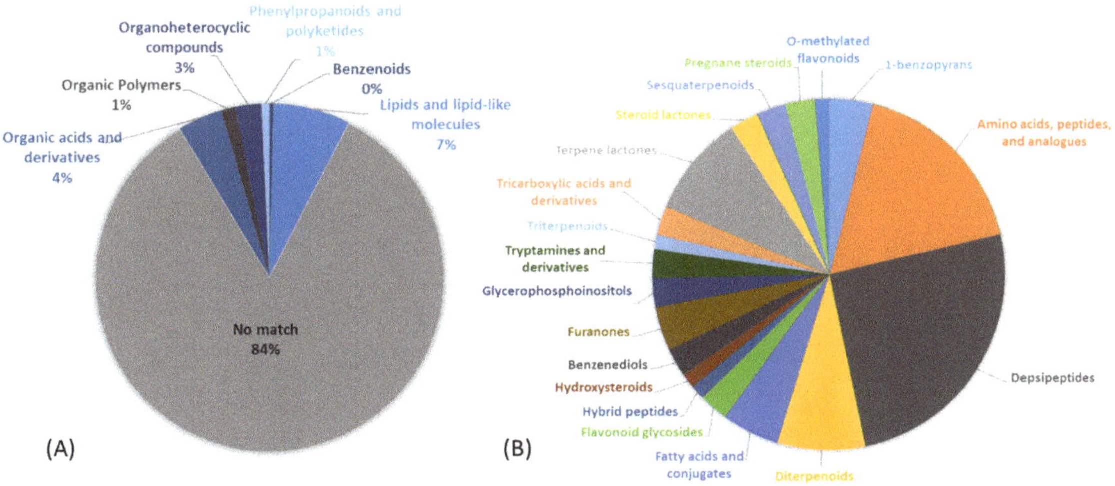

Figure 3. Chemical space of the organic extract of cf. *Neolyngbya* sp. HAINAN-19SEP17-3 as evaluated by data-dependent LC-MS/MS. Samples were analyzed via the GNPS platform using NAP, Dereplicator and MolNetEnhancer workflows to yield putative annotations of (**A**) SuperClasses and (**B**) SubClasses of annotated molecular features based on observed fragmentation patterns.

2.2. Inhibition Activity on Human Colon Cancer Cells In Vitro

The inhibitory effect of the organic extract and fractions of cf. *Neolyngbya* sp. HAINAN-19SEP17-3 were evaluated using HCT116 human colorectal cancer cells (Figure S23A). This allowed for the targeted discovery of new bioactive natural products akin to a published method [43]. Cells were treated for 24 h and analyzed using an XTT cell viability assay to detect fast-acting fractions and compound constituents [44]. It is understood that extended duration exposure (e.g., to 48 or 72 h) will typically increase the observed efficacy or potency of cytotoxicity due to the relatively prolonged accumulation of dead cells. While the crude extract was not cytotoxic at the concentrations tested (200 and 400 μg/mL) in this 24 h experiment, fraction C demonstrated high potency (94–97% mortality) in treated cells versus untreated at both concentrations tested (Figure S23A). After further separation into 6 sub-fractions, a more marked concentration-dependent activity was observed for C3 (Figure S23B). Additional chromatography yielded sub-fractions that were also shown to act concentration-dependently, i.e., C3–5 and C3–7 (Figure S24). While the active fraction C3–7 was observed to be an impure mixture of compounds, fraction C3–5 was found to be a pure molecule (**1**) that was active in this in vitro test model (24 h IC_{50} = 38 μM), and noticeably active even after only 8 h of treatment (Figure S25). This sample was thus evaluated further.

To clarify the cell viability decrease following 24 h treatment with C3 and **1** (30 μg/mL), cell cycle distribution analysis was examined. A FACS analysis demonstrated that treatment with C3 and **1** resulted in the accumulation of cells in the sub-G1 phase of the cell cycle at 3.9% and 12.4%, respectively, compared to 2.2% in the untreated (control) cells (Figure 4A). Furthermore, the cells were observed to be accumulating at the G2/M phase following treatment with **1** (34.7% vs. 26.2% in the control), indicating suppression of cell proliferation. Normal, non-cancerous colon cell lines are unavailable. However, the same pattern of cell cycle arrest was not observed when the samples were tested in normal human dermal fibroblasts (NHDF; Figure 4B).

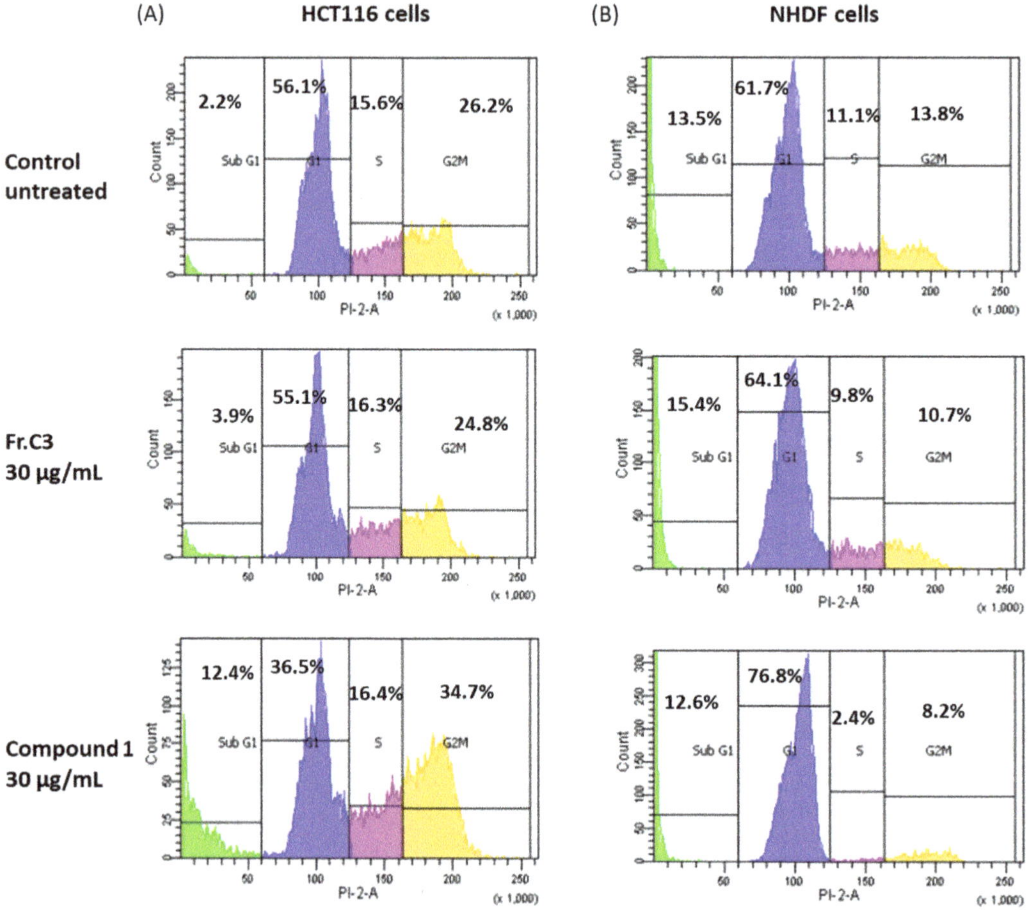

Figure 4. In vitro effects of fraction C3 and compound **1** on cell cycle progression after 24 h treatment. Distribution of (**A**) HCT116 human colon cancer cells and (**B**) NHDF normal human dermal fibroblasts at the different cell cycle phases as determined by FACS.

The cell cycle arrest at the G2/M phase accompanied by an accumulation in the sub-G1 phase observed due to treatment with C3 or **1** is suggestive of apoptotic cell death, since this has been reported previously for human colon cancer cells [45]. In order to confirm this hypothesis, HCT116 cells were treated with 30 μg/mL C3 or **1** for 24 h, stained with FITC labeled Annexin-V and PI, and analyzed by flow cytometry (Figure 5A). The results indicated an increase of approximately 4.4% in apoptotic cells (Q2 + Q4) following treatment with C3, and about 11.3% after exposure to **1**. Annexin/PI double staining analysis of NHDF cells in vitro showed a similar increase in accumulation of apoptotic cells after treatment with fraction C3, of about 4.8%, but a much smaller increase following treatment with compound **1**, of about 1.3%, in comparison to untreated cells (Figure 5B).

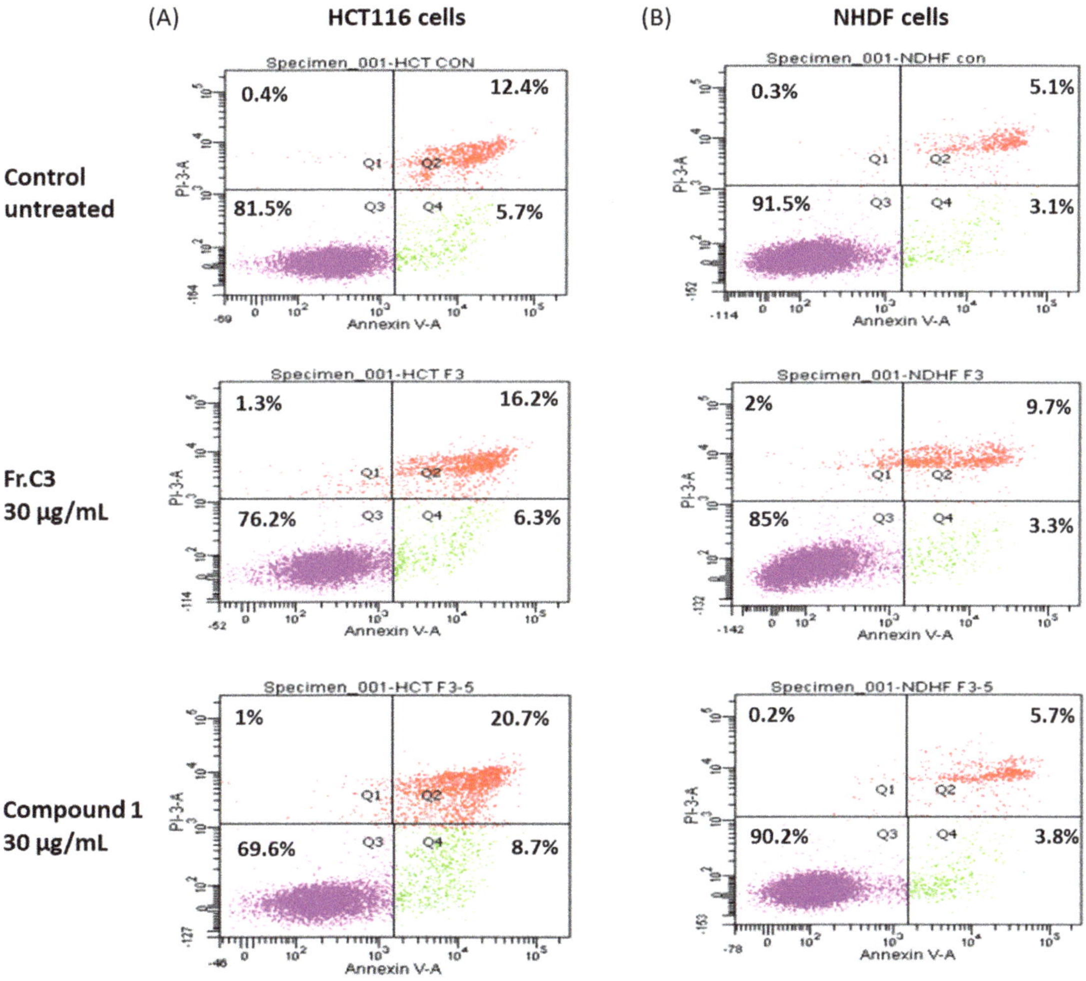

Figure 5. Annexin-V/PI double staining and flow cytometry evaluation of mechanistic in vitro cytotoxicity of fraction C3 and compound **1** after 24 h treatment of (**A**) HCT116 human colon cancer cells and (**B**) NHDF normal human dermal fibroblasts. For each plot, the lower left quadrant (Q3) represents viable cells, the upper left quadrant (Q1) indicates necrotic cells, the lower right quadrant (Q4) denotes early apoptotic cells, and the upper right quadrant (Q2) represents necrotic or late apoptotic cells.

2.3. Natural Product Structure Elucidation

Compound **1** was obtained as a white powder and assigned the molecular formula $C_{64}H_{106}N_8O_{14}$ based on a sodium adduct peak in the HRESIMS spectrum at *m/z* 1233.7748 $[M + Na]^+$ (calcd. for $C_{64}H_{106}N_8O_{14}Na^+$, 1233.7721). This formula indicated that **1** possessed 16 degrees of unsaturation. The ^{1}H and ^{13}C NMR data of **1** (Table 1) were suggestive of a lipopeptide scaffold with seven sets of signals characteristic of amino acid α protons, as well as two aromatic rings, two oxygenated methylenes, three oxygenated methines, one methoxy and three *N*-methyl groups, along with many alkyl moieties and eight amide carbonyls. The region measured from δ_H 3.8 to 4.9 ppm had sufficient peak resolution to nucleate seven amino acid and derivative substructures that were able to be constructed using 1D and 2D NMR data. For example, an "α proton" signal at δ_H 3.91 (H-2) was connected to a carbon at δ_C 52.4 (C-2) with the evidence of a peak in the ^{1}H-^{13}C HSQC spectrum. After examination of the ^{1}H-^{1}H COSY spectrum and HSQC data, this methine was determined to be adjacent to an oxygenated methylene group, CH_2-1 (δ_C 62.7, δ_H 3.35), and a benzylic methylene group, CH_2-3 (δ_C 35.6, δ_H 2.77 and 2.53). The assignment of the aromatic ring connected to C-3 was completed by further inclusion of long-range coupling data obtained from the ^{1}H-^{13}C HMBC spectrum. As shown in Figure 6, this *para*-methoxy-substituted phenyl group was characterized by correlations observed between H_2-3 and C-5/9, H-5/9 and C-7, H_3-7-*O*-Me and C-7, as well as H-6/8 and C-4. The planar structure of this subunit was thus established as 2-amino-3-(4-methoxyphenyl)propan-1-ol; "Amp".

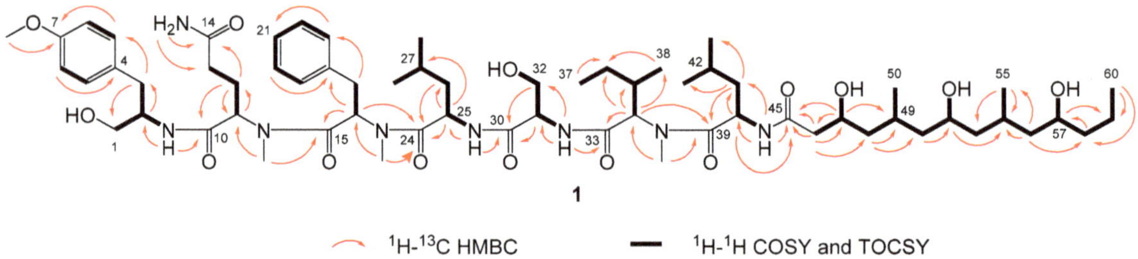

Figure 6. Selected correlations used to determine the planar structure of wenchangamide A (**1**). Red single-sided arrows represent cross peaks from the ^{1}H-^{13}C HMBC spectrum. Black bolded bonds show protons correlated in the ^{1}H-^{1}H COSY and TOCSY spectra.

Much of the remaining NMR data for **1** could be further assigned to a series of standard or *N*-methyl amino acid residues that were determined by similar methods as for the Amp group, including two Ile residues, an *N*-Me-Gln, *N*-Me-Phe, *N*-Me-Ile, and Ser. Several of the aliphatic groups had partially overlapping signals in the ^{1}H NMR spectrum, e.g., H_2-12 (δ_H 1.97 and 1.61) and H-42 (δ_H 1.61), as well as H_2-13 (δ_H 1.90 and 1.83) and H-35 (δ_H 1.9), which complicated their assignment using NMR data from the COSY or even ^{1}H-^{1}H TOCSY spectra. However, these groups were differentiated and assigned conclusively by the resolution of their corresponding signals in the HSQC and HSQC-TOCSY spectra, e.g., C-12 (δ_C 23.8) and C-42 (δ_C 24.3), as well as C-13 (δ_C 31.3) and C-35 (δ_C 32.6). Since the signals from TOCSY and HSQC-TOCSY result from extended or even complete ^{1}H-^{1}H spin system couplings, the signals observed from the well-resolved region (δ_H 3.8 to 4.9 ppm) in the f2 dimension were sufficient to support the assignment of the structural subunits described above. Each of the three *N*-methyl groups was able to be assigned to a defined amino acid residue based on correlations observed in the HMBC spectrum, i.e., from H_3-11-*N*-Me (δ_H 2.42) to C-11 (δ_C 56.0), H_3-16-*N*-Me (δ_H 2.89) to C-16 (δ_C 54.0), and H_3-34 *N*-Me (δ_H 2.94) to C-34 (δ_C 59.9). Amide NH protons were similarly able to be assigned by correlations observed in the COSY and TOCSY spectra, i.e., from 2-NH (δ_H 7.27) to H-2, 25-NH (δ_H 8.04) to H-25 (δ_H 4.49), 31-NH (δ_H 7.53) to H-31 (δ_H 4.23), and 40 NH (δ_H 8.15) to H-40 (δ_H 4.72). As further shown in Figure 6, the sequence of amide or "peptide" bonds was able to be deduced from the HMBC correlations observed between *N*-Me, NH, and "α proton" signals to the carbonyl of the adjacent residue. The sequence order of these structural subunits was further supported by characteristic amide bond "y" fragmentation masses that were detected in the MS/MS spectrum of **1** (Figure 7).

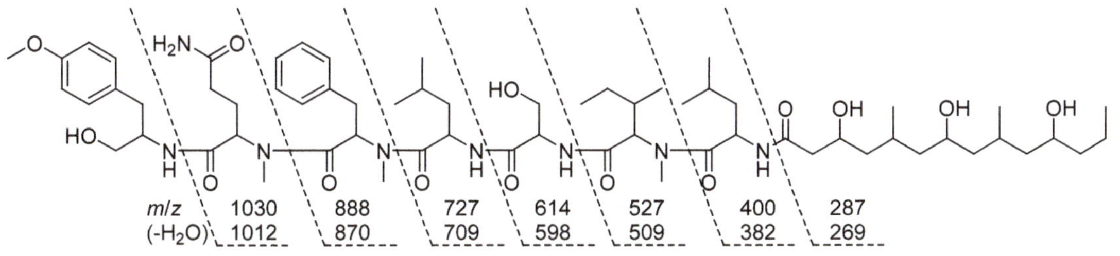

Figure 7. Selected MS/MS fragmentation ions observed that supported the amino acid and derivative residue sequence in the planar structure of wenchangamide A (**1**).

All of the NMR data that remained unassigned was proposed to result from a polyhydroxylated fatty acid moiety (FA), since this corresponded to three oxygenated methines, six downfield methylenes, and three alkyl methyl groups and one carbonyl. Due to diagnostic HMBC correlations from both H-40 and 40-NH to the remaining unassigned carbonyl (δ_C 171.0; C-45), the attachment point for this structural subunit was able to be assigned to the nitrogen of the Leu-2 residue. Further HMBC correlations to C-45 were observed from a deshielded methylene (δ_H 2.22 and 2.13, δ_C 43.8; CH_2-46) and a more deshielded, oxygenated, methine (δ_H 3.87, δ_C 65.7; CH-47). This allowed for the generation of a growing alkyl carbon chain that was able to be extended by COSY correlations, i.e., from CH-47 to CH_2-48 (δ_H 1.23 and 0.92) and then CH-49 (δ_H 1.76), as well as signals in the HMBC spectrum, including from H_2-46 to C-48 (δ_C 45.2) and H-47 to C-49 (δ_C 25.6). CH-49 was connected to and had a COSY correlation with a methyl group (δ_H 0.82, δ_C 20.3; CH_3-50). This PKS-like subunit, –CH_2–(CH–OH)–CH_2–(CH–CH_3)–, was found to repeat two more times in the linear alkyl chain of the FA moiety, and terminated the molecule with an alkyl methyl group (δ_H 0.85, δ_C 14.2; CH_3-60) adjacent to a penultimate methylene unit (δ_H 1.35 and 1.26, δ_C 18.6; CH_2-59). In sum, this yielded the planar structure of **1** as shown in Figure 6. Compound **1** is a new natural product, here assigned the trivial name wenchangamide A due to the location of the geographical collection site that yielded this discovery.

The structure of **1** has many features that resemble minnamide A, a cyanobacterial natural product recently reported from a sample of *Okeania hirsuta* that was collected in Minna island, Okinawa Prefecture, Japan [46]. However, noteworthy differences in the structures (Figure 8) include a different length polypeptide core scaffold, where minnamide A has an *N*-Me-Val–Ser–*N*-Me-Val moiety instead of the *N*-Me-Phe group present in **1**, as well as a longer fatty acid tail that contains an additional PKS-like repeating unit described above (repeats 3x in **1** and 4x in minnamide A). Accordingly, the molecular weight of minnamide A is 238 Da higher than that of **1**, and these molecules have significantly different MS/MS spectra due to the multiple structural differences. However, the hydrolysis of an aliquot of **1**, and subsequent analysis by chiral HPLC along with standard compounds, supported the assignment of the same configuration for all shared amino acid residues and derivatives from minnamide A, specifically (*S*)-Amp, *N*-Me-L-Gln, D-Leu-1, D-Ser, *N*-Me-D-*allo*-Ile, and L-Leu-2. Comparison of the NMR data obtained for **1** in pyridine-*d*5 (see Supplementary Table S1) with published values for minnamide further supported these assignments [46]. The *N*-Me-Phe residue (present in **1** and absent in minnamide A) was determined to be that of the L form by the same protocol. It is hypothesized that the configuration of the repeating PKS-like subunits of the fatty acid chain in **1** match with those reported for minnamide A; however, this has not been established empirically in the present study. In total, this information was used to assign the absolute configuration of the peptide core scaffold of **1** as presented in Figures 1 and 8.

Table 1. ^{1}H and ^{13}C NMR Spectroscopic Data for **1** in DMSO-d_6 [a,b].

Moiety	Position	δ_C	Type	δ_H, Mult (*J* in Hz)	Moiety	Position	δ_C	Type	δ_H, Mult (*J* in Hz)
AMP	1	62.7	CH_2	3.35, m [c]	*N*-Me-Ile	33	169.4	C	
	2	52.4	CH	3.91, ddd (9.4, 5.1, 4.9)		34	59.9	CH	4.67, d (10.7)
	3	35.6	CH_2	2.77, dd (14.0, 5.1); 2.53, dd (14.0, 4.9)		35	32.6	CH	1.9, m [c]
	4	130.9	C			36	25.5	CH_2	1.35, m [c]; 0.99, m
	5, 9	130.0	CH	7.04, d (8.6)		37	11.3	CH_3	0.81, m [c]
	6, 8	113.5	CH	6.79, d (8.6)		38	14.6	CH_3	0.68, d (6.7)
	7	157.6	C			34-*N*-Me	30.5	CH_3	2.94, s
	7-*O*-Me	55.0 [c]	CH_3	3.71, s					
	2-NH			7.27, m [c]	Leu-2	39	173.0	C	
						40	47.4	CH	4.72, m
N-Me-Gln	10	169.2	C			41	40.5	CH_2	1.46, m [c]; 1.35, m [c]
	11	56.0	CH	4.84, dd (5.1, 10.4) [c]		42	24.3	CH	1.61, m [c]
	12	23.8	CH_2	1.97, m; 1.61, m [c]		43	23.1	CH_3	0.87, d (6.6) [c]
	13	31.3	CH_2	1.90, m [c]; 1.83, m [c]		44	21.5	CH_3	0.87, d (6.6) [c]
	14	173.7	C			40-NH			8.15, d (7.8)
	14-NH_2			7.28, m [c]; 6.71, br s					
	11-*N*-Me	29.8	CH_3	2.42, s	FA	45	171.0	C	
						46	43.8	CH_2	2.22, dd (14.0, 5.4)
N-Me-Phe	15	170.3	C						2.13, dd (14.0, 7.4)
	16	54.0	CH	5.62, dd (10.0, 5.9)		47	65.7	CH	3.87, m
	17	34.6	CH_2	2.99 m; 2.94 m		48	45.2	CH_2	1.23, m; 0.92, m [c]
	18	137.3	C			49	25.6	CH	1.76, m
	19, 23	129.5	CH	7.26, m		50	20.3	CH_3	0.82, d (6.7)
	20, 22	128.0	CH	7.23, m		51	45.3	CH_2	1.35, m [c]; 0.92, m [c]
	21	126.3	CH	7.17, t (6.7)		52	64.9	CH	3.55, m
	16-*N*-Me	30.1	CH_3	2.89, s		53	46.7	CH_2	1.26, m [c]; 1.04, m
						54	25.3	CH	1.83, m [c]
Leu-1	24	171.4	C			55	19.2	CH_3	0.81, d (6.6) [c]
	25	46.9	CH	4.49, m		56	45.7	CH_2	1.25 m [c]; 1.02 m [c]
	26	39.7 [c]	CH_2	0.95, m; 0.73, m		57	67.0	CH	3.46, m [c]
	27	23.7	CH	1.12, m		58	40.4	CH_2	1.46, m [c]; 1.26, m [c]
	28	23.0	CH_3	0.70, d (6.7)		59	18.6	CH_2	1.35, m [c]; 1.26, m [c]
	29	21.7	CH_3	0.69, d (6.7)		60	14.2	CH_2	0.85, t (6.8)
	25-NH			8.04, d (7.9)		47-OH			4.53, m
						52-OH			4.11, br s
Ser	30	170.0	C			57-OH			4.17, br s
	31	55.0 [c]	CH	4.23, dt (7.8, 5.7)					
	32	61.6	CH_2	3.43, m [c]					
	31-NH			7.53, d (7.8)					
	32-OH			4.84, m [c]					

[a] Data recorded at 298 K, 600 MHz (^{1}H) and 150 MHz (^{13}C). [b] Assignments supported by 2D NMR. [c] Signal partially overlapped.

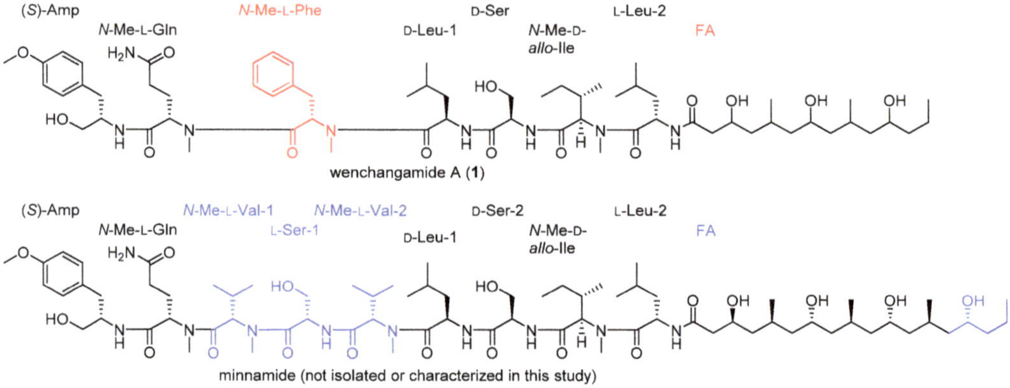

Figure 8. Structural comparison of wenchangamide A (**1**) and minnamide. Shared structural motifs are drawn in black. Differences in **1** are highlighted in red. Differences in minnamide are highlighted in blue. Configurations from the shared part of the FA residue in **1** are hypothesized to match those of minnamide.

2.4. Additional Structure Hypothesis Generation

The GNPS-produced LC-MS/MS molecular network highlights molecules with a potential structural similarity as "molecular families", based on fragmentation patterns. The cluster that contained wenchangamide A (**1**) suggested the presence of further analogue molecules in the extract. One of these compounds presented an *m/z* value of 1297, which is 86 Da higher than that of **1** in the same experiment. Upon closer examination of the MS/MS spectra and fragmentation ions related to the "y" ions produced from amide bond backbone cleavages, it was determined that the entire difference of 86 Da between the *m/z* 1297 molecule and **1** was located on the FA residue. Since this same mass difference corresponds to one additional repeating unit of a PKS-like moiety present 3x in **1**, akin to the 4x in minnamide A, the corresponding "hybrid" molecule, wenchangamide B, is here hypothesized (Figure 9). While the structure of this molecule contains the same FA moiety from minnamide A, it has the same polypeptide core as **1**, and is accordingly assigned the trivial name, wenchangamide B. Although fragmentation data from mass spectrometry cannot distinguish between configurational isomers of peptides, and even some constitutional isomers (e.g., Ile, Leu, and *N*-Me-Val), the structure of wenchangamide B is proposed as drawn, based on biosynthetic logic. This molecule was not able to be isolated in pure form in sufficient quantity for empirical structural characterization in this study, and is suggested for targeted isolation, structure elucidation, and more accurate pharmacological characterization in future research. This strategy of structure proposal based on MS/MS fragmentation analysis and molecular networking for compounds beyond isolation in the initial study, later followed by targeted isolation or synthesis for confirmation and structure-activity relationship (SAR) study, has been recently exemplified by Gerwick, Luesch, and coworkers in the expansion of the cyanobacterial natural product family of doscadenamides [47–49].

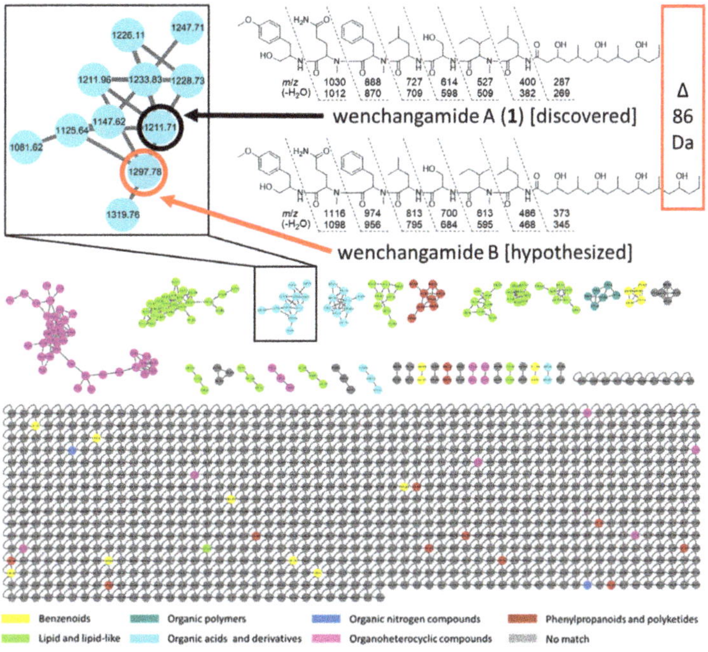

Figure 9. GNPS-based LC-MS/MS molecular network analysis of fraction C3 and active sub-fractions. Enlarged network highlights the structural similarity based on MS/MS fragmentation patterns of the discovered molecule **1** (wenchangamide A; node circled in black) and the proposed analogue (wenchangamide B; circled in red).

The reported activities of minnamide and **1** have been demonstrated in discrete cell lines, with different conditions, and using alternative temporal end points for measurement. In terms of activity, minnamide A was reported to be a potent inhibitor of HeLa cells that led to necrosis in a 72 h incubation assay (IC_{50} 0.17 μM); it was also suggested to act via the generation of lipid ROS facilitated by specific metal ions including copper and manganese [46]. Wenchangamide B remains of particular interest because the parent subfraction (C3-7) was here found to inhibit HCT116 cells in vitro (Figure S24). Future research on new natural products and synthetic analogues may contribute relatable SAR data for the growing class of cytotoxic minnamide and wenchangamide lipopeptides.

3. Materials and Methods

3.1. General Experimental Procedures

Analytical separations were performed on a Waters ACQUITY UPLC instrument employing a UPLC Kinetex C18 column (1.7 μm, 2.1 × 50 mm, Phenomenex) and an HPLC Kinetex C18 column (5 μm, 5 × 250 mm, Phenomenex), respectively, combined with a Waters 2998 photodiode array detector (PDA) (Waters, Milford, MA, USA). Medium pressure liquid chromatography (MPLC) was carried out on a Biotage-Isolera One system (SE-751 03 Uppsala, Sweden) equipped with a YMC-Pack ODS-A column (500 mm × 50 mm, 50 μm, YMC, Tokyo, Japan). All LC/MS data were obtained on a Phenomenex Kinetex C18 analytical column (1.7 μm, 2.1 × 50 mm, Phenomenex) using an Agilent HPLC equipped with a Bruker Maxis impact QTOF system mass spectrometer. Chromatographic analyses for configuration analysis were performed using an HPLC system consisting of a pump (model PU-2080, JASCO, Easton, MD, USA) and a UV detector (model UV-2075, JASCO). The NMR data were recorded using standard pulse programs on a Bruker AVANCE NEO 600 spectrometer equipped with a 5 mm inverse detection triple resonance (H-P/C/N-D) QCI 600S3 cryoprobe, capable of applying z-gradients. The chemical shifts were calibrated relative to the residual solvent peak in DMSO-d_6 (δ_H 2.50 and δ_C 39.52). High-resolution electrospray ionization mass spectra (HRESIMS) were measured on an Agilent (Santa Clara, CA, USA) 6545 Q-TOF instrument. Optical rotations were measured with a JASCO P-2000 automatic polarimeter.

3.2. Cyanobacterial Collection and Taxonomy

The biomass of the environmental sample of marine filamentous cyanobacteria used in this research was collected by hand by several of the co-authors on 17 September 2019 from the intertidal zone (0–2 m deep water) near Bangtang Bay, Wenchang District, Hainan Province, China (N 19°31′43.9″, E 110°51′02.7″). A voucher specimen for this organism was encoded as HAINAN-19SEP17-3 and deposited in the repository of the Department of Marine Pharmacy, Ningbo University (available from C.B.N., Ningbo, China). A small sample of this material was preserved in RNAlater solution for molecular analysis, and the rest was directly frozen at −18 °C for transportation to the lab and storage in the same condition until the time of chemical extraction. The majority of the biomass present was tentatively identified as a marine filamentous cyanobacterium belonging to the *Lyngbya*-like and *Phormidium*-like morphotype based on its macroscopic colonial appearance and morphological features observed under light microscopy (Figure 2). The taxonomy of this organism was further refined to a cf. *Neolyngbya* sp. by independent 16S rRNA gene sequencing at Beijing Genomics Institute, using universal bacteria PCR primers for the 16S-V3-V4 region and Operational Taxonomic Unit mapping using USEARCH. Data were visualized using the Krona Tools web browser [50]. Phylogenetic tree by neighbor joining was generated via SILVA [51].

3.3. Extraction and Isolation

The freeze-dried and powdered biomass (dry weight 600 g) of the above environmental collection was exhaustively extracted in 2:1 CH_2Cl_2/MeOH (8×). The extracts were dried under vacuum and then rinsed with H_2O (3×) to remove residual sea salt, affording 3.1 g of an organic crude extract. This material was subjected to vacuum liquid chromatography (VLC) separation over normal-phase silica gel column chromatography (200–300 mesh) using a stepwise gradient (10% EtOAc/hexanes, 20% EtOAc/hexanes, 40% EtOAc/hexanes, 60% EtOAc/hexanes, 80% EtOAc/hexanes, 100% EtOAc, 10% MeOH/EtOAc, and 20% MeOH/EtOAc). The column was eluted to provide 8 fractions: A (200.9 mg), B (300.5 mg), C (316.4 mg), D (250.6 mg), E (150.9 mg), F (707.5 mg), G (506.7 mg), and H (259.6 mg). Fraction C was further separated by RP-18 MPLC with a 120 g Biotage SNAP Cartridge, KP-C18-HS, and a gradient solvent system (60% to 100% MeOH/H_2O in 60 min) to generate subfractions C1–C6 with yields of 40 mg, 40 mg, 60 mg, 30 mg, 20 mg, and 70 mg, respectively. Subfraction C3 was additionally fractionated using a Waters ACQUITY UPLC equipment instrument equipped with a PDA detector on a reversed-phase Phenomenex Kinetex C18 column (5 μm, 5 × 250 mm, Phenomenex) using MeCN/H_2O as a mobile phase, at a flow rate of 1 mL/min. The gradient program was 50–100% MeCN/H_2O in 20 min with a linear gradient elution. The eluent was delivered to an automatic fraction collector for timed sampling every 0.75 min from 6.2 min to 15.2 min, and all the fractions were dried in glass tubes and weighed. In total, 12 fractions, Fr.C3−1−C3–12 were obtained from the subfraction C3 with the yields 1 mg, 6 mg, 1 mg, 2 mg, 3 mg, 2 mg, 3 mg, 1 mg, 1 mg, 1 mg, 2 mg, and 2 mg, respectively. Fraction C3–5, corresponding to a 3 mg sample collected around a UV 210 nm peak at t_R = 9.6, was found to contain the pure compound **1** after it was analyzed by LC-MS and 1D NMR.

3.4. Isolated Materials (New Natural Products)

*Wenchangamide A (**1**)*: white powder; $[\alpha]_D^{17}$ −315 (*c* 0.1, MeOH); UV (MeOH) λ_{max} (log ε) = 218 (3.92), 275 (3.04) nm; IR (KBr) ν_{max} 3350 (br), 2921, 2815, 2742, 1612, 1515, 1505, 1487, 1416, 1235 cm^{-1};for ^1H NMR and ^{13}C NMR data see Table 1; HR-ESI-MS $[M + Na]^+$ *m/z* 1233.7748 (calcd. for $C_{64}H_{106}N_8O_{14}Na^+$, 1233.7721).

3.5. Determination of the Absolute Configuration of Wenchangamide A (1)

Wenchangamide A (**1**, 1.0 mg) was treated with 6 M HCl (100 μL) for 24 h at 110 °C. The hydrolyzed product was evaporated to dryness for purification of the individual structural components. Using HPLC separation and a Cosmosil $5C_{18}$-PAQ column [(ϕ4.6 × 250 mm); flow rate, 1.0 mL/min; UV detection at 215 nm; solvent H_2O], the components; Ser (t_R = 2.6), Leu and *N*-Me-Ile (t_R = 5.2), and *N*-Me-Phe (t_R = 12.3) were collected. In another HPLC separation using the Cosmosil $5C_{18}$-PAQ column [(ϕ4.6 × 250 mm); flow rate, 1.0 mL/min; UV detection at 215 nm; solvent 0.1% aqueous TFA], *N*-Me-Glu (t_R = 3.4) was obtained. In a final HPLC separation using the Cosmosil $5C_{18}$-PAQ column [(ϕ4.6 × 250 mm); flow rate, 1.0 mL/min; UV detection at 215 nm; solvent 40% aqueous MeOH], Amp (t_R = 3.7) was collected.

Each hydrolyzed fraction, except for Amp, was dissolved in H_2O and analyzed by chiral HPLC, and the retention times were compared to those of authentic standards. For this analysis, a DAICEL CHIRALPAK MA(+) column [(ϕ4.6 × 50 mm); flow rate 1 mL/min; detection, UV 254 nm; solvent 2.0 mM $CuSO_4$, 2.0 mM $CuSO_4$/MeCN = 95/5] was used. With 2.0 mM $CuSO_4$ as a solvent, the retention times of *N*-Me-Glu and Leu hydrolyzed from **1** matched those of the authentic standards of *N*-Me-L-Glu (20.2 min; *N*-Me-D-Glu, 18.6 min), D-Leu (9.6 min) and L-Leu (18.7 min). With 2.0 mM $CuSO_4$/MeCN = 95/5 as a solvent, the retention time of *N*-Me-Phe hydrolyzed from **1** matched that of the authentic standard of *N*-Me-L-Phe (19.8 min; *N*-Me-D-Phe, 16.5 min). Increased resolution was required for the Ser residue, and a series of two DAICEL CHIRALPAK MA(+) columns [(ϕ4.6 × 50 mm); flow rate 1 mL/min; detection, UV 254 nm; solvent 2.0 mM $CuSO_4$] was used. The retention time of Ser hydrolyzed from **1** matched those of the authentic standards of D-Ser (2.5 min; L-Ser, 3.2 min).

For analysis of the Amp and *N*-Me-Ile residues, Marfey's method was used to clarify the absolute configurations. To each isolated residue was added 1.0% L-FDLA acetone sol. (100 μL) and 1 M $NaHCO_3$ (25 μL). The mixtures were heated at 80 °C for 3 min, cooled to room temperature, and neutralized with 1 M HCl. The products were analyzed by HPLC and the retention time was compared with those of authentic standards. A Cosmosil Cholester column [(ϕ4.6 × 250 mm); flow rate 1 mL/min; detection, UV 340 nm; solvent MeCN/H_2O/TFA = 70/30/0.1] was used to evaluate the Amp derivatives. The retention time of Amp-L-FDLA from hydrolysate of **1** matched that of the authentic standard (*S*)-Amp-L-FDLA (t_R = 4.9 min; (*S*)-Amp-D-FDLA, 5.6 min). A Cosmosil PBr column [(4.6 × 250 mm); flow rate 1 mL/min; detection, UV 340 nm; solvent MeCN/H_2O/TFA = 55/45/0.1] was used to evaluate the *N*-Me-Ile derivatives. The retention time of *N*-Me-Ile-L-FDLA from hydrolysate of **1** matched that of the authentic standard *N*-Me-D-*allo*-Ile-L-FDLA (t_R = 17.8 min; *N*-Me-L-Ile-L-FDLA 14.2 min; *N*-Me-D-Ile-L-FDLA 17.3min; *N*-Me-D-*allo*-Ile-D-FDLA 14.7 min).

3.6. LC−MS Analysis and Molecular Networking Generation

The crude extract and fractions A−H were dissolved in MeOH at 0.5 mg/mL. A 50 μL aliquot of each sample was injected via LC−MS/MS on a Thermo Dionex Ultimate 3000 LC-PDA system coupled to a Bruker Maxis impact QTOF system in an ESI positive mode and eluted with a gradient of H_2O with 0.1% formic acid and CH_3CN with a gradient method as follows: 10% CH_3CN/H_2O for 2 min, 10% CH_3CN/H_2O to 45% in 8 min, held at 45% CH_3CN/H_2O for 2 min, 45% CH_3CN/H_2O to 99% in 4 min, held at 99% CH_3CN/H_2O for 1 min, then 99% CH_3CN/H_2O to 10% CH_3CN/H_2O in 1 min, and finally held at 10% CH_3CN/H_2O for 2 min with the flow rate of 0.6 mL/min at room temperature. The UV chromatogram was measured at 210, 230, 280, 360 nm by photodiode array detection. Data-dependent (automated) MS/MS spectra were collected during the same run. The raw data of MS/MS spectra from the all fractions were converted to mzXML format using the ProteoWizard tool MSConvertGUI, and the processed files were uploaded to the GNPS website (http://gnps.ucsd.edu) to generate a molecular network that was visualized using Cytoscape 3.8 software (Weblinks S1 and S2). A molecular network was created using the online workflow on the GNPS website (https://ccms-ucsd.github.io/GNPSDocumentation). The precursor ion mass tolerance was set to 1 Da and a MS/MS fragment ion tolerance of 0.5 Da. The spectra in the network were then searched against available GNPS spectrometric libraries. The library spectra were filtered in the same manner as the input data. All matches kept between network spectra and library spectra were required to have a score above 0.7 and at least 4 matched peaks [33].

3.7. Cell Culture

The human colorectal cancer cell line, HCT116, was purchased from American Type Culture Collection (ATCC; Bethesda, MD, USA). Cells were maintained in DMEM medium, supplemented with 1% L-glutamine, 10% fetal bovine serum (FBS), 1% sodium pyruvate and 1% PenStrep (penicillin + streptomycin) (Biological Industries, Beit Haemek, Israel). Cells were grown in a humidified incubator at 37 °C with 5% CO_2 in air, and served twice a week with fresh medium.

3.8. XTT Cell Proliferation Assay

Evaluation of the effect of each crude organic extract and fractions A-H, as well as subfractions C1-C6 and C3–1–C3–12 on cell viability was performed using the standard XTT assay and an established protocol [44]. In brief, HCT116 cells were seeded in 96-well plates (10^4 cell/well) and 24 h later were treated for a period of 24 h with two doses from the crude extract and fractions A-H; 200 and 400 μg/mL, and with 4 doses for each subfraction; 15, 25, 50, and 100 μg/mL. Medium and DMSO were added to control wells. For sub-fraction C3–5, the XTT assay was additionally conducted using 30 μg/mL for 24 h. Following treatment, cell viability was determined by the XTT assay (Biological Industries, Beit Haemek, Israel) according to the manufacturer's instructions using a plate reader (version, BioTek, Winooski, VT, USA). Experiments were repeated 3 times. Data were presented as the average proliferation percentage of the respective control.

3.9. Cell Cycle Analysis

A cell cycle evaluation experiment was carried out as described previously [44]. Briefly, 10^6 cells were treated with 30 μg/mL of C3 or C3–5 for 24 h. At the end of treatment time, cells were trypsinized, harvested and centrifuged at 2000 rpm for 5 min at 4 °C. Cells were washed with cold PBS and fixed with 70% EtOH for 1 h at −20 °C. Cells were incubated with 0.1% NP-40 on ice for 5 min, followed by 30 min of incubation on ice with 100 μg/mL RNase (Sigma-Aldrich, St. Louis, MO, USA). Finally, 50 μg/mL propidium iodide (PI) was added to cells for 20 min. Cell cycle analysis was carried out by flow cytometry using a FACSCantoII with FACSDiva software (Becton Dickenson, San Jose, CA, USA); 10^4 cells were counted for each the control and the treatment groups.

3.10. Annexin-V/PI Double Staining

Apoptotic cell death was evaluated and quantified using an Annexin-V FITC and PI double staining kit (Mebcyto® Apoptosis Kit, MBL, Nagoya, Japan) according to the manufacturer's instructions. In brief, 2×10^5 HCT116 cells were seeded in 25 cm^2 flasks. The next day, cells were treated with 30 μg/mL of C3 or **1** for 24 h. Both adherent and floating cells were collected in order to detect early and late apoptotic cells. Treated and untreated cells (control) were harvested by trypsinization, washed and suspended in ice-cold PBS. The washed cell pellets were re-suspended in an ice-cold binding buffer containing FITC-conjugated Annexin-V and PI. Samples were incubated at room temperature for 15 min in the dark before analysis by FACS, managed with FACSDiva software. The Annexin V-FITC-negative/PI negative, which are the normal healthy cells population are represented by quadrants Q3. Annexin V-FITC-positive/PI negative cells, which are defined as early apoptotic cells (Q4), whereas the Annexin V-FITC-positive/PI positive are the cells found in late apoptosis (Q2). The Annexin V-FITC-negative/PI-positive cells (Q1) include the necrotic cells. The percentage distributions of normal, early apoptotic, late apoptotic, and necrotic cells were calculated using FACSDiva software (Becton Dickenson, San Jose, CA, USA).

4. Conclusions

Cyanobacteria are vastly abundant organisms in various ecological niches, and marine filamentous cyanobacteria are a subset known to produce a treasure trove of natural products. Until challenges are overcome for using molecular biology tools to predict and realize the potential chemical arsenal of filamentous cyanobacteria via their biosynthetic gene clusters, a more complete chemical diversity of these organisms can be studied using large environmental collections. The chemical space of extracts produced from these assemblages is largely affected by external factors, such as the associated microbial consortia and environmental conditions, and thus increases the complexity of studying assemblages for new molecule discovery. Metabolomics-based approaches can be used to unravel the chemical potential of such complex samples, and minimize the rediscovery of previously reported compounds. The South China Sea harbors largely untapped filamentous cyanobacteria biodiversity that may be investigated to yield new pharmaceutical lead molecules. In this study, the investigation of a cf. *Neolyngbya* sp. cyanobacterium that was collected near Wenchang, Hainan, China led to the discovery of wenchangamide A (**1**) and characterization of its new chemical scaffold. Compound **1** was found to be a fast-acting and concentration-dependent inducer of apoptosis in HCT116 human colon cancer cells in vitro. Further untargeted LC-MS/MS-based metabolomics suggested the occurrence of an additional analogue, wenchangamide B, for which a structure has been proposed with high confidence. Bioassay results from the fraction containing this related molecule also showed in vitro apoptotic activity using HCT116 cells, suggesting that the core polypeptide-derived scaffold may be a pharmacophore and that the length of the polyketide chain could be tailoring molecules of this class for variable potency or solubility. The further expansion of this chemical class and structure–activity relationship should be evaluated for natural products anticancer drug discovery and development.

Supplementary Materials: The following are available online at https://www.mdpi.com/article/10.3390/md19070397/s1: ^{1}H, ^{13}C, DEPT135, COSY, TOCSY, HSQC-TOCSY, HSQC, HMBC, and ROESY NMR, UV, and IR for compound **1**. Tabulated NMR data for **1** in pyridine-d_5. MS/MS spectra for compound **1** and the proposed analogue, wenchangamide B. Chiral HPLC chromatograms of hydrolysates of **1** and authentic standards. In vitro bioassay data. Weblinks for the GNPS metabolomic data used to produce Figures 3 and 9. 16S rRNA gene V3–V4 amplicon used to prepare Figure 2C.

Author Contributions: Conceptualization, C.B.N. and T.L.-K.; Methodology, L.D., R.B.-S., N.K., S.L., A.I.; Data Analysis, R.B.-S., D.A., A.I., C.B.N., T.L.-K.; Resources, G.P., A.I., K.S., C.Z., H.L., F.T., C.B.N.; Writing—Original Draft Preparation, L.D., R.B.-S., A.I., C.B.N., T.L.-K.; Writing—Review and Editing, all authors; Project Administration, F.F., C.B.N., T.L.-K.; Funding Acquisition, L.D., C.B.N., S.H., X.Y. All authors have read and agreed to the published version of the manuscript.

Funding: This study was supported by the National Key Research and Development Program of China, funded through MOST (the Ministry of Science and Technology of China; grant 2018YFC0310900 to X.Y., S.H. and C.B.N.), NSFC (The National Natural Science Foundation of China; grants 81850410553 and 82050410451 to C.B.N.), the National 111 Project of China (D16013), CSC (China Scholarship Council; no. 201908330173 to L.D.), and the Li Dak Sum Yip Yio Chin Kenneth Li Marine Biopharmaceutical Development Fund of Ningbo University.

Institutional Review Board Statement: Not applicable.

Data Availability Statement: The datasets generated for this study can be found in the online supplementary materials. Metabolomics data are archived on the GNPS platform and can be found in the following links: https://gnps.ucsd.edu/ProteoSAFe/status.jsp?task=f62b23918fb24bca9f4a234f3555df50; https://gnps.ucsd.edu/ProteoSAFe/status.jsp?task=0e36af9bc15d4d6c901292d5be8ff32b.

Acknowledgments: We thank Meirav Avital Shacham, Head of analytical and chromatography unit, the Faculty of Natural Sciences, University of Haifa, Israel and Sagie Schif-Zuck for the use of FACSCanto II (BD) equipment, Faculty of Natural Sciences, University of Haifa. We also thank Larisa Panz, Mass spectrometry Center, Schulich Faculty of Chemistry, Technion, Israel and Shai Zaid, Department of Marine Biology, The Charney School of Marine Sciences, University of Haifa, Israel for their help in MS data acquisition.

Conflicts of Interest: The authors declare no conflict of interest. The funders had no role in the design of the study; in the collection, analyses, or interpretation of data; in the writing of the manuscript, or in the decision to publish the results.

References

1. Salvador-Reyes, L.A.; Luesch, H. Biological targets and mechanisms of action of natural products from marine cyanobacteria. *Nat. Prod. Rep.* **2015**, *32*, 478–503. [CrossRef] [PubMed]
2. Demay, J.; Bernard, C.; Reinhardt, A.; Marie, B. Natural products from cyanobacteria: Focus on beneficial activities. *Mar. Drugs* **2019**, *17*, 320. [CrossRef] [PubMed]
3. Tan, L.T.; Phyo, M.Y. Marine cyanobacteria: A source of lead compounds and their clinically-relevant molecular targets. *Molecules* **2020**, *25*, 2197. [CrossRef] [PubMed]
4. Mayer, A.M.S.; Guerrero, A.J.; Rodríguez, A.D.; Taglialatela-Scafati, O.; Nakamura, F.; Fusetani, N. Marine pharmacology in 2014–2015: Marine compounds with antibacterial, antidiabetic, antifungal, anti-inflammatory, antiprotozoal, antituberculosis, antiviral, and anthelmintic activities; affecting the immune and nervous systems, and other miscellaneous mechanisms of action. *Mar. Drugs* **2020**, *18*, 5. [CrossRef]
5. Jang, M.-H.; Ha, K.; Lucas, M.C.; Joo, G.-J.; Takamura, N. Changes in microcystin production by *Microcystis aeruginosa* exposed to phytoplanktivorous and omnivorous fish. *Aquat. Toxicol.* **2004**, *68*, 51–59. [CrossRef] [PubMed]
6. Jiang, X.; Gao, H.; Zhang, L.; Liang, H.; Zhu, X. Rapid evolution of tolerance to toxic *Microcystis* in two cladoceran grazers. *Sci. Rep.* **2016**, *6*, 25319. [CrossRef] [PubMed]
7. Leao, T.; Castelão, G.; Korobeynikov, A.; Monroe, E.A.; Podell, S.; Glukhov, E.; Allen, E.E.; Gerwick, W.H.; Gerwick, L. Comparative genomics uncovers the prolific and distinctive metabolic potential of the cyanobacterial genus *Moorea*. *Proc. Natl. Acad. Sci. USA* **2017**, *114*, 3198–3203. [CrossRef]
8. Moss, N.A.; Leao, T.; Glukhov, E.; Gerwick, L.; Gerwick, W.H. Collection, Culturing, and Genome Analyses of Tropical Marine Filamentous Benthic Cyanobacteria. In *Methods in Enzymology*; Moore, B.S., Ed.; Elsevier: Cambridge, UK, 2018; Volume 604, pp. 3–43, ISBN 9780128139592.
9. Crnkovic, C.M.; May, D.S.; Orjala, J. The impact of culture conditions on growth and metabolomic profiles of freshwater cyanobacteria. *J. Appl. Phycol.* **2018**, *30*, 375–384. [CrossRef]

10. Pye, C.R.; Bertin, M.J.; Lokey, R.S.; Gerwick, W.H.; Linington, R.G. Retrospective analysis of natural products provides insights for future discovery trends. *Proc. Natl. Acad. Sci. USA* **2017**, *114*, 5601–5606. [CrossRef]
11. Hašler, P.; Dvořák, P.; Johansen, J.R.; Kitner, M.; Ondřej, V.; Poulíčková, A. Morphological and molecular study of epipelic filamentous genera *Phormidium, Microcoleus* and *Geitlerinema* (Oscillatoriales, Cyanophyta/cyanobacteria). *Fottea-Olomouc* **2012**, *12*, 341–356. [CrossRef]
12. Stoyanov, P.; Moten, D.; Mladenov, R.; Dzhambazov, B.; Teneva, I. Phylogenetic relationships of some filamentous cyanoprokaryotic species. *Evol. Bioinform.* **2014**, *10*, 39–49. [CrossRef] [PubMed]
13. Nuryadi, H.; Sumimoto, S.; Teruya, T.; Suenaga, K.; Suda, S. Characterization of macroscopic colony-forming filamentous cyanobacteria from Okinawan coasts as potential sources of bioactive compounds. *Mar. Biotechnol.* **2020**, *22*, 824–835. [CrossRef]
14. Anagnostidis, K. Nomenclatural changes in cyanoprokaryotic order Oscillatoriales. *Preslia Praha* **2001**, *73*, 359–375.
15. Hoffmann, L.; Komárek, J.; Kaštovský, J. System of cyanoprokaryotes (cyanobacteria) state in 2004. *Arch. Hydrobiol. Suppl. Algol. Stud.* **2005**, *117*, 95–115. [CrossRef]
16. Komárek, J.; Johansen, J.R. Filamentous Cyanobacteria. In *Freshwater Algae of North America: Ecology and Classification*, 1st ed.; Academic Press: Cambridge, MA, USA, 2003; pp. 117–196. ISBN 9780123858771.
17. Komárek, J.; Johansen, J.R. Filamentous Cyanobacteria. In *Freshwater Algae of North America: Ecology and Classification*, 2nd ed.; Academic Press: Cambridge, MA, USA, 2015; pp. 135–235. ISBN 9780123858771.
18. Komárek, J.; Kaštovský, J.; Mareš, J.; Johansen, J.R. Taxonomic classification of cyanoprokaryotes (cyanobacterial genera) 2014, using a polyphasic approach. *Preslia* **2014**, *86*, 295–335.
19. Engene, N.; Paul, V.J.; Byrum, T.; Gerwick, W.H.; Thor, A.; Ellisman, M.H. Five chemically rich species of tropical marine cyanobacteria of the genus *Okeania* gen. nov. (Oscillatoriales, Cyanoprokaryota). *J. Phycol.* **2013**, *49*, 1095–1106. [CrossRef]
20. Tronholm, A.; Engene, N. *Moorena gen. nov.*, a valid name for "*Moorea* Engene & *al.*" nom. inval. (*Oscillatoriaceae, Cyanobacteria*). *Not. Algarum* **2019**, *122*, 122.
21. Caires, T.A.; de Mattos Lyra, G.; Hentschke, G.S.; de Gusmão Pedrini, A.; Sant'Anna, C.L.; de Castro Nunes, J.M. *Neolyngbya* gen. nov. (Cyanobacteria, Oscillatoriaceae): A new filamentous benthic marine taxon widely distributed along the Brazilian coast. *Mol. Phylogenet. Evol.* **2018**, *120*, 196–211. [CrossRef]
22. Caires, T.A.; da Silva, A.M.S.; Vasconcelos, V.M.; Affe, H.M.J.; de Souza Neta, L.C.; Boness, H.V.M.; Sant'Anna, C.L.; Nunes, J.M.C. Biotechnological potential of *Neolyngbya* (Cyanobacteria), a new marine benthic filamentous genus from Brazil. *Algal Res.* **2018**, *36*, 1–9. [CrossRef]
23. Lydon, C.A.; Mathivathanan, L.; Sanchez, J.; dos Santos, L.A.H.; Sauvage, T.; Gunasekera, S.P.; Paul, V.J.; Berry, J.P. Eudesmacarbonate, a eudesmane-type sesquiterpene from a marine filamentous cyanobacterial mat (Oscillatoriales) in the Florida Keys. *J. Nat. Prod.* **2020**, *83*, 2030–2035. [CrossRef] [PubMed]
24. Guan, H.; Wang, S. Algae. In *Chinese Marine Materia Medica*; Shanghai Scientific and Technical Publishers, China Ocean Press, and Chemical Industry Press: Shanghai, Beijing, China, 2009; pp. 37–304. ISBN 978-7-5323-9958-1.
25. Titlyanov, E.A.; Titlyanova, T.V.; Li, X.; Huang, H. Chapter 2—Marine Plants of Coral Reefs. In *Coral Reef Marine Plants of Hainan Island*; Titlyanov, E.A., Titlyanova, T.V., Li, X., Huang, H., Eds.; Academic Press: Cambridge, MA, USA, 2017; pp. 5–39, ISBN 978-0-12-811963-1.
26. Sun, W.; Wu, W.; Liu, X.; Zaleta-Pinet, D.A.; Clark, B.R. Bioactive compounds isolated from marine-derived microbes in China: 2009-2018. *Mar. Drugs* **2019**, *17*, 339. [CrossRef]
27. Demarque, D.P.; Dusi, R.G.; de Sousa, F.D.M.; Grossi, S.M.; Silvério, M.R.S.; Lopes, N.P.; Espindola, L.S. Mass spectrometry-based metabolomics approach in the isolation of bioactive natural products. *Sci. Rep.* **2020**, *10*, 1051. [CrossRef]
28. Luzzatto-Knaan, T.; Garg, N.; Wang, M.; Glukhov, E.; Peng, Y.; Ackermann, G.; Amir, A.; Duggan, B.M.; Ryazanov, S.; Gerwick, L.; et al. Digitizing mass spectrometry data to explore the chemical diversity and distribution of marine cyanobacteria and algae. *eLife* **2017**, *6*, e24214. [CrossRef]
29. Luzzatto-Knaan, T.; Melnik, A.V.; Dorrestein, P.C. Mass spectrometry tools and workflows for revealing microbial chemistry. *Analyst* **2015**, *140*, 4949–4966. [CrossRef]
30. Yang, J.Y.; Sanchez, L.M.; Rath, C.M.; Liu, X.; Boudreau, P.D.; Bruns, N.; Glukhov, E.; Wodtke, A.; de Felicio, R.; Fenner, A.; et al. Molecular networking as a dereplication strategy. *J. Nat. Prod.* **2013**, *76*, 1686–1699. [CrossRef] [PubMed]
31. Olivon, F.; Allard, P.-M.; Koval, A.; Righi, D.; Genta-Jouve, G.; Neyts, J.; Apel, C.; Pannecouque, C.; Nothias, L.-F.; Cachet, X.; et al. Bioactive natural products prioritization using massive multi-informational molecular networks. *ACS Chem. Biol.* **2017**, *12*, 2644–2651. [CrossRef]
32. Nothias, L.F.; Nothias-Esposito, M.; da Silva, R.; Wang, M.; Protsyuk, I.; Zhang, Z.; Sarvepalli, A.; Leyssen, P.; Touboul, D.; Costa, J.; et al. Bioactivity-based molecular networking for the discovery of drug leads in natural product bioassay-guided fractionation. *J. Nat. Prod.* **2018**, *81*, 758–767. [CrossRef] [PubMed]
33. Wang, M.; Carver, J.J.; Phelan, V.V.; Sanchez, L.M.; Garg, N.; Peng, Y.; Nguyen, D.D.; Watrous, J.; Kapono, C.A.; Luzzatto-Knaan, T.; et al. Sharing and community curation of mass spectrometry data with Global Natural Products Social Molecular Networking. *Nat. Biotechnol.* **2016**, *34*, 828–837. [CrossRef] [PubMed]
34. Wolfender, J.L.; Litaudon, M.; Touboul, D.; Queiroz, E.F. Innovative omics-based approaches for prioritisation and targeted isolation of natural products—New strategies for drug discovery. *Nat. Prod. Rep.* **2019**, *36*, 855–868. [CrossRef]

35. Fox Ramos, A.E.; Evanno, L.; Poupon, E.; Champy, P.; Beniddir, M.A. Natural products targeting strategies involving molecular networking: Different manners, one goal. *Nat. Prod. Rep.* **2019**, *36*, 960–980. [CrossRef]
36. Ernst, M.; Kang, K.B.; Caraballo-Rodríguez, A.M.; Nothias, L.F.; Wandy, J.; Wang, M.; Rogers, S.; Medema, M.H.; Dorrestein, P.C.; van der Hooft, J.J.J. MolNetEnhancer: Enhanced molecular networks by integrating metabolome mining and annotation tools. *Metabolites* **2019**, *9*, 144. [CrossRef]
37. Cornet, L.; Bertrand, A.R.; Hanikenne, M.; Javaux, E.J.; Wilmotte, A.; Baurain, D. Metagenomic assembly of new (sub)polar cyanobacteria and their associated microbiome from non-axenic cultures. *Microb. Genom.* **2018**, *4*, 212. [CrossRef]
38. Gris, B.; Treu, L.; Zampieri, R.M.; Caldara, F.; Romualdi, C.; Campanaro, S.; La Rocca, N. Microbiota of the therapeutic Euganean thermal muds with a focus on the main cyanobacteria species. *Microorganisms* **2020**, *8*, 1590. [CrossRef] [PubMed]
39. Gogineni, V.; Hamann, M.T. Marine natural product peptides with therapeutic potential: Chemistry, biosynthesis, and pharmacology. *Biochim. Biophys. Acta Gen. Subj.* **2018**, *1862*, 81–196. [CrossRef]
40. Gross, H.; König, G.M. Terpenoids from marine organisms: Unique structures and their pharmacological potential. *Phytochem. Rev.* **2006**, *5*, 115–141. [CrossRef]
41. Sorokina, M.; Steinbeck, C. Review on natural products databases: Where to find data in 2020. *J. Cheminform.* **2020**, *12*, 1–51. [CrossRef]
42. Wang, H.; Fewer, D.P.; Holm, L.; Rouhiainen, L.; Sivonen, K. Atlas of nonribosomal peptide and polyketide biosynthetic pathways reveals common occurrence of nonmodular enzymes. *Proc. Natl. Acad. Sci. USA* **2014**, *111*, 9259–9264. [CrossRef]
43. Naman, C.B.; Rattan, R.; Nikoulina, S.E.; Lee, J.; Miller, B.W.; Moss, N.A.; Armstrong, L.; Boudreau, P.D.; Debonsi, H.M.; Valeriote, F.A.; et al. Integrating molecular networking and biological assays to target the isolation of a cytotoxic cyclic octapeptide, samoamide A, from an American Samoan marine cyanobacterium. *J. Nat. Prod.* **2017**, *80*, 625–633. [CrossRef]
44. Bar-Shalom, R.; Bergman, M.; Grossman, S.; Azzam, N.; Sharvit, L.; Fares, F. *Inula viscosa* extract inhibits growth of colorectal cancer cells *in vitro* and *in vivo* through induction of apoptosis. *Front. Oncol.* **2019**, *9*, 227. [CrossRef]
45. Zheng, Q.; Hirose, Y.; Yoshimi, N.; Murakami, A.; Koshimizu, K.; Ohigashi, H.; Sakata, K.; Matsumoto, Y.; Sayama, Y.; Mori, H. Further investigation of the modifying effect of various chemopreventive agents on apoptosis and cell proliferation in human colon cancer cells. *J. Cancer Res. Clin. Oncol.* **2002**, *128*, 539–546. [CrossRef]
46. Sumimoto, S.; Kobayashi, M.; Sato, R.; Shinomiya, S.; Iwasaki, A.; Suda, S.; Teruya, T.; Inuzuka, T.; Ohno, O.; Suenaga, K. Minnamide A, a linear lipopeptide from the marine cyanobacterium *Okeania hirsuta*. *Org. Lett.* **2019**, *21*, 1187–1190. [CrossRef]
47. Liang, X.; Matthew, S.; Chen, Q.Y.; Kwan, J.C.; Paul, V.J.; Luesch, H. Discovery and total synthesis of doscadenamide A: A quorum sensing signaling molecule from a marine cyanobacterium. *Org. Lett.* **2019**, *21*, 7274–7278. [CrossRef]
48. Leber, C.A.; Naman, C.B.; Keller, L.; Almaliti, J.; Caro-Diaz, E.J.E.; Glukhov, E.; Joseph, V.; Sajeevan, T.P.; Reyes, A.J.; Biggs, J.S.; et al. Applying a chemogeographic strategy for natural product discovery from the marine cyanobacterium *Moorena bouillonii*. *Mar. Drugs* **2020**, *18*, 515. [CrossRef]
49. Liang, X.; Chen, Q.-Y.; Seabra, G.M.; Matthew, S.; Kwan, J.C.; Li, C.; Paul, V.J.; Luesch, H. Bifunctional doscadenamides activate quorum sensing in gram-negative bacteria and synergize with TRAIL to induce apoptosis in cancer cells. *J. Nat. Prod.* **2021**, *84*, 779–789. [CrossRef]
50. Ondov, B.D.; Bergman, N.H.; Phillippy, A.M. Interactive metagenomic visualization in a Web browser. *BMC Bioinform.* **2011**, *12*, 385. [CrossRef]
51. Pruesse, E.; Peplies, J.; Glöckner, F.O. SINA: Accurate high-throughput multiple sequence alignment of ribosomal RNA genes. *Bioinformatics* **2012**, *28*, 1823–1829. [CrossRef]

marine drugs

MDPI

Article

Anti-Infective and Antiviral Activity of Valinomycin and Its Analogues from a Sea Cucumber-Associated Bacterium, *Streptomyces* sp. SV 21

Joko T. Wibowo [1,2,*], Matthias Y. Kellermann [1], Matthias Köck [3], Masteria Y. Putra [2], Tutik Murniasih [2], Kathrin I. Mohr [4], Joachim Wink [4], Dimas F. Praditya [2,5,6], Eike Steinmann [5,6] and Peter J. Schupp [1,7,*]

1 Institute for Chemistry and Biology of the Marine Environment (ICBM), Carl-von-Ossietzky University Oldenburg, Schleusenstraße 1, D-26382 Wilhelmshaven, Germany; matthias.kellermann@uni-oldenburg.de
2 Research Center for Biotechnology, Indonesian Institute of Science, Jl. Raya Bogor KM 46, Cibinong 16911, Indonesia; mast001@lipi.go.id (M.Y.P.); tuti007@lipi.go.id (T.M.); Dimas.Praditya@ruhr-uni-bochum.de (D.F.P.)
3 Alfred-Wegener-Institut für Polar- und Meeresforschung in der Helmholtz-Gemeinschaft, Am Handelshafen 12, 27570 Bremerhaven, Germany; Matthias.Koeck@awi.de
4 Helmholtz Centre for Infection Research, Inhoffenstraße 7, 38124 Braunschweig, Germany; kathrinmohr4@gmail.com (K.I.M.); joachim.wink@helmholtz-hzi.de (J.W.)
5 TWINCORE-Centre for Experimental and Clinical Infection Research (Institute of Experimental Virology) Hannover, Feodor-Lynen-Str. 7-9, 30625 Hannover, Germany; Eike.Steinmann@ruhr-uni-bochum.de
6 Department of Molecular and Medical Virology, Ruhr-University Bochum, 44801 Bochum, Germany
7 Helmholtz Institute for Functional Marine Biodiversity at the University of Oldenburg (HIFMB), Ammerländer Heerstrasse 231, D-26129 Oldenburg, Germany
* Correspondence: joko.tri.wibowo@uni-oldenburg.de (J.T.W.); peter.schupp@uni-oldenburg.de (P.J.S.); Tel.: +49-4421-944-100 (P.J.S.)

Citation: Wibowo, J.T.; Kellermann, M.Y.; Köck, M.; Putra, M.Y.; Murniasih, T.; Mohr, K.I.; Wink, J.; Praditya, D.F.; Steinmann, E.; Schupp, P.J. Anti-Infective and Antiviral Activity of Valinomycin and Its Analogues from a Sea Cucumber-Associated Bacterium, *Streptomyces* sp. SV 21. *Mar. Drugs* **2021**, *19*, 81. https://doi.org/10.3390/md19020081

Academic Editors: Vassilios Roussis and Max Crüsemann

Received: 4 December 2020
Accepted: 28 January 2021
Published: 2 February 2021

Publisher's Note: MDPI stays neutral with regard to jurisdictional claims in published maps and institutional affiliations.

Abstract: The manuscript investigated the isolation, characterization and anti-infective potential of valinomycin (**3**), streptodepsipeptide P11A (**2**), streptodepsipeptide P11B (**1**), and one novel valinomycin analogue, streptodepsipeptide SV21 (**4**), which were all produced by the Gram-positive strain *Streptomyces cavourensis* SV 21. Although the exact molecular weight and major molecular fragments were recently reported for compound **4**, its structure elucidation was not based on compound isolation and spectroscopic techniques. We successfully isolated and elucidated the structure based on the MS^2 fragmentation pathways as well as ^1H and ^{13}C NMR spectra and found that the previously reported structure of compound **4** differs from our analysis. Our findings showed the importance of isolation and structure elucidation of bacterial compounds in the era of fast omics technologies. The here performed anti-infective assays showed moderate to potent activity against fungi, multi drug resistant (MDR) bacteria and infectivity of the Hepatitis C Virus (HCV). While compounds **2**, **3** and **4** revealed potent antiviral activity, the observed minor cytotoxicity needs further investigation. Furthermore, the here performed anti-infective assays disclosed that the symmetry of the valinomycin molecule is most important for its bioactivity, a fact that has not been reported so far.

Keywords: cyclodepsipeptides; marine Actinobacteria; *Streptomyces* spp.; antibiotic; sea cucumber; HCV

1. Introduction

Natural products play a dominant role in the discovery of leads for the development of novel drugs to treat human diseases [1]. For the past 30 years, there has been an increasing effort by scientists from many disciplines to identify novel natural products from marine organisms, including marine bacteria, due to their rich biological and chemical diversity [2,3]. With the strong demand to find new antibiotics to solve the antibiotic resistance crisis, research on marine natural products expanded in the last decade to include marine bacteria. Several studies have shown that many novel bioactive compounds were often derived from marine Gram-positive Actinobacteria [3,4].

Recently, the isolation and fast identification of putatively new bioactive compounds from sea cucumber-associated bacteria have been reported in [5]. Extracts of *Streptomyces* sp. SV 21 showed potent anti-infective activities. Bio-guided fractionation of the bacterial extracts and subsequent MS/MS and NMR experiments revealed valinomycin (**3**), two of its analogues, namely streptodepsipeptide P11B (**1**), streptodepsipeptide P11A (**2**) [6], and one putative new valinomycin analogue named streptodepsipeptide SV21 (**4**). All the compounds (**1–4**) exhibited inhibitory activities against bacteria, fungi, and the Hepatitis C Virus (HCV). Streptodepsipeptide SV21 (**4**) had recently been characterized based on exact mass and MS/MS analysis [7]; however, it was neither isolated nor elucidated via NMR nor tested for its bioactivities.

Valinomycin is a common cyclodepsipeptide produced by various soil-derived Actinobacteria, such as *Streptomyces fulvissimus*, *S. roseochromogenes*, and *S. griseus* var. *flexipartum* [8], as well as from marine *Streptomyces* species associated with the sponges *Axinella polypoides* and *Aplysina aerophoba* [9]. Valinomycin is considered as one of the ionophore antibiotics. This bioactive compound has both a hydrophobic and hydrophilic moiety, which is necessary to bind and shield ions, but also allows the molecule to transport those ions through the lipophilic membrane barrier of living cells. Valinomycin is known to be highly selective for binding potassium ions and thus has the potential to disrupt the intracellular ion concentration of the cell. The probability to transport ions through membranes not only affects osmoregulatory processes, but also affects the homeostasis of the cell, which in turn may result in an increased level of toxicity or even death for the organism [10,11]. Therefore, this cyclodepsipeptide was reported to have many bioactivities, such as antitumor, antibacterial, antibabesia, and antifungal activity [6,9,12,13]. Another interesting bioactivity of valinomycin was its potency against the causative agent of the world's first pandemic in the 21st century, the SARS-CoV virus. Unfortunately, valinomycin also showed enhanced cytotoxicity that prevented the drug to enter the clinical phase [14]. Besides the pharmacological potential, an ecological role also has been reported, as valinomycin is used in chemical defense against pathogens by the leafcutter ant *Acromyrmex echinatior* [15].

In this study, valinomycin (**3**) and its three analogues (**1**, **2**, and **4**) were isolated and characterized based on MS/MS and NMR analysis. In addition, the anti-infective activities of compounds **1–4** against multi drug-resistant (MDR) bacteria (*Bacillus subtilis*, *Staphylococcus aureus*), fungi (*Candida albicans*, *Mucor hiemalis*, *Rhodoturula glutinis*) and the Hepatitis C Virus (HCV) were identified.

2. Results and Discussion

The exact masses of the compounds (MS^1 data, Figure S1) were compared with compounds in the MarinLit database (Table 1). The results showed that exact masses of compounds **1–3** closely matched with streptodepsipeptide P11B ([M] = 1082.5988), P11A ([M] = 1096.6142), and valinomycin ([M] = 1110.6315), respectively. While, streptodepsipeptide SV21 (**4**), having a precursor ion of *m/z* 1142.6804 $[M + NH_4]^+$, had not been reported yet in the MarinLit database. Further analysis, using the GNPS MASST database, on the precursor (MS^1) and product ion (MS^2) spectral data (Figures S2–S5) showed that compounds **1–4** were related to valinomycin with cosine scores ranking all above 0.7, while considering more than 40 major product ion peaks. This result indicated that **4** was also a valinomycin analogue.

Table 1. MS^1 data analysis results of the isolated compounds. The exact masses from the MS^1 spectra of compounds **1–4** were compared against the MarinLit database (±0.01 Dalton).

Compound	Exact Mass, Observed MS^1	Results in MarinLit	References
1	1100.6332 $[M + NH_4]^+$ 1082.5988 [M]	Streptodepsipeptide P11B ([M] = 1082.5999)	[6]
2	1114.6486 $[M + NH_4]^+$ 1096.6142 [M]	Streptodepsipeptide P11A ([M] = 1096.6155)	[6]
3	1128.6659 $[M + NH_4]^+$ 1110.6315 [M]	valinomycin ([M] = 1110.6311)	[6,9]
4	1142.6804 $[M + NH_4]^+$ 1124.6460 [M]	Not yet reported	

To have an overview of the structure for all four valinomycin analogues, we analyzed and compared the MS^2 spectra of compounds **1**, **2**, and **4** with valinomycin (**3**). Valinomycin consists of the enantiomers *D*- and *L*-valine (Val), *D*-α-hydroxyisovaleric acid (Hiv), and *L*-lactic acid (Lac) [6]. One valinomycin molecule consists out of three repeating units of Val–Hiv–Val–Lac, where one unit has an exact mass of 370.208 Da.

Compound identification started by comparing the precursor ion of each compound (cf. Table 1) as well as the fragment ions in the mass region between *m/z* 600 and *m/z* 1150 (Figure S6). Both, the precursor ion and the fragment ions showed a consecutive mass increase of 14 Da from compound **1** to **4**. However, the fragment ion *m/z* 713.4 was found to be in all valinomycin analogues. Based on the molecular mass, the fragment ion at *m/z* 713.4 is represented by two units of Val–Hiv–Val–Lac after the loss of a unit of C=O for the initial opening of the ring structure. To crosscheck the existence of a unit Val–Hiv–Val–Lac in all compounds, the neutral loss of 370.208 Da was observed in all compound spectra after the loss of a C=O unit, which initially opened the ring structure. The neutral loss of two units of Val–Hiv–Val–Lac, with an exact mass of *m/z* 740.419 Da, was also observed in compounds **1–4**, indicating that all four molecular species contained at least two units of Val–Hiv–Val–Lac.

Despite the similar smaller fragment ions that occurred in the mass spectra at *m/z* 50–*m/z* 600, further analysis showed some unique fragment ions for each valinomycin analogue. For example, the fragment ion at *m/z* 315.192 was only present in streptodepsipeptide P11B (**1**). This compound represents a monomer and dimer of depsipeptide (Val–Hiv–Val–Lac) as well as a monomer of Val–Hiv–Val–Lac minus 28 Da. Based on the previous studies, the mass difference of 28 Da might be the result of the substitution of a Hiv with a Lac [6,7]. Therefore, the fragment ion at *m/z* 315.192 is likely a unit of Val–Lac–Val–Lac. This is further supported by the neutral loss of 171 Da (Val–Lac) from *m/z* 315.192 to *m/z* 144.103 (shown as black arrow in Figure S6A). The fragment ion at *m/z* 144.103 is a unit of Val–Lac with a loss of C=O.

Another example is represented by the fragment ion at *m/z* 329.208, which was only found in streptodepsipeptide P11A (**2**). This compound has a mass of about 14 Da lower than a unit of Val–Hiv–Val–Lac. By comparing out the MS^2-based analysis with previous studies, there are at least two possible explanations: first, a substitution of a Hiv with a hydroxybutanoic acid (Hba) [6]; or second, a substitution of a Val with an isoleucine or a leucine (Ile/Leu) in a unit of Val–Lac–Val–Lac [7]. Both scenarios would be possible since the ion for Val–Hba–Val–Lac and Ile/Leu–Lac–Val–Lac create a fragment mass of *m/z* 329.207. Furthermore, the fragment ion at *m/z* 186.113 in **2** might be the protonated ion of Val–Hba or Ile/Leu–Lac. However, after the fragmentation pathway of the compound was simulated for both substitutions, a peak for Val–Lac–Val–Lac around *m/z* 315.191 could not be found in the spectra, if a Val was substituted with Ile/Leu. Therefore, the most suitable substitution in **2** is a Hiv with a Hba, as also mentioned in [6].

A fragment ion at *m/z* 357.239 occurred in the spectra for streptodepsipeptide SV21 (**4**). It has a molecular mass of 14 Da higher than a unit Val–Hiv–Val–Lac. In a previous study, the additional 14 Da were suggested to result from a substitution of a Val with either an Ile or Leu unit [7]. However, when we simulated the fragmentation of Val–Hiv–Ile/Leu–Lac, we were unable to detect the peak at *m/z* 158.118 in the MS^2 spectra. Fragmentation of

Val–Hiv–Ile/Leu–Lac should have resulted in Val–Hiv and Ile/Leu–Lac with the calculated *m/z* 172.133 and *m/z* 158.118, respectively. Therefore, we propose the structure of **4** to have a substitution of Hiv with hydroxymethylpentanoic acid (Hmpa), since we detected the fragment ions *m/z* 186.150 (Val–Hmpa) and *m/z* 144.103 (Val–Lac), thus indicating a single unit of Val–Hmpa–Val–Lac. In summary, the difference between compounds (**1–4**) is only a substitution of a Hiv with either a Lac, a Hba or Hmpa within a single unit of Val–Hiv–Val–Lac (cf. Figure 1).

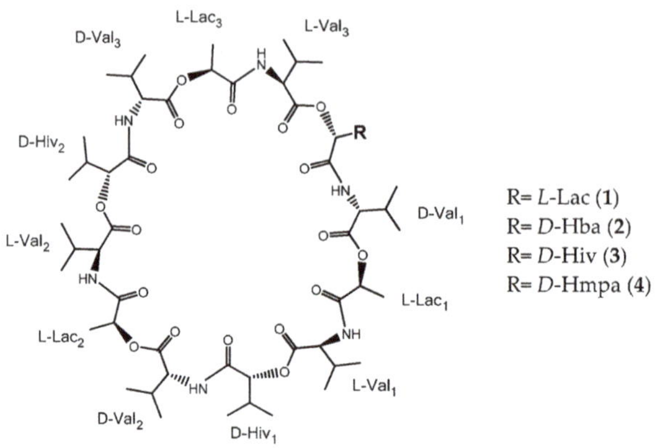

Figure 1. Identified structures of the four valinomycin analogues **1–4**. Based on our NMR and MS^2 experiments, we assumed the absolute configuration to be identical to the one reported by Ye and colleagues [6].

The configuration of the compounds **1–3** in Figure 1 was assumed to be identical with [6], while configuration of **4** was derived from the biosynthetic pathway of valinomycin. The structure of compounds **1–4** were quite similar, therefore we agreed with [7] that valinomycin and their analogues are derived from the same biosynthetic pathway. Biosynthesis of valinomycin is accomplished by nonribosomal peptides (NRPS) that are composed of two proteins, namely, VLM1 and VLM2. Those proteins are divided into four modules, each one responsible for incorporation of one unit of *D*-Hiv, *D*-Val, *L*-Lac, and *L*-Val. The depsipeptide chain (*D*-Hiv–*D* -Val–*L*-Lac–*L*-Val) is linked to the C-terminal iterative thioesterase (TE) domain at the last module in VLM2. The terminal TE domain controls the termination, release and cyclization of the growing chains in the biosynthetic process [16].

Biosynthesis of *D*-Hiv in valinomycin is occurring in module 1 in VLM1 [16]. The study also explained that module 1 contains four functional domains: adenylation (A; designated as VLM1A1), hypothetical transaminase (TA), hypothetical dehydrogenase (DH2) and peptidyl carrier protein (PCP). Extracted NRPS codes from VLM1A1 did not yield any predictable substrate, leading to the assumption that VLM1A1 might have adapted to select and activate hydroxyl acids independently [16]. However, the adenylation domain is a core of each module that recognize the cognate substrate [17]. Therefore, feeding experiments using different substrates, i.e., *D*-Hiv, *D*-Hba, or *D*-Hmpa, are needed to verify which substrates are needed to produce valinomycin and its analogues. In turn, substitution of *D*-Hiv with *L*-Lac in streptodepsipeptide P11B (**1**) could be explained as a variation in the linearity within modules 3 and 4 instead of modules 1 and 2 in one round of the tetradepsipetide assembly [7].

Streptodepsipeptide P11B (**1**) proved to be the known depsipeptide based on the comparison of the measured MS, NMR, and optical rotation data with the references [6,7]. To crosscheck the structure with the MS^2 data, we simulated the fragmentation pathways for each compound. The fragmentation pathway of compound **1** started with the ring opening and the loss of a C=O unit of 27.995 Da. After the ring opened, the fragment ion *m/z* 1055.611 (calc. *m/z* 1055.612) (Figure 2) continued to lose either a unit of Val–Lac or Val–Hiv with 171.089 and 199.121 Da, respectively (cf. Figure S7). The sequential loss of a unit of Val–Lac or Val–Hiv explained the occurrence of fragment ions *m/z* 884.520 (calc. *m/z* 884.523) or *m/z* 856.491 (calc. *m/z* 856.491; fragment ions from MS^2 spectra *cf.* Figure S7).

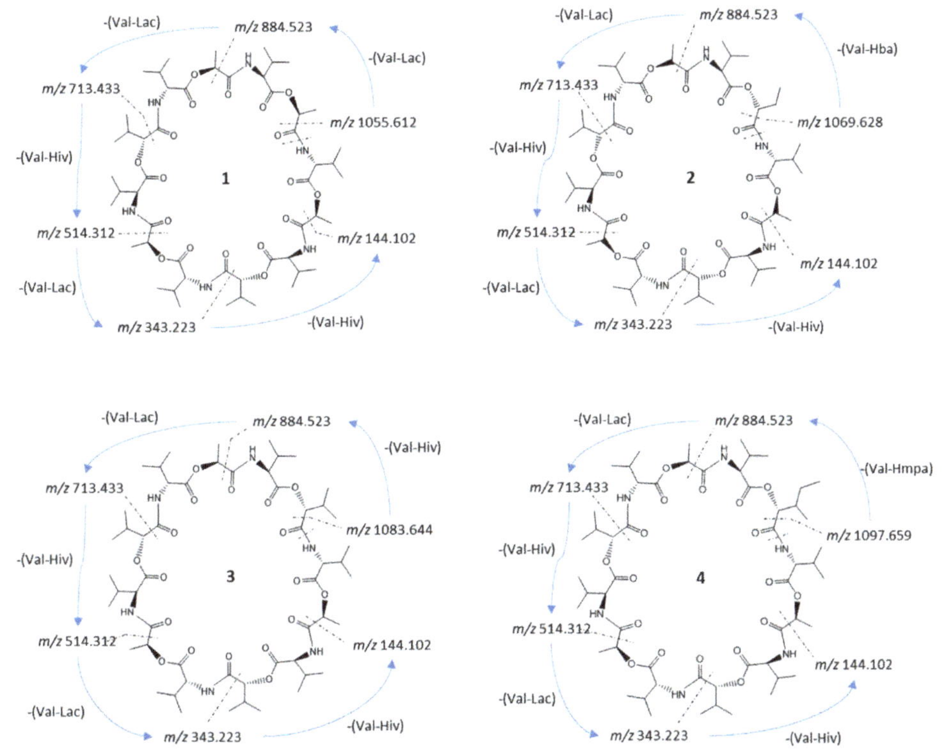

Figure 2. Scheme of the fragmentation pathways of compounds **1**–**4**. The *m/z* ratios were calculated and then compared with the MS^2 fragment ions. The fragmentation started from the loss of a C=O unit.

In total, the fragmentation pathway of streptodepsipeptide P11B (**1**) took five major steps of losing either a unit of Val–Lac or Val–Hiv. However, since **1** has one substitution of Hiv with a Lac residue, one of the fragmentation steps is the repetition of losing a unit of Val–Lac, which is indicated by the consecutive tan arrows in Figure S7.

Besides a thorough mass spectral analysis, the four valinomycin analogues were also compared by their Hα/Cα region of the HSQC spectra (Figure 3). Every residue showed a distinct fingerprint region in the HSQC spectrum and thus allows counting the different residues. For example, in the spectra of streptodepsipeptide P11B (**1**), all 12 Hα/Cα correlations can be observed. The *D*-Val/*L*-Val plot indicates no changes since there are three signals for *L*-Val and three signals for *D*-Val. However, the plot on the left side indicates a loss of a Hiv residue and an increase of a Lac residue, which is in accordance with the molecular formula of **1** (valinomycin minus 2 × CH_2). In case of streptodepsipeptide SV21 (**4**), there is quite some overlap in the four regions of the HSQC spectrum. Two of the three *L*-Val and two of the three *D*-Val residues overlapped. The same is true for the two Hiv residues. The three Lac residues all appear in one signal. The only signal without any overlap is the new Hmpa residue (5.17 ppm/76.7 ppm).

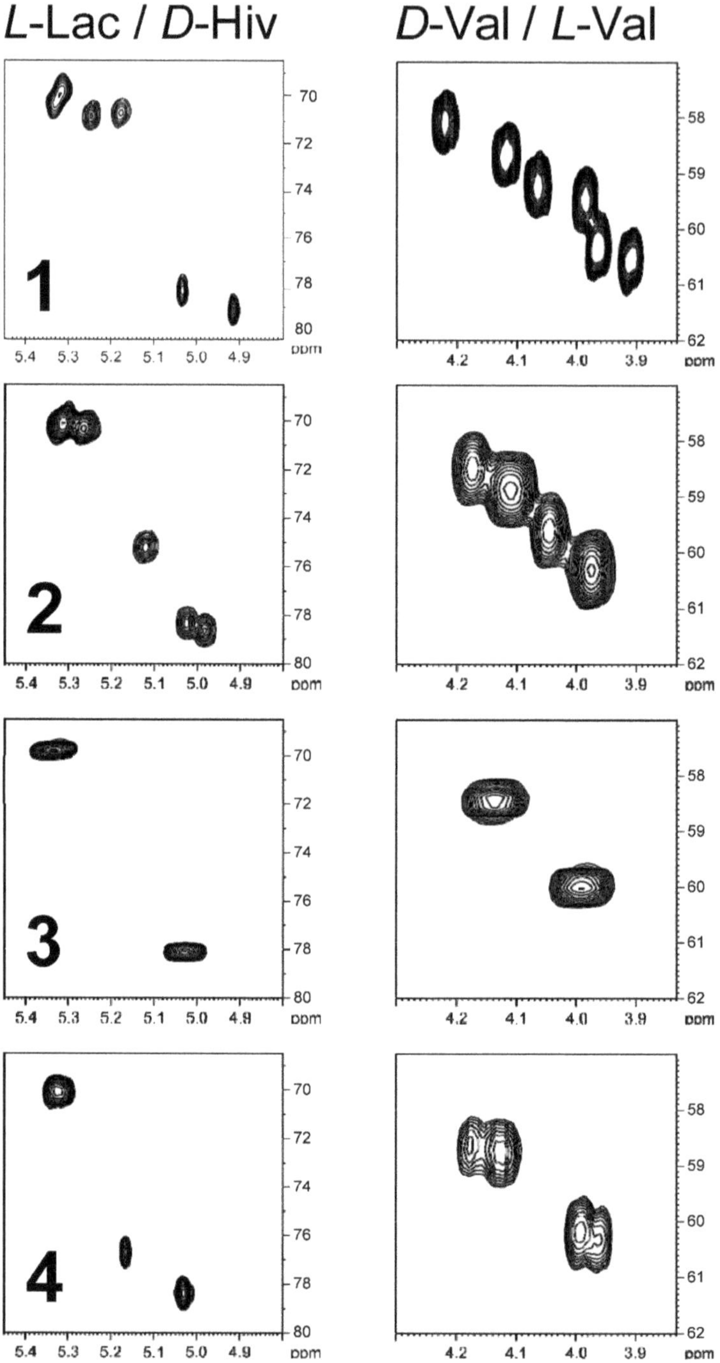

Figure 3. The Hα/Cα region of the HSQC spectra of compounds **1–4** for *D*-Hiv/*L*-Lac on the left side and *D*-Val/*L*-Val on the right side. The spectra on the top represent the ones for streptodepsipeptide P11B (**1**) and the ones on the bottom for **4**, respectively. The *D*-Hiv/*L*-Lac plots (left side) are divided into two subgroups: appr. 71 ppm (*L*-Lac) and appr. 79 ppm (*D*-Hiv). The same is true for the *D*-Val/*L*-Val plot (right side): appr. 59 ppm (*D*-Val) and appr. 60 ppm (*L*-Val).

The precursor ion of streptodepsipeptide P11A (**2**) was 1114.649 [M + NH_4]$^+$. It has 14 Da more compared to streptodepsipeptide P11B (**1**). Most of the fragment ions of **2** also have a 14 Da difference to fragment ions of **1** (cf. Figure S6). Therefore, the fragment ion at *m/z* 1069.627 (calc. 1069.628) resulted from a neutral loss of a C=O (Figure 2). The loss of a C=O may have happened anywhere in the structure; therefore, fragmentation of **2** then continued with a loss of a unit of Val–Lac, Val–Hiv, or Val–Hba at any positions near the opened ring. It explains the occurrence of the fragment ion *m/z* 898.536 (calc. 898.538), *m/z* 884.524 (calc. 884.523), *m/z* 870.509 (calc. 870.507), etc. (cf. Figure S8). Fragmentation pathways for **2** in Figure S8 seems to be more complex than **1**. However, the pathways still consist of five major steps of losing intermittently a unit of Val–Lac then Val–Hiv, or Val–Lac then Val–Hba, with only the loss of one Val–Hba for each possible pathway (blue arrows in Figure S8).

The reported fragmentation pattern for streptodepsipeptide P11A (**2**) in [7] did not fit well with our measured fragment ions of compound **2**. However, the NMR data for streptodepsipeptide P11A (**2**) (Figure 3) matched closely with the published data in [6] and also resembled our fragmentation pattern (cf. Figure S8).

The exact mass and also precursor ion ($\pm$0.01 Da) of the isolated valinomycin (**3**) matched the reported mass data in [6,7,9]. The fragmentation of **3** is initiated by the loss of a C=O at any position in the ring to produce the fragment ion *m/z* 1083.643 (calc. 1083.644). The fragmentation process is then followed by the loss of a unit of Val–Lac or Val–Hiv. Following the same five major fragmentation steps as for streptodepsipeptide P11B (**1**) and P11A (**2**), fragment ions *m/z* 912.549 (calc. 912.554), *m/z* 884.524 (calc. 884.523), *m/z* 713.433 (calc. 713.433), etc., were detected (cf. Figure S9).

Streptodepsipeptide SV21 (**4**) had a precursor ion of *m/z* 1142.680 [M + NH_4]$^+$ and did not match any reported data in MarinLit. However, MS^2 analysis of **4** using the MASST GNPS database showed that **4** was strongly related to valinomycin based on a cosine score of 0.77 and 42 shared peaks (Figure S5). A cosine score has a value between 0 and 1, with 1 indicating 100% similarity. A sample is considered an analogue of a reported compound if the cosine score is >0.7 [18]. Several measured peaks of **4** were identical to the fragment ions of valinomycin (**3**) (visualized by green lines, see Figures S2–S5). Fragment ion *m/z* 1097.660 (calc. *m/z* 1097.659) resulted from the loss of a C=O group via ring opening. The fragmentation process then followed the previous reported pattern via loss of Val–Lac, Val–Hiv, or Val–Hmpa, resulting in peaks of *m/z* 926.566 (calc. *m/z* 926.570), *m/z* 898.540 (calc. *m/z* 898.538), and *m/z* 884.523 (calc. *m/z* 884.523), respectively (cf. Figure S10).

For the ^{13}C and ^{1}H NMR assignments of valinomycin (**3**), please see Figure 3. The structure of valinomycin consisted of four units: *L*-Val (appr. 60 ppm), *D*-Val (appr. 59 ppm), *L*-Lac (appr. 71 ppm), and *D*-Hiv (appr. 79 ppm). Each unit showed characteristic NMR signals, which were useful for the characterization of the analogues (**1**, **2**, and **4**). The ^{1}H NMR spectra showed the purity of compounds **1**–**4** and allowed the comparison with the reported compounds from [6] (cf. Figures S11–S15 and Tables S1–S4).

The ^{13}C NMR signals for streptodepsipeptide SV21 (**4**) displayed 55 carbon signals for 12 carbonyls (δ_C 169.9–172.4), six oxymethines (δ_C 19.1–19.3), six nitrogenated methines (δ_C 118.0–118.8), nine methines (δ_C 19.0–26.1), a methylene (δ_C 14.0), and 21 methyls (Table 2 and Figure S16). The ^{1}H NMR spectrum of **4** showed six signals for NH at δ_H 7.88, 7.83, 7.80, 7.75, 7.69, and 7.67 ppm (Table 2 and Figure S17). Those data indicated that **4** consisted of 6 esters and 6 amino acids residues.

Table 2. ^{1}H and ^{13}C NMR data for compound **4**.

Position	NH		CO	Cα		Cβ		Cγ1		Cγ2		Cδ		Cβ-Me	
	δ_C	δ_H (J in Hz)	δ_C	δ_C	δ_H (J in Hz)	δ_C	δ_H (J in Hz)	δ_C	δ_H (J in Hz)	δ_C	δ_H (J in Hz)	δ_C	δ_H (J in Hz)	δ_C	δ_H (J in Hz)
D-Val (1)	118.4	7.88	169.9	58.5	4.19	28.4	2.34	19.0	1.05	19.1	0.96				
D-Val (2)	118.4	7.83	170.2	58.7	4.13	28.4	2.33	19.0	1.05	19.1	0.96				
D-Val (3)	118.0	7.80	170.1	58.7	4.14	28.4	2.32	19.0	1.05	19.1	0.96				
L-Lac (1)			172.4	70.2	5.30	17.0	1.45								
L-Lac (2)			172.4	70.2	5.30	17.0	1.45								
L-Lac (3)			172.4	70.2	5.30	17.0	1.45								
L-Val (1)	118.8	7.75	171.5	60.2	4.00	28.3	2.26	19.6	1.08	19.3	0.96				
L-Val (2)	118.8	7.69	171.8	60.3	3.97	28.3	2.23	19.6	1.07	19.3	0.95				
L-Val (3)	118.7	7.67	171.7	60.2	3.99	28.3	2.24	19.6	1.08	19.3	0.96				
D-Hiv (1)			170.5	78.5	5.02	30.2	2.35	16.5	0.98						
D-Hiv (2)			170.7	78.5	5.02	30.2	2.35	16.5	0.98						
Hmpa			170.9	76.7	5.17	36.7	2.11	26.1	1.41	26.1	1.29	11.7	0.93	14.0	0.96

The MS results clearly indicate that compound **4** has an additional methylene group compared to valinomycin (**3**). In principle, the additional CH_2 group could be added to each of the four residues. The inspection of the four Hα/Cα regions in the HSQC spectrum (cf. Figure 3) clearly shows a loss of a Hiv residue, which means that the extra CH_2 group of **4** was added to this residue. There are two possibilities how to add a methylene group: First, a transition from Hiv to Hmpa would be possible. Second, from an "amino acid" point of view, it could be the transition from Val to Leu or Ile. However, the Hmpa unit was established by analysis of the COSY and HMBC spectra. The complete spin system of Hmpa could be assigned by the TOCSY spectrum without the determination of the explicit positions. Starting from Hα, the Hβ can be assigned by the COSY correlation, and the corresponding Cβ (36.7 ppm) is accessible by the HSQC (Figure 3 and Figure S18). Furthermore, three HMBC correlations can be observed starting from Hα (36.7 ppm, 26.1 ppm, and 14.0 ppm). This already indicates the existence of a Hmpa residue. For the constitutional isomer "Leu" only two HMBC correlations would have been expected and no correlation to a methyl group (here 14.0 ppm). The complete assignment of the Hmpa residue is given in Table 2.

Valinomycin (**3**) and its analogues (**1**, **2**, and **4**) showed a narrow spectrum of antimicrobial activities (Table 3). Compounds **1–4** showed that all antifungal activity against *Mucor hiemalis (Mh)* and *Ruegeria glutinis (Rg)*, with streptodepsipeptide P11A (**2**) and valinomycin (**3**) being the most active ones, revealed similar or lower MIC values compared to the commercial antifungal compound nystatin (cf. Table 3). Valinomycin was eight times stronger than nystatin against *Mh* and as strong as nystatin against *Rg*. Previous studies had also shown antifungal activity of valinomycin against the plant pathogens *Phytophthora capsici* and *Botrytis cinerea* [13,14]. Only valinomycin (**3**) and streptodepsipeptide SV21 (**4**) also exhibited activities against the Gram-positive bacterium *Staphylococcus aureus (Sa)* and *Bacillus subtilis* (*Bs*) (only (**4**) had activity). However, the activity of valinomycin on *Bs* was strongly affected by the pH regime in the conducted assay. At the different pH values from 5.5 to 9.5, valinomycin showed an increase in antibacterial activity against *Bs* at higher pH values [19]. To the best of our knowledge, this is the first report on the antimicrobial activity of compounds **1**, **2**, and **4**.

Table 3. Minimum inhibitory concentration (MIC) of valinomycin (**3**) and analogues (**1**, **2**, and **4**) against different human pathogenic MDR bacteria and fungi. The activities of the tested compounds were compared to the positive controls oxytetracyclin, kanamycin, gentamycin, and nystatin.

Tested Strains:	MIC (μg mL^{-1})							
	Gram-Positive			Gram-Negative		Fungi		
	Bs	*Sa*	*Ms*	*Ec*	*Pa*	*Ca*	*Mh*	*Rg*
Compound:								
Streptodepsipeptide P11B (**1**)	-	-	-	-	-	-	16.6	33.3
Streptodepsipeptide P11A (**2**)	-	-	-	-	-	-	8.3	8.3
Valinomycin (**3**)	-	4.2	-	-	-	-	2.1	4.2
Streptodepsipeptide SV21 (**4**)	33.3	16.6	-	-	-	-	16.6	16.6
Positive controls:								
Oxytetracycline	8.3	0.2	n.t.	1.7	n.t.	n.t.	n.t.	n.t.
Kanamycin	n.t.	n.t.	3.3	n.t.	n.t.	n.t.	n.t.	n.t.
Gentamycin	n.t.	n.t.	n.t.	n.t.	0.4	n.t.	n.t.	n.t.
Nystatin	n.t.	n.t.	n.t.	n.t.	n.t.	33.3	16.6	4.2

Abbreviation for MDR bacterial strains and fungi: *Bs*: *Bacillus subtilis* (DSM 10); *Ca*: *Candida albicans* (DSM 1665); *Ec*: *Eschericia coli* (DSM 1116); *Mh*: *Mucor hiemalis* (DSM 2656); *Ms*: *Mycobacterium smegmatis* (ATCC 700084); *Pa*: *Pseudomonas aeruginosa* (PA14); *Sa*: *Staphylococcus aureus* (DSM 346); *Rg*: *Rhodoturula glutinis* (DSM 10134); -: not active; n.t.: not tested.

Furthermore, we tested all 4 compounds (**1**–**4**) against the Hepatitis C Virus (HCV, Figure 4). Although structurally closely related, only the compounds **2**–**4** showed pronounced infectivity against HCV compared to the positive control epigallocatechin gallate (EGCG). Streptodepsipeptide P11B (**1**) significantly less affected the HCV. This finding indicated that valinomycin (**3**) and its analogues (**2** and **4**) have a strong potential to function as potent ani-HCV agents. However, viability of the Huh7.5 cells for valinomycin (**3**) and its analogues (**2** and **4**) were lower than for the positive control, meaning these compounds also slightly affected the host cell as well.

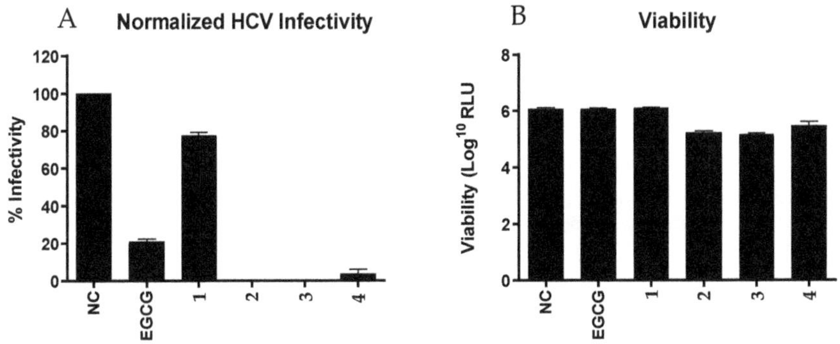

Figure 4. Activity of compounds **1**–**4** to Huh7.5 cells that were infected with Hepatitis C Virus (HCV). (**A**) The percentage of HCV-infected hepatoma cells. (**B**) The viability of Huh7.5 cells after exposure to the test compounds. NC: negative control; and EGCG: epigallocatechin gallate as positive control.

The isolation and structure assignment of valinomycin and the three derivatives, including the new streptodepsipeptide SV21 (**4**), allowed us for the first time to conduct a structure activity relationship (SAR) analysis to determine the essential functional groups for the observed antimicrobial and newly reported antiviral activities. The symmetry of the ring system seems to be key for the activity of valinomycin and its analogues. Compounds **1**–**4** have the same number of carbonyl groups and share the same two units of Val–Hiv–Val–Lac. The difference is only in one unit of the depsipeptide, which affects the symmetry of the molecule. Valinomycin affects the cells by dissipating the electrochemical gradient, which is essential for cell life through influx of the potassium ions into the cell. Valinomycin can change its conformation, allowing it to dissolve in aqueous but also lipophilic environments. The carbonyl groups in valinomycin form the hydrophilic site, while the methyl and isopropanyl groups form the hydrophobic site. A previous study on the antibiotic mechanism of valinomycin indicated that potassium was released from the hydrophilic site after forming a complex with valinomycin. At the hydrophobic membrane interface, the potassium ion is selectively released through the substitution with water molecules at the Lac rather than Hiv site [20].

Valinomycin (**3**) was the most active of the four tested compounds. Deletion of one or two CH_2 groups in the valinomycin structure resulted in weaker antifungal activity, while addition of a CH_2 group gave weaker antifungal but broader antibacterial activity. Thus, it seems likely that the symmetry of valinomycin is important for the observed higher bioactivity.

The antiviral activity of valinomycin (**3**) and its analogues (**2** and **4**) against HCV amplifies the potential of these compounds to be developed as or used a scaffold for the development of anti-viral agents. In a previous study, valinomycin also showed promising activity against the SARS-CoV virus [21]. Therefore, it will be interesting to conduct experiments with valinomycin and its analogues against the new strain of Coronavirus (SARS-CoV-2).

3. Materials and Methods

3.1. Bacterium Culture Condition, Isolation, and Identification of Bioactive Compounds

Streptomyces sp. SV 21 was isolated from the sea cucumber *Stichopus vastus* in Lampung, Indonesia. Sequences from the 16S rRNA of the bacterium has been submitted to the NCBI database under the accession number MK696479. It showed 100% similarity sequence to *Streptomyces cavourensis* with the type strain accession number NR_043851.1. Further information on bacterial isolation can be found in [5]. After successful isolation, the bacterium was grown from the glycerol stock on Marine Agar that was made from Marine Broth (MB, Carl Roth, Karlsruhe, Germany) according to manufacturer's instruction, with addition of 9 g/L agar (Agar-agar Bacteriological, Carl Roth, Karlsruhe, Germany). A single colony of the bacterium was transferred into 10 mL of MB and incubated at room temperature (~22 °C) for three days and used as seeding broth. For that, 1 mL of the seed broth was used to inoculate 800 mL of fresh MB media stored in a sterile 2 L Erlenmeyer flask. The culture was grown for 14 days at room temperature (~22 °C) under constant shaking (100 rpm) to keep the media aerated.

A total of 2.4 L of broth culture were filtered through a 65 g/m^2 paper filter grade 3 hw (Sartorius, Goettingen, Germany) to separate the cell mass from the remaining MB media. Subsequently, the resulting cellular material on the paper filter was extracted exhaustively with methanol (MeOH; HPLC grade VWR International GmbH, Darmstadt, Germany). The remaining broth media was extracted with ethyl acetate (EtOAc; HPLC grade VWR International GmbH, Darmstadt, Germany) in a 1 to 1 ratio by using an Ultra-Turrax (T25, IKA, Staufen, Germany) set at 12,000 rpm and applied for approximately 30 s. Both organic extracts were finally mixed and dried using a rotary evaporator (Rotavapor R II, Büchi, Flawil, Switzerland).

The bacterial crude extract was fractionated into seven fractions (Fr.) using a C_{18}-based solid phase extraction (SPE) cartridge (10 g) with a column capacity of 75 mL (HyperSep C_{18}, Fischer Scientific, Leicestershire, UK) with a mixture of DI water (Arium 611, Sartorius, Goettingen, Germany) and MeOH in different ratios starting with 70% and ending with 100% MeOH. However, only Fr. 3, 4 and 5 (85, 90, and 95% MeOH) showed high anti-infective activities. The target compounds were further purified by high-performance liquid chromatography (HPLC) (Agilent 1260 Infinity, Agilent, Santa Clara, SA, USA), using a C_{18} (Pursuit XRs 5 µm C_{18} 250 × 10.0 mm, Agilent, Santa Clara, SA, USA) semi-preparative column. A linear gradient (sequence: 10 min from 70:30 MeCN:H_2O to 100:0

$MeCN:H_2O$, 30 min 100:0 $MeCN:H_2O$, then 20 min 70:30 $MeCN:H_2O$) was applied. Formic acid (FA, 98%, Carl Roth, Karlsruhe, Germany) was added at a concentration of 0.1% to both the solvent MeCN and H_2O. The flow rate was set at 1.5 mL min^{-1}, the column temperature was set at 40 °C, and the detection wavelength of the Diode Array Detector (DAD; Agilent 1260 Infinity Diode Array Detector (G4212-60008), Agilent, Santa Clara, SA, USA) was set to 210 nm. With each semi-preparative run, 100 µL of a 10 mg mL^{-1} solution was injected. The target compounds eluted between 28 and 36 min. Each individual compound was collected: compound **1** (0.6 mg, RT 29.1 min), compound **2** (1.3 mg, RT 30.4 min), compound **3** (23.2 mg, 32.5 min), and compound **4** (1.8 mg, 34.6 min).

Analysis of the SPE fractions was performed on an ultra-high-performance liquid chromatography–high-resolution mass spectrometer (UPLC-HRMS; Waters Synapt G2-Si, Milford, MA, USA). Chromatographic separation was achieved on a BEH C_{18} column (Waters ACQUITY, Milford, MA, USA; 1.7 µm, 2.1 × 50 mm) with the column temperature set to 40 °C. The mobile phase was a linear gradient (sequence: 30 min from 5:95 $MeCN:H_2O$ to 95:5 $MeCN:H_2O$, 10 min 95:5 $MeCN:H_2O$, then 10 min 5:95 $MeCN:H_2O$). The flow rate was set at 0.3 mL min^{-1}. Formic acid (FA, 98%, Carl Roth, Karlsruhe, Germany) was added at a concentration of 0.1% to both the solvent MeCN and H_2O. Analytes were detected by ESI-MS in the positive ionization mode (POS) by monitoring the mass range of *m/z* 50 to 2000 Dalton (Da). The target compounds showed clear peaks in the total ion chromatogram (TIC), with *m/z* of 1100.633, 1114.650, 1128.673, and 1142.685 Da.

For structure verification purposes, we analyzed the MS^2 data by using MASST GNPS to identify the likely fragments of the target compounds or its analogues with the set parameters described in [5]. In addition, we also measured the NMR spectra on a Bruker 700 MHz cryo NMR spectrometer (Avance III HD) with Topspin 3.6.2 for analysis. For compounds **1** to **3**, the structures were verified with the following NMR experiments: 1D proton, $^1H,^{13}C$-HSQC (pulse program: hsqcedetgpsisp2.3) and $^1H,^{13}C$-HMBC (pulse program: hmbcgplpndqf). For structure elucidation of compound **4**, the following additionally experiments were conducted: 1D carbon, $^1H,^1H$-COSY (pulse program: cosygpppqf) and $^1H,^1H$-TOCSY (pulse program: mlevphpp). The following parameters were used for compound **4**: COSY (data acquisition: 2K/512 points, relaxation delay D1 1.5 s, acquisition time AQ 133 ms, number of scans NS 32), TOCSY (data acquisition: 2K/512 points, relaxation delay D1 2 s, acquisition time AQ 133 ms, number of scans NS 32), HSQC (data acquisition: 2K/256 points, relaxation delay D1 2 s, acquisition time AQ 146 ms, number of scans NS 16, delay $^1J_{CH}$ 145 Hz) and HMBC (data acquisition: 2K/256 points, relaxation delay D1 1.5 s, acquisition time AQ 146 ms, number of scans NS 40, delay $^nJ_{CH}$ 8 Hz). All samples were dissolved in 0.6 mL $CDCl_3$. Optical rotation was measured on a polarimeter (Anton Paar, Graz, Austria) with a 100 mm path length and sodium D line at 589 nm.

Streptodepsipeptide P11B (**1**): white amorphous powder; molecular formula $C_{52}H_{86}N_6O_{18}$; UV (MeOH, photodiode array), λmax 220 nm; $[\alpha]_D^{20}$ +23.3° (*c* 0.03, $CHCl_3$) (lit. +26.7°, [6]); HR-ESI-MS *m/z* 1100.6332 $[M + NH_4]^+$ (calcd. for $C_{52}H_{90}N_7O_{18}{}^+$, 1100.6337).

Streptodepsipeptide P11A (**2**): white amorphous powder; molecular formula $C_{53}H_{88}N_6O_{18}$; UV (MeOH, photodiode array), λmax 220 nm; $[\alpha]_D^{20}$ +34.0° (*c* 0.05, $CHCl_3$) (lit. +21.6°, [6]); HR-ESI-MS *m/z* 1114.6486 $[M + NH_4]^+$ (calcd. for $C_{53}H_{92}N_7O_{18}{}^+$, 1114.6493).

Valinomycin (**3**): white amorphous powder; molecular formula $C_{54}H_{90}N_6O_{18}$; UV (MeOH, photodiode array), λmax 210 nm; $[\alpha]_D^{20}$ +29.7° (*c* 0.60, $CHCl_3$) (lit. +18.6°, [6]); HR-ESI-MS *m/z* 1128.6659 $[M + NH_4]^+$ (calcd. for $C_{54}H_{94}N_7O_{18}{}^+$, 1128.6650).

Streptodepsipeptide SV21 (**4**): white amorphous powder; molecular formula $C_{55}H_{92}N_6O_{18}$; UV (MeOH, photodiode array), λmax 210 nm; $[\alpha]_D^{20}$ +15.0° (*c* 0.10, $CHCl_3$); HR-ESI-MS *m/z* 1142.6804 $[M + NH_4]^+$ (calcd. for $C_{55}H_{96}N_7O_{18}{}^+$, 1142.6806); for the ^{13}C and ^1H NMR data, see Table 2.

3.2. Antimicrobial Assay

The panel of test microorganisms consisted of the following multi drug-resistant (MDR) bacteria: Gram-negative *Escherichia coli* (DSM 1116) and *Pseudomonas aeruginosa*

(PA16); Gram-positive *Bacillus subtilis* (DSM 10), *Staphylococcus aureus* (DSM 346), and *Mycobacterium smegmatis* (ATCC 7000048); yeasts *Candida albicans* (DSM 1665) and *Rhodotorula glutinis* (DSM 10134); and filamentous fungi *Mucor hiemalis* (DSM 2656). The positive controls were nystatin, oxytetracyclin, kanamycin, and gentamycin, with a concentration of 1 mg/mL. Compounds **1–4** were prepared in a concentration of 1 mg/mL MeOH. The activity of the samples was observed by using the microdilution technique in 96 well plates for tissue cultures (TPP). As much as 20 μL of the MeOH solution of each compound (1 mg/mL) was mixed with 300 μL of bacterial or fungal suspension, except for the positive controls where 2 μL of either oxytetracycline, kanamycin, and gentamycin in 300 μL of bacterial suspension was used. The samples were tested in seven 1:2 serial dilution steps (concentrations A to H) in 96-well plates. Bacteria were cultivated in Mueller–Hinton bouillon (Roth) and fungi/yeasts in MYC medium (1.0% phytone peptone, 1.0% glucose, and 1.19% HEPES, pH 7.0). Start OD_{600} was 0.01 for *B. subtilis*, *E. coli*, and *S. aureus*; start OD_{548} was 0.1 for *M. hiemalis*, *C. albicans*, *R. glutinis*, *M. smegmatis*, and *P. aeruginosa*. The test organisms were cultivated at 30 °C and 160 rpm overnight.

3.3. Inhibitory Effects on Hepatitis C Virus (HCV) Infectivity

The anti-HCV assay was performed as mentioned in [5]. In brief, Huh7.5 cells stably expressing Firefly luciferase (Huh7.5 Fluc) were cultured in Dulbecco's modified minimum essential medium (DMEM, Gibco, Thermo Fisher Scientific, Schwerte, Germany) and maintained in a 37 °C environment with 5% CO_2 supply. Samples were added to the cells, and then the cells were infected with Jc1-derived *Renilla* reporter viruses. Compounds and the positive control (Epigallocatechin gallate, EGCG) were tested at a concentration of 10 μg/mL. *Renilla* and *Firefly luciferase* activities from the infected cells were measured on a Berthold Technologies Centro XS3 Microplate Luminometer (Bad Wildbad, Germany) as indicators of viral genome replication and cell viability, respectively.

Supplementary Materials: The following are available online at https://www.mdpi.com/1660-3397/19/2/81/s1. Figure S1. The HRMS spectra of compounds **1–4**; Figures S2–S5. Mirror-match of compounds **1–4** with valinomycin from the MASST GNPS database; Figures S6–S10. MS^2 spectra of the compounds **1–4**; Tables S1–S4. ^{1}H-NMR from [6]; Figures S11–S15. ^{1}H-NMR of compounds **1–4** in $CDCl_3$; Figure S16. 1D ^{13}C-NMR spectrum of streptodepsipeptide SV21 (**4**) in $CDCl_3$; Figure S17. 1D ^{1}H-NMR spectrum of streptodepsipeptide SV21 (**4**) in $CDCl_3$; Figure S18. Full HSQC spectrum of streptodepsipeptide SV21 (**4**).

Author Contributions: J.T.W., M.Y.K., M.K., E.S., K.I.M., J.W., and P.J.S. conceived and designed the experiments; J.T.W., M.Y.K., D.F.P., M.K., and K.I.M., performed the experiments; J.T.W., M.Y.K., M.K., D.F.P., K.I.M., and P.J.S. analyzed the data; J.T.W., M.Y.K., and P.J.S. wrote the paper; J.W., T.M., M.Y.P., and D.F.P. reviewed and edited the paper. All authors have read and agreed to the published version of the manuscript.

Funding: JTW acknowledges funding by DAAD special program Germany-Indonesia Anti-infective Cooperation. P.J.S. acknowledges funding by the Federal Ministry of Education and Research (BMBF) for the GINAICO project, grant 16GW0106 and DFG funding INST 1841147.1FUGG for the high-resolution mass spectrometer Waters Synapt G2-Si.

Data Availability Statement: The data presented in this study are available on request from the corresponding authors.

Acknowledgments: We are grateful to DAAD for the PhD scholarship special program Biodiversity and Health (2016 for J.T.W., 2017 for D.F.P.), to the University of Oldenburg for a STIBET short term scholarship, and to Indonesian Institute of Sciences (LIPI) for granting a study leave (J.T.W.) and for the support in taking samples. Research was carried out under the GINAICO Cooperation Agreement from July 2015 and respective MTA and MOU between University of Oldenburg and RCO LIPI, Jakarta. P.J.S. acknowledges research permit by Ristekdikti Jakarta, Indonesia, number 1493/FRP/E5/Dil.K!/VII/2017. We also like to thank the editor and two reviewers for their valuable comments which helped to improve the manuscript.

Conflicts of Interest: The authors declare no conflict of interest.

References

1. Newman, D.J.; Cragg, G.M. Natural products as sources of new drugs from 1981 to 2014. *J. Nat. Prod.* **2016**, *79*, 629–661. [CrossRef] [PubMed]
2. Pye, C.R.; Bertin, M.J.; Lokey, R.S.; Gerwick, W.H.; Linington, R.G. Retrospective analysis of natural products provides insights for future discovery trends. *Proc. Natl. Acad. Sci. USA* **2017**, *114*, 5601–5606. [CrossRef] [PubMed]
3. Wiese, J.; Imhoff, J.F. Marine bacteria and fungi as promising source for new antibiotics. *Drug Dev. Res.* **2019**, *80*, 24–27. [CrossRef] [PubMed]
4. Schinke, C.; Martins, T.; Queiroz, S.C.; Melo, I.S.; Reyes, F.G. Antibacterial compounds from marine bacteria, 2010–2015. *J. Nat. Prod.* **2017**, *80*, 1215–1228. [CrossRef] [PubMed]
5. Wibowo, J.T.; Kellermann, M.Y.; Versluis, D.; Putra, M.Y.; Murniasih, T.; Mohr, K.I.; Wink, J.; Engelmann, M.; Praditya, D.F.; Steinmann, E.; et al. Biotechnological Potential of Bacteria Isolated from the Sea Cucumber Holothuria leucospilota and Stichopus vastus from Lampung, Indonesia. *Mar. Drugs* **2019**, *17*, 635. [CrossRef]
6. Ye, X.; Anjum, K.; Song, T.; Wang, W.; Liang, Y.; Chen, M.; Huang, H.; Lian, X.-Y.; Zhang, Z. Antiproliferative cyclodepsipeptides from the marine actinomycete Streptomyces sp. P11-23B downregulating the tumor metabolic enzymes of glycolysis, glutaminolysis, and lipogenesis. *Phytochemistry* **2017**, *135*, 151–159. [CrossRef]
7. Paulo, B.S.; Sigrist, R.; Angolini, C.F.; De Oliveira, L.G. New Cyclodepsipeptide Derivatives Revealed by Genome Mining and Molecular Networking. *ChemistrySelect* **2019**, *4*, 7785–7790. [CrossRef]
8. Brockmann, H.; Schmidt-Kastner, G. Valinomycin I, XXVII. Mitteil. über antibiotica aus actinomyceten. *Chem. Ber.* **1955**, *88*, 57–61. [CrossRef]
9. Pimentel-Elardo, S.M.; Kozytska, S.; Bugni, T.S.; Ireland, C.M.; Moll, H.; Hentschel, U. Anti-parasitic compounds from Streptomyces sp. strains isolated from Mediterranean sponges. *Mar. Drugs* **2010**, *8*, 373–380. [CrossRef]
10. Moore, C.; Pressman, B.C. Mechanism of action of valinomycin on mitochondria. *Biochem. Biophys. Res. Commun.* **1964**, *15*, 562–567. [CrossRef]
11. Berezin, S.K. Valinomycin as a classical anionophore: Mechanism and ion selectivity. *J. Membr. Biol.* **2015**, *248*, 713–726. [CrossRef] [PubMed]
12. Yamasaki, M.; Nakamura, K.; Tamura, N.; Hwang, S.-J.; Yoshikawa, M.; Sasaki, N.; Ohta, H.; Yamato, O.; Maede, Y.; Takiguchi, M. Effects and mechanisms of action of ionophorous antibiotics valinomycin and salinomycin-Na on Babesia gibsoni in vitro. *J. Parasitol.* **2009**, *95*, 1532–1539. [CrossRef] [PubMed]
13. Lim, T.H.; Oh, H.C.; Kwon, S.Y.; Kim, J.H.; Seo, H.W.; Lee, J.H.; Min, B.S.; Kim, J.C.; Lim, C.H.; Cha, B.J. Antifungal activity of valinomycin, a cyclodepsipeptide from Streptomyces padanus TH-04. *Nat. Prod. Sci.* **2007**, *13*, 144–147.
14. Park, C.N.; Lee, J.M.; Lee, D.; Kim, B.S. Antifungal activity of valinomycin, a peptide antibiotic produced by *Streptomyces* sp. Strain M10 antagonistic to Botrytis cinerea. *J. Microbiol. Biotechnol.* **2008**, *18*, 880–884.
15. Van der Meij, A.; Worsley, S.F.; Hutchings, M.I.; van Wezel, G.P. Chemical ecology of antibiotic production by actinomycetes. *FEMS Microbiol. Rev.* **2017**, *41*, 392–416. [CrossRef]
16. Cheng, Y.Q. Deciphering the biosynthetic codes for the potent anti-SARS-CoV cyclodepsipeptide valinomycin in Streptomyces tsusimaensis ATCC 15141. *ChemBioChem* **2006**, *7*, 471–477. [CrossRef]
17. Stachelhaus, T.; Mootz, H.D.; Marahiel, M.A. The specificity-conferring code of adenylation domains in nonribosomal peptide synthetases. *Chem. Biol.* **1999**, *6*, 493–505. [CrossRef]
18. Wang, M.; Carver, J.J.; Phelan, V.V.; Sanchez, L.M.; Garg, N.; Peng, Y.; Nguyen, D.D.; Watrous, J.; Kapono, C.A.; Luzzatto-Knaan, T. Sharing and community curation of mass spectrometry data with Global Natural Products Social Molecular Networking. *Nat. Biotechnol.* **2016**, *34*, 828–837. [CrossRef]
19. Tempelaars, M.H.; Rodrigues, S.; Abee, T. Comparative analysis of antimicrobial activities of valinomycin and cereulide, the Bacillus cereus emetic toxin. *Appl. Environ. Microbiol.* **2011**, *77*, 2755–2762. [CrossRef]
20. Forester, T.R.; Smith, W.; Clarke, J.H. Antibiotic activity of valinomycin molecular dynamics simulations involving the water/membrane interface. *J. Chem. Soc. Faraday Trans.* **1997**, *93*, 613–619. [CrossRef]
21. De Clercq, E. Potential antivirals and antiviral strategies against SARS coronavirus infections. *Expert Rev. Anti-Infect. Ther.* **2006**, *4*, 291–302. [CrossRef] [PubMed]

marine drugs

MDPI

Article

Micrococcin P1 and P2 from Epibiotic Bacteria Associated with Isolates of *Moorea producens* from Kenya

Thomas Dzeha [1,2,*], Michael John Hall [3] and James Grant Burgess [3]

[1] D. John Faulkner Centre for Marine Biodiscovery and Biomedicine, P.O. Box 4, Kinango 80405, Kenya
[2] Department of Pure and Applied Sciences, Technical University of Mombasa, P.O. Box 90420, Mombasa 80100, Kenya
[3] School of Natural and Environmental Sciences, Newcastle University, Newcastle upon Tyne NE1 7RU, UK; michael.hall@newcastle.ac.uk (M.J.H.); grant.burgess@newcastle.ac.uk (J.G.B.)
* Correspondence: thomas.dzeha@gmail.com

Abstract: Epibiotic bacteria associated with the filamentous marine cyanobacterium *Moorea producens* were explored as a novel source of antibiotics and to establish whether they can produce cyclodepsipeptides on their own. Here, we report the isolation of micrococcin P1 (**1**) ($C_{48}H_{49}N_{13}O_9S_6$; obs. *m/z* 1144.21930/572.60381) and micrococcin P2 (**2**) ($C_{48}H_{47}N_{13}O_9S_6$; obs. *m/z* 1142.20446/571.60370) from a strain of *Bacillus marisflavi* isolated from *M. producens*' filaments. Interestingly, most bacteria isolated from *M. producens*' filaments were found to be human pathogens. Stalked diatoms on the filaments suggested a possible terrestrial origin of some epibionts. $CuSO_4 \cdot 5H_2O$ assisted differential genomic DNA isolation and phylogenetic analysis showed that a Kenyan strain of *M. producens* differed from *L. majuscula* strain CCAP 1446/4 and *L. majuscula* clones. Organic extracts of the epibiotic bacteria *Pseudoalteromonas carrageenovora* and *Ochrobactrum anthropi* did not produce cyclodepsipeptides. Further characterization of 24 Firmicutes strains from *M. producens* identified extracts of *B. marisflavi* as most active. Our results showed that the genetic basis for synthesizing micrococcin P1 (**1**), discovered in *Bacillus cereus* ATCC 14579, is species/strain-dependent and this reinforces the need for molecular identification of *M. producens* species worldwide and their epibionts. These findings indicate that *M. producens*-associated bacteria are an overlooked source of antimicrobial compounds.

Keywords: *Moorea producens*; $CuSO_4 \cdot 5H_2O$ assisted; differential gDNA isolation; filamentous bacteria; micrococcin P1 and P2; stalked diatoms

Citation: Dzeha, T.; Hall, M.J.; Burgess, J.G. Micrococcin P1 and P2 from Epibiotic Bacteria Associated with Isolates of *Moorea producens* from Kenya. *Mar. Drugs* **2022**, *20*, 128. https://doi.org/10.3390/md20020128

Academic Editors: Max Crüsemann and Ipek Kurtboke

Received: 8 July 2021
Accepted: 14 January 2022
Published: 7 February 2022

1. Introduction

Global health care is continually facing new challenges from human pathologies including cancers, diseases of old age (e.g., Alzheimer's and Parkinson's), rare orphan diseases, emerging infectious diseases, and, increasingly, the threat of drug-resistant infectious diseases. Infectious diseases claim over 13 million lives worldwide each year, with over 700,000 deaths currently attributed to antibiotic-resistant infections [1]. Drug resistance threatens to overturn the gains in antibiotic discovery since penicillin. Thus, there is an overwhelming urgency to discover new antibiotics, especially to fight antibiotic-resistant strains of MRSA, *Pseudomonas aeruginosa*, and *Klebsiella pneumoniae*. New natural products are needed not only to address antibiotic resistance, but also the aforementioned healthcare challenges.

To date, bacteria have provided the majority of the antimicrobial agents so far discovered [2,3]. Historically, the main source of bacteria for isolation of antibiotics has been soils [4] and, more recently, marine sediments [5,6]. Spore-forming actinomycetes that are defined as "chemically diverse bacteria" due to their ubiquitous production of antibiotics are abundant in soils but are also found in the marine environment. It is uncertain if they originate in the ocean or are washed into the sea in large numbers [6,7]. The study of bacteria that live on the surfaces of other organisms or symbiotically within other organisms has also been fruitful [8,9]. There is evidence that some organisms such as seaweeds and cyanobacteria harbor interesting holobionts, which are capable of producing bioactive compounds [10]. Cyanobacteria are also well known as sources of a diverse range of bioactive compounds. On the other hand, the study of cyanobacteria-associated bacteria in the discovery of novel antibiotics is in its infancy.

Bacteria–cyanobacteria associations are pre-historic at 440 Ma years ago, according to fossil evidence [11]. Bacteria attach themselves to cyanobacteria for buoyancy and to obtain nutrients released during photosynthesis; there is often a symbiotic relationship between these prokaryotes. Cyanobacterial filaments can be surrounded by a tough polysaccharide sheath that can harbor a multitude of heterotrophic bacteria that are difficult to remove [12]. The dominating heterotrophic bacteria associated with these sheaths are Gram-negative species from the phyla Proteobacteria and Bacteroidetes [13].

The association of bacteria with a cyanobacterial host is quite diverse and encompasses all phyla including Firmicutes, Actinobacteria, and γ-proteobacteria [14]. These assemblages constitute highly specific symbiotic relationships. Four specific strains of highly colored bacteria producing a quinone antibiotic were associated with *Lyngbya majuscula* from Puerto Rico [15]. The isolation of two minor hydroxyquinone compounds, quinone alkaloid 1 and 2 from a Curacao strain of *L. majuscula*, led to the speculation that these compounds may be synthesized by associated bacteria [16]. In a later study, the filamentous non-heterocystous marine cyanobacteria *Lyngbya* sp. was shown to harbor a maximum of six isolates of cultivable bacteria [12]. A study of other species of the order Oscillatoriales, comprising *Oscillatoria pseudogeminata, O. subtilissima, O. amphibian, O. cortiana; Phormidium lucidum, Phormidium* sp., *P. valderianum, P. tenue, P. foveolarum; Lyngbya confervoides* BDU 140301, *Lyngbya* sp. BDU 91711, and *Lyngbya* sp. BDU 141561, led to the isolation of 46 cultivable bacterial isolates [12].

The filamentous marine cyanobacterium *Moorea producens* is known to grow symbiotically with a number of other microorganisms, some of which are difficult to isolate [17]. *M. producens* has also been linked with swimmers' itch arising from debromoaplysiatoxin (DAT) [18]. In common with other Oscillatoriales, a Kenyan isolate of the filamentous marine cyanobacteria *M. producens* has associated bacteria including those with the ability to resist UV radiation [19]. Taxonomically, Moorea has recently been renamed Moorena [20]. This cyanobacterium is also a source of the cyclodepsipeptides homodolastatin 16 and antanapeptin A [21] and the potent anticancer molecule, dolastatin 16 (this study). The quest for a sustainable supply of these compounds generated an interest in obtaining the metagenomic DNA (gDNA) of the cyanobacteria/bacterial community. The immense diversity of the *Oscillatoriales* suggests that morphological identification is unreliable [13]. By contrast, molecular identification is accurate and specific as it is based on the genomic content of the organism. Whereas the latter method works efficiently for axenic species, its use for the speciation of non-axenic cyanobacteria is inadequate due to intragenomic gene heterogeneity arising from the presence of bacteria and other microorganisms [13,22,23]. Currently, molecular identification of non-axenic cyanobacteria utilizes the multiple displacement amplification (MDA) method, which has a limited total genomic coverage [24,25].

Various approaches for obtaining axenic cultures of cyanobacteria from non-axenic strains are documented [26]. However, they do not elaborate on how to isolate gDNA from non-axenic strains. Bacteria, yeast, and viruses are easily killed on contact with Cu^{2+} ions by reactive hydroxyl ions and hydroxy radicals that damage the cell while denaturing DNA in a Fenton-type reaction [27].

$$Cu^{+} + H_2O \rightarrow Cu^{2+} + OH^{-} + OH^{\bullet}$$

The use of copper and its alloys in "contact" killing of microorganisms dates back to both the Sumerian and Akkadian civilizations and only lost its prominence in medicine at the advent of commercially available antibiotics in 1932 [28]. However, the contact killing of microbes by copper is still being applied in Agriculture to control bacterial and fungal diseases [27]. Thus, we report here a novel method for the $CuSO_4{\cdot}5H_2O$ assisted differential gDNA isolation of non-axenic filamentous marine cyanobacteria. It is based on the treatment of cyanobacterial biomass with $CuSO_4{\cdot}5H_2O$ prior to exhaustive differential isolation of bacterial gDNA from cyanobacterial biomass to provide a residual substrate for isolation of the cyanobacteria gDNA. $CuSO_4{\cdot}5H_2O$ provides the Cu^{2+} ions needed for the contact killing of bacteria on the cyanobacteria biomass during treatment. A Kenyan isolate of *M. producens* was used for these studies. In addition, this method was used to confirm the identity of *L. majuscula* CCAP 1446/4 from the Culture Collection, Oban, Scotland, and to delineate the Kenyan *M. producens* from other species elsewhere. Bacteria associated with *M. producens*, including those associated with the filaments of *M. producens*, are described. The current study also highlights the first isolation of the antibiotics micrococcin P1 (**1**) and micrococcin P2 (**2**) from organic extracts of *B. marisflavi* and establishes an IC_{50} value of micrococcin P1 (**1**) against *Staphylococcus aureus*.

2. Results and Discussion

2.1. Detection of Homodolastatin 16, Dolastatin 16, and Antanapeptin A in Kenyan Isolates of a Filamentous Cyanobacterium, Moorea producens

Besides morphological appearance, the identity of the filamentous Kenyan marine cyanobacterium *M. producens* [21] was supported by the detection of a number of natural products known to be associated with this species. Following organic extraction of the sample and fractionation on C-18 silica, comparative HRFABMS against a dolastatin 15 standard, showed the presence of homodolastatin 16 (m/z $[M + Na]^+$ $C_{48}H_{72}O_{10}N_6Na$ (calcd. 915.5202)), dolastatin 16 ($[M + Na]^+$ $C_{47}H_{70}O_{10}N_6Na$ (calcd. 901.5046)), and antanapeptin A ($C_{41}H_{60}O_8N_4$ (calcd. 759.4314)) (Figure 1).

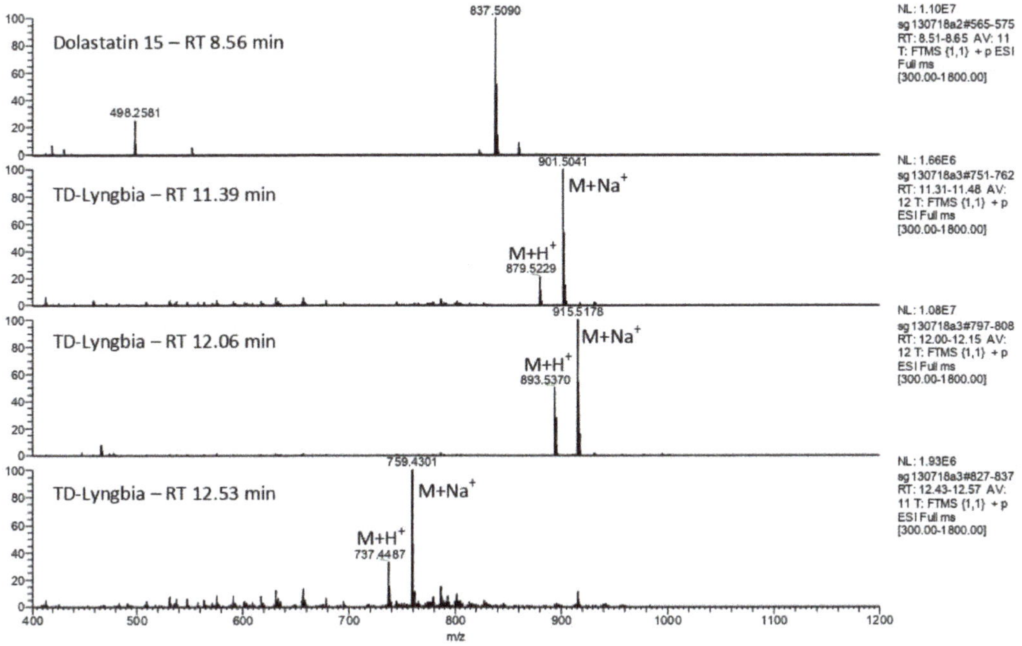

Figure 1. Electrospray mass spectrometry showing molecular ions of dolastatin 16, homodolastatin 16, and antanapeptin A from LCMS analysis of Kenyan *M. producens'* extracts at retention times of 11.39 min, 12.06 min, and 12.53 min, respectively. Note: dolastatin 15 included as standard. LCMS conditions: gradient of 10% 0.1% formic acid in water/90% 0.1% formic acid in acetonitrile to 5% 0.1% formic acid in water/95% formic acid in acetonitrile at 0.3 mL min^{-1}.

The detection of molecular ions corresponding to homodolastatin 16 from *M. producens* in the current study was consistent with that of the HRFABMS m/z $[M+Cs]^+$ 1025.4364 (calcd for $C_{48}H_{73}N_6O10Cs$, 1025.4364) obtained earlier [21]; however, this work represents the first report of the detection of dolastatin 16 in the Kenyan *M. producens*. The dolastatins are a group of antineoplastic pseudopeptides initially isolated from the sea hare *Dolabela auricularia* but that originate from the marine cyanobacterium *M. producens* distributed pan-tropically worldwide. Debromoaplysiatoxin (DAT) that is associated with *M. producens'* swimmers' itch was not detected by LCMS in the Kenyan strain of *M. producens*. The non-axenic nature of the Kenyan *M. producens* has been reported earlier [19] and was consistent with the isolation of the filament bacteria *Pseudoalteromonas carrageenovora* and *Ochrobactrum anthropi* from detached *M. producens'* filaments on marine agar 2216 (10% w/v).

2.2. Phylogenetic Divergence of M. producens from L. majuscula

L. majuscula CCAP 1446/4 strain from the Culture Collection, Oban, Scotland, United Kingdom, and 16S rDNA analysis were used to delineate the Kenyan *M. producens* from other *L. majuscula* species elsewhere. Treatment of the cyanobacteria with cycloheximide, several rinses with phosphate buffered saline (PBS), and nitrogen liquefaction ensured that detached filaments were free from eukaryotic cells, protozoa, and fungi. Further, the cyanobacteria were treated with copper sulphate powder ($CuSO_4{\cdot}5H_2O$) and left to stand for 10 min, 30 min, and 60 min, respectively, to kill any available bacteria. The control was untreated. Pooled detached filaments of both *L. majuscula* CCAP 1446/4 strain and the Kenyan *M. producens* biomass, free from eukaryotic cells, protozoa, and fungi, respectively, but with dead bacteria afforded sufficient biomass for gDNA extraction and genome sequencing. Crushing and homogenization of the biomass using a bench top bead-based homogenizer (PowerLyzer^{TM}, 5 min) (MO BIO LABORATORIES Inc., California, USA) produced a homogenate from which bacterial gDNA was exhaustively extracted and the residue retained. $CuSO_4{\cdot}5H_2O$ assisted differential bacterial gDNA isolation of the residue of pre-extracted non-axenic filamentous cyanobacteria biomass followed by nitrogen liquefaction and sonication generated quality gDNA of *M. producens* for genome sequencing. The gDNA isolated from the residue provided high-purity DNA with 260/280 and 260/230 ratios of between 1.90 and 2.29 in the qubit assay, respectively. Treatment of the cyanobacteria biomass for times greater than 60 min denatured the *M. producens* DNA (Figure S1). The untreated *M. producens* control did not generate any pure DNA. Sequences of the Kenyan *M. producens* at the aforementioned times of 10 min, 30 min, and 60 min were synonymous with Kenyan *Moorea producens* Rep 1, Kenyan *Moorea producens* Rep 2, and Kenyan *Moorea producens* Rep 3, respectively, shown on the phylogeny diagram (Figure 2).

Initial NCBI blasts matched the cyanobacterium with *Aminobacterium colombiense*. However, there was a distinct difference in the sizes of DNA for bacteria and cyanobacteria observable in an electrophoresis gel. Moreover, mismatches arising from the primer CYA 106F were not unusual [29]. To validate the method, it was used to identify *L. majuscula* CCAP 1446/4. Further NCBI blasts of the generated sequence of the Kenyan *M. producens*, without restricting organism identity, matched the sequence at 99% identity with an uncultured *Aminanaerobia bacterium*. With the blast restriction to cyanobacteria, the sequences matched with an uncultured cyanobacterium at 98% identity. The 16S rDNA sequences obtained from *L. majuscula* strain CCAP 1446/4 by the aforesaid method for five replicates did not show any matches to *Aminanaerobia bacteria* but consistently matched with *L. majuscula* at 100% identity. The phylogenetic divergence of Kenya *M. producens* from *L. majuscula* and its clones is shown in Figure 2 and the blasted sequences are shown in Figure S2.

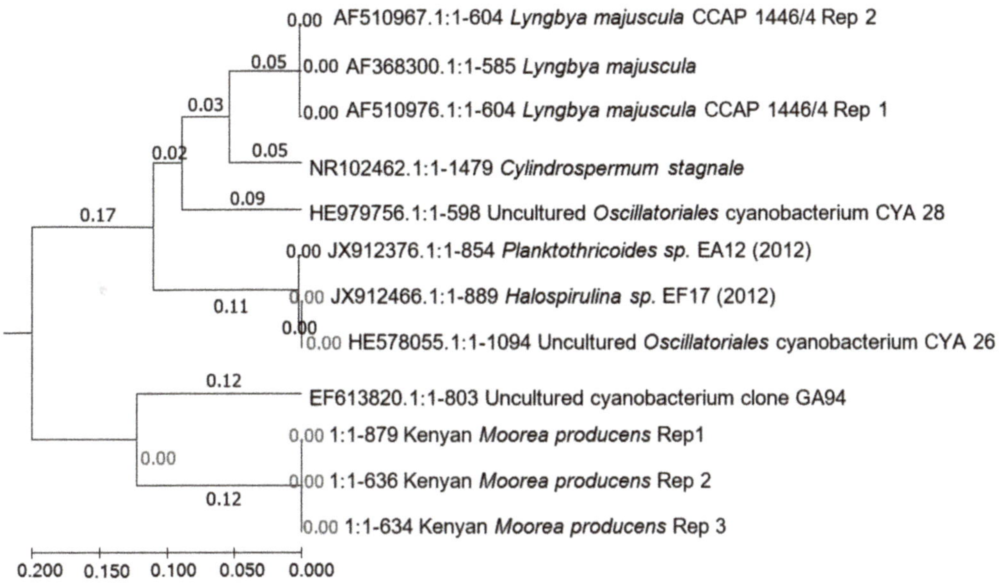

Figure 2. Phylogeny of Kenyan *M. producens* relative to *Lyngbya majuscula* and *Lyngbya majuscula* CCAP 1446. Both *L. majuscula* and *L. majuscula* CCAP 1446 are phylogenetically far distant from the Kenyan *M. producens*. Kenyan *M. producens* Rep 1 ($CuSO_4 \cdot 5H_2O$, 10 min), Kenya *M. producens* Rep 2 ($CuSO_4 \cdot 5H_2O$, 30 min), Kenyan *M. producens* Rep 3 ($CuSO_4 \cdot 5H_2O$, 60 min). Rep 1 and Rep 2 of *L. majuscula* CCAP 1446 are sequence replicates of the biomass treated with $CuSO_4 \cdot 5H_20$ at 10 min.

2.3. Bacterial Isolates from M. producens' Filaments

In the quest to establish if *M. producens'* filaments could have their associated bacteria completely removed, detached filaments were stained with acridine orange to establish cyanobacteria-bacteria association of the filament and with nigrosin to study cell wall and DNA degradation of the filament by bacteria.

Clearly, despite treatment of the cyanobacteria with cycloheximide, several rinses with phosphate buffered saline (PBS) and nitrogen liquefaction, microscopy and the isolation of the live filament bacteria (LFB) and dead filament bacteria (DFB) from the filament surface indicated that bacteria are always associated with *M. producens* (Figure 3A). Treatment of the cyanobacteria biomass with $CuS0_4 \cdot 5H_2O$ killed all bacteria except *Pseudoalteromonas carrageenovora* and *Ochrobactrum anthropi*. These surviving bacteria associated with the filament were plated on marine agar and identified through 16S rDNA gene partial sequence. The association of bacteria with cyanobacteria was regardless of the cyanobacteria getting actively involved with phototropism or on the verge of dying. Oxygen is acknowledged to be poisonous towards cyanobacteria including *M. producens*. Bacteria utilize oxygen for respiration and cyanobacteria capture carbon dioxide during photosynthesis, creating an energy balance on the cyanobacteria–bacteria interface. This close metabolic dependency may explain the close physical association of bacteria with the protective sheath surrounding the *M. producens'* filaments. When bacteria on the surface of an untreated filament were left overnight to die, it was observed that they did not enter the core of the filament targeting the DNA material. Nevertheless, there was considerable loss of cell wall material (Figure 3B), leading to the speculation that some of the bacteria on the surface survive on organic carbon from the cyanobacteria. These findings overnight were corroborated by a broken cell wall, as observed on a nigrosine-stained filament similarly left to die.

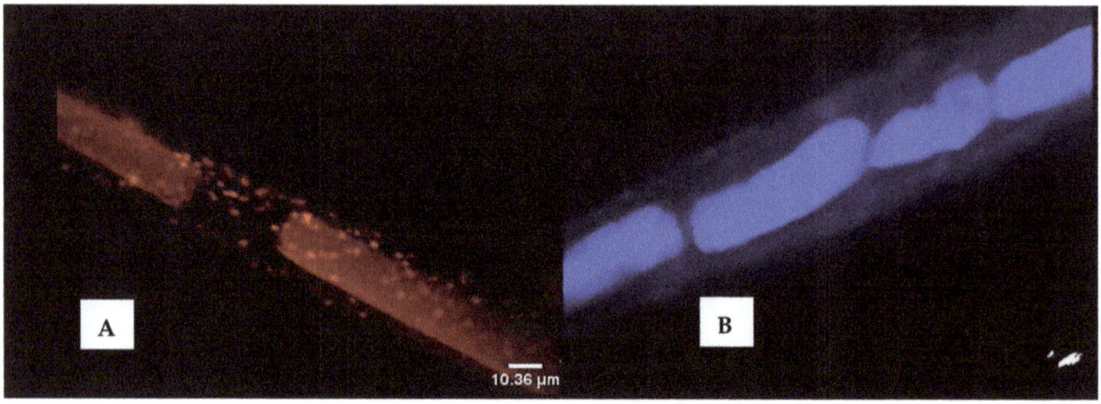

Figure 3. Bacteria on the surface of a live *M. producens'* filament (**A**) and DNA in blue at the center and cell wall material outside (**B**). The images of the filaments on a # 1.5 (~170-μm-thick) glass cover slip were acquired by the author using a Leica DMIRB inverted microscope fitted with a color and black-and-white cooled digital camera. Acridine orange was used to stain the filament shown in (**A**) and nigrosin stained the filament shown in (**B**). Scale bar = 10.36 μm.

Most bacteria isolated from the filaments of *M. producens* are close relatives of human pathogenic bacteria. The presence of Firmicutes and Actinobacteria on the filaments that are ubiquitous with antimicrobial agents suggested that within the consortium some bacterial species, in addition to other roles, may provide chemical defense molecules, which benefit the bacterial cells as well as the host cyanobacterial cells. However, it was unclear how the living filament retained its cylindrical shape, despite the presence of many species of bacteria, some of which were cellulose degraders, as exhibited by the bacteria on a dying filament (Figure 4B).

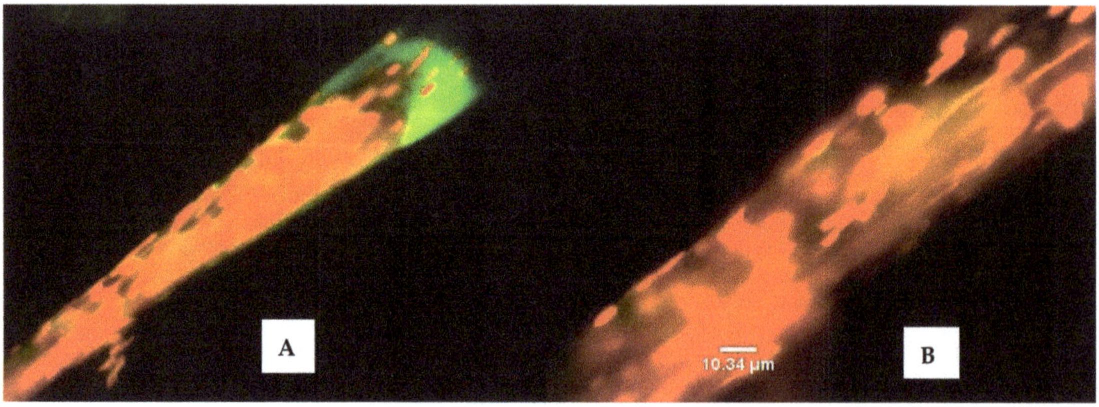

Figure 4. A non-uniform near-dead filament with congregation of live bacteria on the dead filament shown by the red color (**A**). Bacteria embedded in surface of a dying filament (**B**). The green and brown areas in (**A**,**B**) are the live and dead parts of the filament, respectively. The images were acquired by the author, as in Figure 3 above. Staining of the filament was with acridine orange. Scale bar = 10.34 μm.

Further, microscopy of the Kenyan *M. producens* also showed that this cyanobacterium is associated with stalked diatoms (Figure 5). The apparent presence of stalked diatoms on the *M. producens'* filaments indicated that microbes from estuarine and freshwater habitats may have colonized their surfaces [30]. Stalked diatoms, in particular, are found in marshes, rivers, and lagoons and are characteristically in freshwater. In the present study, *M. producens'* samples were taken from an area around the Shimoni creek. This creek is a freshwater river inlet into Shimoni Bay.

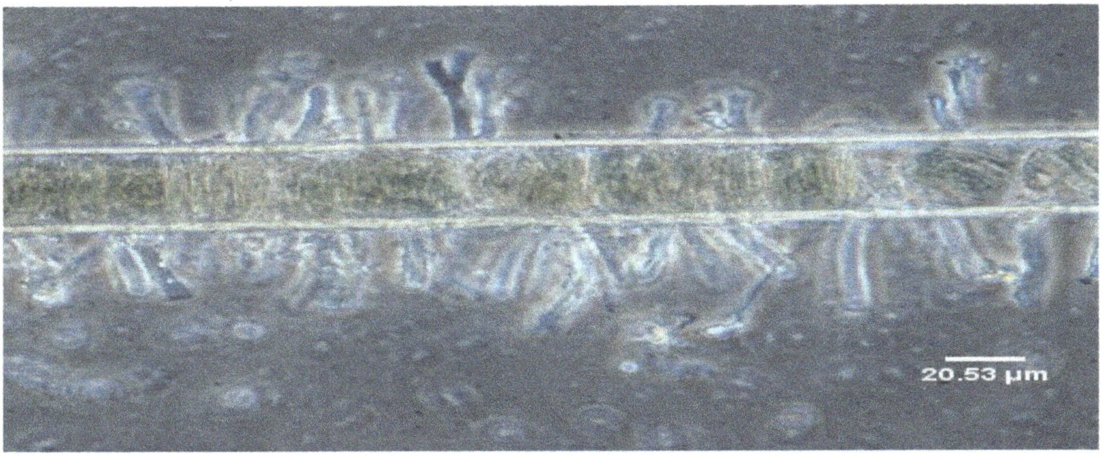

Figure 5. Filament of the Kenyan *M. producens* with stalked diatoms protruding from both its sides. Light microscopy of the filament with an OLYMPUS BX 51 equipped with inter-differential contrast optics and digital camera. The image was acquired by the author. Scale bar = 20.53 µm. Stalked diatoms were confirmed as being of a terrestrial nature by Prof. Brian Whitton of Durham University, United Kingdom.

2.4. Isolation of Bacteria from M. producens and Their Antimicrobial Activities

2.4.1. Isolation and Identification of Bacteria from *M. producens'* Sheath

The collection of *Moorea producens'* biomass at Shimoni (4°38′55″ S, 39°22′35″ E) and Wasini (4°39′18″ S, 39°22′14″ E), Kenya, at low tide was reported previously [19]. Bacterial isolates from the Kenyan *M. producens'* biomass were streaked directly onto marine agar 2216 (10% *w*/*v*). This consistently led to the isolation of colored colonies that were re-streaked to obtain pure strains. The concentration of marine broth was altered between 1% and 10% to differentiate between bacteria growing under poor and rich nutrient conditions, respectively. *Pseudomonas stutzeri* (yellow) was isolated from the sub-culturing of colonies growing together with colonies of *Enterobacter cloacae* (creamy), a mixture that was characterized by a green pigment. There were diverse morphologies of bacterial isolates after overnight incubation including tiny colonies of *Bacillus subtilis*, glassy *Pseudomonas putida*, large soft *Shewanella algae* (purple), and *Pseudomonas stutzeri* (yellow), respectively. Hard colonies were observed, which were identified as *Bacillus licheniformis* (red). A list of representative epibiotic bacterial isolates from the Kenyan *M. producens* is shown in Table 1.

Nearly 70% of all isolates were γ-proteobacteria. Firmicutes were isolated in reasonable quantities (17%), whereas α-proteobacteria and Actinobacteria were minimal. It is possible that the cyanobacterium appropriated pathogenic bacteria of terrestrial origin at low tide. Direct streaking led to the isolation of 137 bacterial strains, from which 24 strains were selected for further study and their organic extracts examined for antimicrobial activities. In common with the *M. producens'* filament, most bacteria isolated from the sheath were found to be close relatives of human pathogenic bacteria.

Table 1. A list of representative Kenyan *M. producens* epibiotic bacteria (EB) isolates.

	Accession	Strain	% Similarity of 16S Sequence	Taxon
Shewanella algae	KC660130	SHALG-01	99	γ-proteobacteria
Shewanella algae	KC660131	SHALG-02	99	γ-proteobacteria
Marinobacterium stanieri	KC660132	MARIS-01	99	γ-proteobacteria
Acinetobacter johnsonii	KC660133	ACJ-01	99	γ-proteobacteria
Marinobacterium stanieri	KC660134	MARIS-02	99	γ-proteobacteria
Staphylococcus saprophyticus	KC660135	STAPRO	99	Firmicutes
Pseudomonas stutzeri	KC660136	PST-01	99	γ-proteobacteria
Enterobacter cloacae	KC660137	ENTCLO	99	γ-proteobacteria
Cellulosimicrobium cellulans	KC660138	CCL-01	99	Actinobacteria
Cellulosimicrobium cellulans	KC660139	CCL-02	99	Actinobacteria
Pseudomonas pseudoalcaligenes	KC660140	PPS	99	γ-proteobacteria
Pseudomonas putida	KC660141	PPT	99	γ-proteobacteria
Bacillus aereus	ND	ND	99	Firmicutes
Bacillus licheniformis	KC660142	BLC-01	99	Firmicutes
Bacillus licheniformi	KC660143	BLC-02	99	Firmicutes
Bacillus subtilis	KC660144	BS-00	99	Firmicutes
Pseudomonas stutzeri	KC660145	PST-02	99	γ-proteobacteria
Enterobacter cancerogenus	ND	ND	99	γ-proteobacteria
Klebsiella oxytoca	ND	ND	99	γ-proteobacteria
Yokenella regensburgei	ND	ND	99	γ-proteobacteria
Ochrobactrumanthropi	ND	ND	99	α-proteobacteria
Pseudomonas stutzeri	ND	ND	99	γ-proteobacteria
Pseudoalteromonas carrageenovora	ND	ND	99	γ-proteobacteria

ND–Strain sequences not deposited with Genbank but were inferred from Blast.

2.4.2. Isolation of Brightly Colored Bacteria from *M. producens*' Sheath during Neap Tide

Moorea producens was collected from the sampling sites at a time of minimal tide when the sun and the moon were in quadrature. The growing of sheath bacteria onto marine agar by swab cultures showed the Gram-negative *Pseudoalteromonas* sp. to be the dominant genus. Pseudoalteromonas genus belongs to the sulfur-oxidizing symbiont relatives of γ-*Proteobacteria* commonly associated with sea water. However, this dominance is prevailed by treatment of the *M. producens*' sheath with 70% ethanol (*v*/*v*, 2 min) prior to swab culturing, thereby enhancing the growth of brightly colored colonies of bacteria. The 16S rDNA sequencing identified these brightly colored bacteria as *Nocardia cornyebacterioides* (red), *Paracoccus marcusii* (orange), *Micrococcus* sp. (yellow), *Stappia* sp. (pink), and *Bacillus* sp. BacB3, respectively. Additionally, small colonies of unidentified, creamy, Gram-negative rods were isolated. *Nocardia cornyebacterioides* belongs to the genus *Nocardiopsis*. Prior to 16S rDNA identification techniques, the genus *Nocardiopsis* was defined on the basis of chemotaxonomic markers [31] with phospholipids type III and the phospholipids phosphatidylcholine and phosphatidylmethylethanolamine as salient chemotaxonomic features [31,32]. Previously, *Nocardia cornyebacterioides* was reported as an unpublished strain SAFR-015 with accession number AY167850.1 gi:27497670 in the MWG 16S rDNA data-bank. *Paracoccus marcusii* belongs to the α-3 subclass of the *Proteobacteria* [33], whereas the genus *Stappia* belongs to the ecologically important carboxydotrophic bacteria.

Interestingly, the study established that *Pseudoalteromonas* sp. was inhibited by ethanol (70% *v*/*v*) only during the initial 15 min, after which the bacteria population increased linearly with time. This was against the common belief that 70% ethanol has strong sterilizing activity against common bacteria. The natural microbial environment of bacteria on the surface of *M. producens* was mimicked by growing various strains of bacteria in filter discs (6 mm) over a lawn of the dominant *Pseudoalteromonas* sp. Subsequently, these bacterial antagonism experiments showed *Micrococcus* sp. (yellow) and *Stappia* sp. (pink) to antagonize *Pseudoalteromonas* sp. by slowing the growth of the latter bacteria by a zone of 12 mm to 19 mm and of 6 mm to 8 mm, respectively. The diversity of bacteria associated with the cyanobacterium was higher at low tide and lower during neap tide.

2.4.3. Antimicrobial Activities of Organic Extracts of Bacterial Isolates

Using bacteria isolated from the cyanobacteria, organic extracts of Firmicutes were screened against bacteria, fungi, and known pathogens. Organic extracts were comprised of acetone and methanol, whereupon the acetone extracts were clearly the most active and were, therefore, used for the screens. Aliquots of the extracts and a streptomycin control in methanol (1 mg/mL, 20 μL) were tested against Gram-negative *Escherichia coli* strains JW0451-2 and BW25113, respectively, and Gram-positive *Bacillus subtilis* DSM 10 and *Micrococcus luteus* 1790 in 96-well microtiter plates. The absorbances of the organic extracts of microbial isolates were determined by serial dilution in EBS medium (0.5% casein peptone, 0.5% protease peptone, 0.1% meat extract, 0.1% yeast extract, pH 7.0) for bacteria and MYC medium (1.0% glucose, 1.0% phytone peptone, 50 mM HEPES [11.9 g/L], pH 7.0) for yeast and fungi, and were cultivated (30 °C, 160 rpm, 24–48 h) with cell concentration adjustment to OD_{600} 0.01 for bacteria and OD_{548} 0.1 for yeast and fungi, respectively. Then, they were matched with absorbances of Streptomycin and Nystatin in IC_{50} determinations to afford the levels of inhibitions (antibacterial activities), as shown in Table 2. The antibacterial activities were ranked using a percentage scale with the highest activity being assigned a value of 100% (Table 2).

The % scale activity values were obtained as follows:

$$\frac{\text{Absorbance of microbial organic extract}}{\text{Absorbance of control antibiotic at 1 mg/mL}} \times 100\%$$

Extracts of *B. marisflavi* JC556 (LS974830.1) were active against *Micrococcus luteus* and *B. subtilis*. Those of *Bacillus licheniformis* PB3 (CP025226.1) displayed moderate activity against *Escherichia coli* and *B. subtilis*, whereas organic extracts of *B. subtilis* MJ01 showed very high activity against *E. coli* and *M. luteus*, respectively. Biological activity was strain dependent, as demonstrated by *B. marisflavi* LQ1 (MG025780.1) that was less active compared to *B. marisflavi* JC556 (LS974830.1). Similarly, *Bacillus subtilis* TBS-CBE-BS01 (MK346244.1) had minor activity against *M. luteus* compared with *B. subtilis* MJ01. Organic extracts of the bacterial isolates showed no biological activities against *Pichia anomala* and *Mucor hiemalis*, and neither were biological activities of the extracts observed against the pathogens *Acinetobacter baumannii*, *Citrobacter freundii*, *S. aureus* Newman, *Pseudomonas aeruginosa* PA14, *Mycobacterium smegmatis*, and the yeast *Candida albicans*. Of the 24 strains, 5 that were considered not interesting due to potential pathogenesis were later dropped and are, therefore, not included in Table 2 above. Organic extracts of *B. marisflavi* JC556 (LS974830.1) and *B. subtilis* MJ01 were the most active. *B. marisflavi* extract was selected for bioassay-guided isolation of its natural products. Streptomycin was the reference antibiotic for bacteria and nystatin was a reference against yeast and fungi, respectively.

2.5. Isolation of Micrococcin P1 and Micrococcin P2 and Biological Activities

2.5.1. Isolation of Micrococcin P1 (**1**) and Micrococcin P2 (**2**)

In this study, extracts of a number of cultured Firmicutes were found to inhibit the growth of *Bacillus subtilis* except for those from *B. subtilis*, suggesting that bacteria species can produce antibiotics against pathogens from their own genus. This observation could pave the way for exploring future antibiotics against *Pseudomonas aeruginosa* and *Klebsiella pneumoniae* that are responsible for nosocomial infections from members of the *Pseudomonas* genus and *Klebsiella* spp., respectively. Acetone extracts of *B. marisflavi* cultures were the most biologically active, especially against Gram-positive *Staphylococcus aureus*. The antibacterial compounds identified in these extracts were micrococcin p1 (**1**) and micrococcin p2 (**2**), shown below in Figure 6.

Table 2. Antimicrobial activity of bacterial isolates from a marine cyanobacteria.

Bacterial Strains	Closest Match in GenBank (Accession Number)	% Similarity of 16S Sequence	Antimicrobial Activity	Level of Inhibition
TD1, TD15	*Bacillus marislavi* JC556 (LS974830.1)	100	*M. luteus*, *B. subtilis*	Active
TD2, TD26	*Bacillus marislavi* LQ1 (MG025780.1)	100	*B. subtilis*	Minor activity
TD3, TD6	*Bacillus safensis* 6-11 (MK205159.1)	100	*B. subtilis*	Minor activity
TD10	*Bacillus safensis* 6-11 (MK210556.1)	100	Not Done	
TD11	*Bacillus safensis* D11 (KX068630.1)	100	*B. subtilis*, *P. anomalis*	Minor activity
TD23, 25	*Bacillus safensis* D11 MK337676.1	100	*M. luteus*, *B. subtilis*	Minor activity
TD4	*Bacillus aryabhattai* PYMW (MK346120.1)	100	*B. subtilis*, *P. anomalis*	Minor activity
TD8	*Bacillus aryabhattai* P6 (MK346850.1)	100	*B. subtilis*	Minor activity
TD5, TD22	*Bacillus licheniformis* PB3 (CP025226.1)	99	*E. coli*, *B. subtilis*	Moderately active
TD7	*Bacillus subtilis* MJ01	100	*E. coli*, *M. luteus*	Very active
TD12	*Bacillus subtilis* TBS-CBE-BS01 (MK346244.1)	100	*M. luteus*	Minor activity
TD9	Sequence failed	Not done	*B. subtilis*	Minor activity
TD13	*Arthrobacter* sp. ABCH 95.B (KY327809.1)	100	NA	No activity
TD14	*Bacillus flexus* 00F26 MH542283.1	Not done	NA	No activity

KEY: 0–24%, No activity; 25–49%, Minor activity; 50–74%, Moderate activity; 75–99%, Active; 100%, Very active. Activities were relative to absorbances of Streptomycin and Nystatin in an IC_{50} determination.

C-18 HPLC fractionation of the active fraction of *B. marisflavi* using maXis 2 G (BRUKER DALTONICS, Bremen, Germany) afforded the biologically active antibiotics micrococcin P1 (**1**) and micrococcin P2 (**2**) with the retention times of 9.43 min and 9.67 min, respectively (Figure S3). Using HREIMS, the LCMS-MS fragmentation with maXis 4G (BRUKER DALTONICS, Bremen, Germany) unequivocally isolated the known antibiotics micrococcin P1 and micrococcin P2 from *B. marisflavis* (Figures S4–S7). Molecular formulae were identified by including the isotopic pattern in the calculation (SmartFormula algorithm). Both the fractionation with maXis 2G and the high-resolution MS/MS fragmentation using maXis 4G used an acetonitrile/water gradient system that was buffered with ammonium acetate. Details on how the results were acquired can be found in Section 3.7 of the experimental section.

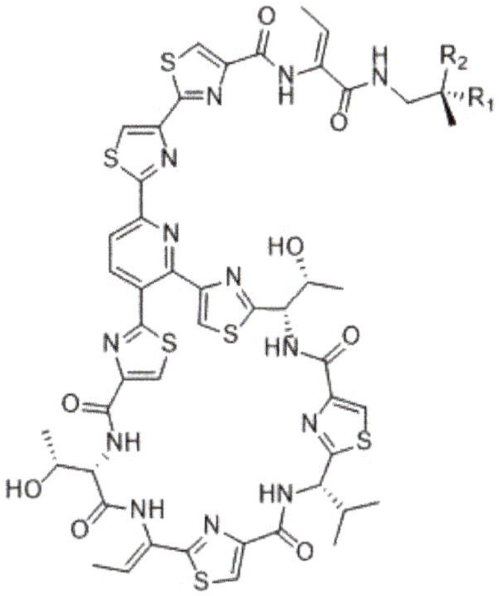

Figure 6. Micrococcin P1 (**1**): R_1 = OH, R_2 = H; Micrococcin P2 (**2**): R_1 = R_2 = O.

Dereplication of the active molecular ions of 571.60/1142.2 and 572.60/1144.2 using MS^2 ions in maXis 4G and the Dictionary of Natural Products linked the strong activity of the *Bacillus marisflavi* strain to its production of micrococcin P1 (**1**) ($C_{48}H_{49}N_{13}O_9S_6$; obs. *m/z* 1144.20227/572.60381) and micrococcin P2 (**2**) ($C_{48}H_{47}N_{13}O_9S_6$; obs. *m/z* 1142.20446/571.60370), respectively. These antibiotics were originally isolated from *Micrococcus* sp. [34]. Their structures were confirmed by spectroscopy in 1978 [35] and the total synthesis and stereochemical assignment was accomplished in 2009 [36]. More recent work includes the ribosomal production of micrococcin P1 and micrococcin P2 antibiotics through prepeptide gene replacement [37]. Most recently, the antibiotic thiopeptide micrococcin P3 was isolated from a marine-derived strain of *Bacillus stratospherius* [38]. In this study, we established the following MS-MS fragmentation pattern for micrococcin P1 (**1**) from the maXis 4G measurements (Table 3) that unequivocally matched with that reported by Walsh et al., in 2010 [37].

Table 3. Fragmentation pattern of micrococcin P1 (**1**) 1144.20227/572.60381.

	Molecular Ion	Expected *m/z* (a.m.u)	Observed *m/z* (a.m.u)
1	M + H	1144.21732	1144.21930
2	M − H_2O + H	1126.20676	1126.20946
3	M − CO	1116.22241	1116.22442
4	M − $2H_2O$ + H	1108.19619	1108.19865
5	M − CO − H_2O	1098.21184	1098.21380
6	M − CO − $2H_2O$	1080.20128	1080.20333
7	b13 + H_2O	1051.13834	1051.14040
8	a13	1041.15399	1041.15222
9	b13 − $2H_2O$	1033.12778	1033.12980
10	b2 + H_2O	1025.15908	1025.16113
11	a13 − H_2O	1023.14343	1023.14492
12	b2 − $2H_2O$	1007.14851	1007.15051
13	a13 − $2H_2O$	1005.13286	1005.13482

Micrococcin P1 and micrococcin P2 are closely related molecules with the former existing as the secondary alcohol and the latter as the ketone congener. The MS/MS fragmentation pattern shown above for micrococcin P1 is the most common pathway followed by thiocillin variants including micrococcin P2 [37]. It could, therefore, be concluded that together with high-resolution mass spectrometry, dereplication of the active molecular ions, and the Dictionary of Natural Products, bioassay-guided fractionation of the extracts of *B. marisflavi* led to the first isolation of the antibiotics micrococcin P1 (**1**) and micrococcin P2 (**2**) from a strain of *B. marisflavi*. Isolation of these known antibiotics was strain dependent since organic extracts of other strains of *B. marisflavi* isolates did not exhibit the activity of *Bacillus marisflavi* JC556 (LS974830.1).

2.5.2. Biological Activity of Micrococcin P1 against *Staphylococcus aureus*

The activity of micrococcin P1 (**1**) against a panel of pathogens, *Acinetobacter baumannii, Citrobacter freundii, S. aureus* Newman, *Pseudomonas aeruginosa* PA14, *Mycobacterium smegmatis,* and the yeast *Candida albicans*, was minimal with activity only observed against *Staphylococcus aureus*. This last activity of micrococcin P1 against *S. aureus* was consistent with that in the literature [33,34,39]. MIC is the lowest concentration of the drug, preventing visible growth of the test organism [40], and IC_{50} is the concentration of the drug at which the growth of half of the test organism (bacteria, fungi or yeast) is inhibited [41]. An MIC value of 0.0157 μM was obtained for micrococcin P1. Using the method of Okanya et al. [41] and its modification as outlined by Jansen et al. [40] and Bader et al. [42], the IC_{50} of micrococcin P1 against *S. aureus* was shown to be 0.357 μM (0.159 mg/mL) (Figure S8). This value is within the range of IC_{50} of micrococcin P1 against an assorted collection of *S. aureus* strains and confirms the activity of micrococcin P1 against *S. aureus* to be strain dependent [39]. The IC_{50} regression curve of the biological activity data of micrococcin P1 against *S. aureus* is shown in Figure S8.

3. Experimental

3.1. *Study Area and Specimen Preparation*

Moorea producens' specimens were collected from Shimoni (4°38′55″ S, 39°22′35″ E) and Wasini (4°39′18″ S, 39°22′14″ E) on the South Coast of Kenya during 2012 (during neap and low tides) and 2018 (low tide). Specimens were preserved in sterile PTFE bottles prior to storage at −20 °C, prior to shipment to the UK (2012) and Germany (2018). Bacteria were isolated from *M. producens* using traditional methods and identified using Gram stain and microscopy in Kenya. At Newcastle University, United Kingdom, and at the Helmholtz Institute, Germany, the bacterial isolates were identified using microscopy and 16S rDNA identification.

3.2. *Detection of Homodolastatin 16, Dolastatin 16, and Antanapeptin A in Kenyan Isolates of a Filamentous Cyanobacterium, Moorea producens*

The detection of homodolastatin 16, dolastatin 16, and antanapeptin A in *M. producens* was confirmed by LCMS analysis of organic extracts of the cyanobacterium. Briefly, *M. producens* (previously known as *L. majuscula*) (2 g) was extracted with 2:1 dichloromethane/methanol (50 mL, 12 h, 25 °C, sonicated) and filtered through glass fiber filters (44 μ). Fractionation of the extracts from the Kenyan "*L. majuscula*" was achieved on C-18 silica to give "TD-Lyng chl" (the first Lyngbya extract fraction to elute from the C-18 column) and "TD-Lyngbia" that eluted immediately after "TD-Lyng chl". TD-Lyng chl and TD-Lyngbia were respectively evaporated and dried under nitrogen. The dried extracts were redissolved in 1:1 methanol/water to a final concentration of 2 mg/mL. Subsequently, 5 μL of the sample was injected onto the column (XBridge C18, 3.5 μm, 2.1 × 150 mm) and separated on a gradient of 10% 0.1% formic acid in water/90% 0.1% formic acid in acetonitrile to 5% 0.1% formic acid in water/95% formic acid in acetonitrile at 0.3 mL/min. Molecular ions for the cyclodepsipeptides were identified by Fourier transform mass spectrometry (FTMS) from ESI Full MS chromatograms. The MS used was a Thermo

Scientific Orbitrap Exactive (THERMO FISHER SCIENTIFIC, Bremen GmbH, Germany); resolution was set to 150,000.

3.3. $CuSO_4 \cdot 5H_2O$ Assisted Differential Genomic DNA (gDNA) Extraction of M. producens

Prior to bacteria genomic DNA (gDNA) isolation, the cyanobacteria cells were treated with cycloheximide (5 mg L^{-1}, overnight) to kill eukaryotic cells, protozoa, and fungi. Thereafter, the cells were rinsed several times with filtered sterile seawater (12 times, 45 µ) and left overnight in phosphate-poor autoclaved seawater [29]. For detaching filaments, clusters of Moorea biomass were submerged in phosphate buffered saline (PBS, pH 7.4). The resulting filaments were rinsed with Millipore water and pooled together, and aliquots were weighed to afford sufficient biomass for gDNA extraction and genome sequencing. Thereafter, the cyanobacteria were treated with copper sulphate powder ($CuSO_4 \cdot 5H_2O$) and left to stand for 10 min, 30 min, and 60 min, respectively, to kill any available bacteria. The control was untreated. For removing the bacteria, biomass of pooled filaments was placed in an Eppendorf tube, freeze-dried with liquid nitrogen, and thawed slowly. The tube contents were sonicated (pulsar 30% of maximal amplitude, 10 min) and the process was repeated 5 times. Representative filaments were stained with acridine to observe the presence of any associated bacteria using a LEICA DMIRB microscope (LEICA DMIRB, Mannheim, Germany) with Media Cybernetics image analysis software Image-Pro Plus 7 (MEDIA CYBERNETICS, Rockville, MA, USA).

Aliquots of the biomass (0.25 g) were weighed in sterile MoBio microfuge tubes into which was added 100 µL of sodium dodecyl sulfate (SDS) and 0.5 mL of RNAse free TE buffer (50 mM Tris HCl, 20 mM EDTA, pH 8.0). The specimen was crushed and homogenized using a bench-top bead-based homogenizer (PowerLyzer™, 5 min). The resulting homogenate was transferred into an Eppendorf tube, freeze-dried in liquid nitrogen, and thawed slowly. The tube contents were sonicated (pulsar 30% maximal amplitude, 10 min) and the process was repeated five times [43]. The sample was centrifuged (10,000× *g*, 3 min) and bacterial gDNA were extracted following the MoBio kit for soil bacteria; the residue was retained. The DNeasy PowerMax Soil Kit used here was formerly sold by MOBIO as PowerMax Soil DNA Isolation Kit, and this is currently sold by Qiagen (QIAGEN, Valencia, CA, USA). The residue was re-extracted for bacterial gDNA until no traces of the gDNA were detected on an electrophoresis gel.

To the bacteria-free residue was added 1 mL of Lysis buffer (TE buffer with RNase) and heated (55 °C, 1 h) prior to adding 300 µL of freshly prepared lysozyme at 50 mg/mL. The mixture was heated (55 °C, 30 min). Into the contents was added 100 µL of a solution containing 450 µL of 10% sarcosyl and 20 µL of 20 µg/mL proteinase k and incubated (55 °C, 30 min). To each of the contents in a 2-mL Eppendorf tube was added 3 volumes of phenol: chloroform: isoamyl alcohol (25:24:1) and the contents of the tubes were mixed with inversion and centrifuged (10,000× *g*, 5 min). The resulting gDNA was isolated and purified following conventional standard methods [44]. Purity and integrity of the gDNA was confirmed using a combination of spectrophotometry (NanoDrop) and agarose gel electrophoresis [44].

PCR amplification of the purified gDNA was done according to the protocol of Nubel et al. [29]. The forward primer is CYA106F (5′-CGGACGGGTGAGTAACGCGT GA-3′), whereas the reverse primer is an equimolar mixture of CYA781Ra (5′-GACTACTG GGGTATCTAATCCCATT-3′) and CYA781Rb (5′-GACTACAGGGGTATCTAATCCCTTT-3′) [29]. Preparatory columns (Invitrogen PCR Preps) were used to clean the PCR products. PCR products were sequenced by Genius labs, UK, and the sequences were annotated using Bioedit 7. Alignment of the sequences and phylogeny of the aligned sequences utilized the MEGA X program [45]. For obtaining gDNA of the cyanobacterium, homogenized *L. majuscula* pellets were exhaustively extracted for bacteria gDNA. The resulting bacterial gDNA of mixed species was degenerated by $CuSO_4 \cdot 5H_2O$ and therefore it did not generate a 16S rDNA sequence.

3.4. Isolation of Bacteria from M. producens' Filaments

Preparation of *M. producens* to detach filaments and to determine its (*M. producens*) gDNA using $CuSO_4{\cdot}5H_2O$ is described in Section 3.3. In another experiment, filaments from cyanobacteria biomass that was treated with $CuSO_4{\cdot}H_2O$ were plated onto marine agar to determine the assemblage of bacteria associated with the filaments on a cyanobacterial sheath. These experiments were repeated for a near-dead *M. producens* mat. Bacteria isolated from the live and dead filaments were designated as LFB and DFB, respectively, prior. These bacterial isolates were identified using 16S rDNA partial gene sequence. Additional filaments from the live and near-dead *M. producens* were thoroughly washed and stained with acridine orange and nigrosin to establish association of the filaments with heterotrophic bacteria.

3.5. The 16S rDNA Identification of Bacterial Isolates

Genomic DNA was extracted from cell pellets of single colony bacterial cultures in marine broth 2216. The Qiagen DNeasy Blood and Tissue kit was used (QIAGEN, Valencia, CA, USA). Specifically, overnight culture containing approximately 1–3 $\times$ 10^9 bacterial cells were transferred to a 1.5-mL Eppendorf tube on ice and centrifuged (13,000$\times$ *g*, 1 min). Prior to the addition of RNase buffer (1.5 µL), the cells were lysed with lysis buffer (300 µL, 65 °C, 15 min), incubated (37 °C, 15 min), and centrifuged. The resulting supernatant from centrifugation (13,000$\times$ *g*, 1 min) was thereafter treated with genomic-binding buffer (0.5 mL), centrifuged (10,000 rpm, 2 min), and passed through a DNA-binding column. Washing the column with genomic wash buffer (1 mL) and three times with 1 mL of 75% ethanol followed by dry spinning afforded purified DNA on the column. The resulting DNA was eluted from the column with milliQ water.

Reacting a mixture containing 10 $\times$ Qiagen buffer (2.5 µL), $MgCl_2$ (0.5 µL), d'NTPS (1 µL), 2.5 µL of primer 27 F (5′-AGAGTTTGATCCTGGCTCAG-3′), and 2.5 µL of primer 1492 R (5′-TACGGYTACCTTGTTACGACTT-3′), DMSO (0.75 µL) and Taq polymerase (0.1 µL) gave the polymerase chain reaction (PCR) product of the 16S rDNA. Sterile Milli Q water was added to adjust the final volume of the PCR mixture to 25 µL. Thermal cycling was performed with an Eppendorf Mastercycler AG 22331 (EPPENDORF, Hamburg, Germany). The sample utilized the standard initial denaturation step (95 °C, 5 min; 95 °C, 30 s) followed by annealing (40 °C, 1 min). Procedurally, the thermal profile used was 30 cycles. This profile consisted of 1 min of primer annealing at 55 °C, 1 min of extension at 72 °C, and 1 min of denaturation at 95 °C. A final extension step consisting of 10 min at 72 °C was also included. PCR products were detected by agarose gel electrophoresis and visualized by UV fluorescence after ethidium bromide staining. The PCR products generated by the 27 F and 1492 R primers were approximately 1 kb in size and purified using the Qiagen genomic DNA as specified by the manufacturer. Sequencing of the final DNA extracts was done by LGC Genomics (Germany).

3.6. Antibacterial and Antifungal Assays

Fifty bacterial strains out of 137 were selected on the basis of color and morphological appearance, from which 24 were sequenced and their respective 16S rDNA sequences were identified by BLAST (BLASTN 2.8.1+) [46]. Cultures were maintained in marine broth, and pre-cultures were grown on medium 5294 [47] in a rotatory shaker incubator (50 mL, 30 °C, XAD resin, 3 days). Precultures were in duplicate. Cultures of the bacteria for secondary metabolite production were grown in Medium 5294 (2% XAD resin, 7 days, 37 °C). The XAD resin was used to sequester secondary metabolites from the media. Specifically, the resin was initially extracted with acetone prior to extraction with methanol. The acetone extracts, being more active than the extracts of methanol, were reconstituted in methanol. Aliquots of the acetone extracts in methanol were used for bioassays against target microbial screens and mass spectrometry profiling. Mass spectrometry profiling is invaluable in this context as it provides all the available masses of the extract.

The antibacterial and antifungal assays adopted the method of Jansen and co-workers [40], briefly described below. Aliquots of the extracts, reference antibiotics, and micrococcin P1 (**1**) (1 mg/mL, 20 µL) were tested against Gram-negative *Escherichia coli* strains JW0451-2 and BW25113, respectively, and Gram-positive *Bacillus subtilis* DSM 10 and *Micrococcus luteus* 1790. Antifungal screens utilized *Pichia anomala* and *Mucor hiemalis*. Streptomycin (SIGMA-ALDRICH) was the reference antibiotic for bacteria and nystatin (SIGMA-ALDRICH) was a reference against yeast and fungi, respectively. *Acinetobacter baumannii*, *Citrobacter freundii*, *S.aureus* Newman, *Pseudomonas aeruginosa* PA14, *Mycobacterium smegmatis*, and the yeast *Candida albicans* were used for assays against pathogens. The % scale activity values were determined in 96-well microtiter plates by 1:1 serial dilution in EBS medium (0.5% casein peptone, 0.5% protease peptone, 0.1% meat extract, 0.1% yeast extract, pH 7.0) for bacteria and MYC medium (1.0% glucose, 1.0% phytone peptone, 50 mM HEPES [11.9 g/L], pH 7.0) for yeasts and fungi. The test organisms were cultivated at 30 °C and 160 rpm for 24−48 h, and the cell concentration was adjusted to OD_{600} 0.01 for bacteria and OD_{548} 0.1 for yeast and fungi before the test. The antibacterial activities were ranked to % scale (Table 2). The activities of micrococcin P1 (**1**) against *S. aureus* were given an activity score relative to their absorbances and matched with their respective concentrations. The lowest concentration of micrococcin P1 inhibiting the growth of *Staphylococcus aureus* was considered to be the MIC. The IC_{50} of micrococcin P1 against *S. aureus* used the method in Okanya et al. [41]. An IC_{50} calculator was used to generate the IC_{50} regression curve and to obtain the IC_{50} of micrococcin P1 (**1**) against *S. aureus*.

*3.7. Isolation of Micrococcin P1 (**1**) and Micrococcin P2 (**2**)*

The active fraction of *B. marisflavi* JC556 (LS974830.1) was cultivated overnight and fractionated according to the respective OD_{600} (0.01 for bacteria and OD_{548} 0.1 for yeast and fungi) using maXis 2 G (BRUKER DALTONICS, Germany); the retention times of the entire 96-well plate were recorded. Fractions with the lowest absorbances were considered to be the most active. LCMS-MS fragmentation of the compounds with the retention times of 9.43 min and 9.67 min, respectively, was realized with maXis 4G (Bruker, Germany). Generally, the methods of Okanya et al. were adopted [41]. Accordingly, HREIMS data were recorded on a maXis spectrometer (BRUKER DALTONICS, Germany). Molecular formulae were identified by including the isotopic pattern in the calculation (SmartFormula algorithm). Analytical RP HPLC utilised an Agilent 1100 HPLC system (AGILENT TECHNOLOGIES, Waldbronn, Germany) equipped with a UV diode-array detector and an evaporative light-scattering (PL-ELS 1000) detector. HPLC conditions were column 125 × 2 mm, Nucleodur C-18, and 5 µm (MACHEREY-NAGEL, Düren, Germany); solvent A, 5% acetonitrile in water, 5 mmol of NH_4Ac, and 0.04 mL of CH_3COOH; solvent B, 95% acetonitrile, 5 mmol of NH_4Ac, and 0.04 mL of CH_3COOH; gradient system, 10% B increasing to 100% in 30 min, 100% B for 10 min, to 10% B post-run for 10 min; 40 °C; and flow rate of 0.3 mL/min. Dereplication of these compounds along with the Dictionary of Natural products were used to identify the known antibiotics micrococcin P1 (**1**) and micrococcin P2 (**2**) from a strain of *B. marisflavi*.

4. Conclusions

The Kenyan isolate of "*Lyngbya majuscula*", also known as *Moorea producens* and recently renamed Moorena, was shown to be phylogenetically distinct from *L. majuscula* CCAP 1446/4 and *L. majuscula* clones. Surprisingly, epibiotic bacteria growing on the surface of *M. producens*' filaments were often found to be human pathogens. A new method for the isolation of genomic DNA (gDNA) from non-axenic filamentous marine cyanobacteria based on the $CuSO_4{\cdot}5H_2O$ assisted differential isolation of bacteria gDNA from a cyanobacteria biomass was reported. Debromoaplysiatoxin (DAT), which is an indicator toxin found earlier in *M. producens*, was not detected in the Kenyan strain of *M. producens*. The phylogenetic divergence, absence of DAT, and the detection of unique cyclodepsipeptides in the Kenyan strain of *M. producens* reinforce a need for molecular identification of non-axenic *M. producens* species worldwide. The IC_{50} of micrococcin P1 against *S. aureus* was within the range of values reported in literature. Our results showed that the genetic basis for synthesizing micrococcin P1 (**1**), originally discovered in *Bacillus cereus* ATCC 14579, is often species or strain dependent and provides evidence for *M. producens*-associated bacteria as an underexplored source of bacterial strains for the discovery of new antibiotics to fight drug resistance.

Supplementary Materials: The following supporting information can be downloaded at: https://www.mdpi.com/article/10.3390/md20020128/s1, Figure S1: Denaturation of *Moorea producens* DNA; Figure S2: Blasted sequences; Figure S3: Micrococcin P1 and P2 chromatogram (MS and UV at 220 nm); Figure S4: Micrococcin P1 MS/MS spectrum; Figure S5: Micrococcin P1 annotated MS/MS spectrum; Figure S6: Micrococcin P2 MS/MS spectrum; Figure S7: Micrococcin P2 annotated MS/MS spectrum; Figure S8: Activity of micrococcin P1 against *S. aureus* Newman.

Author Contributions: T.D. designed and performed the experiments and wrote the manuscript. M.J.H. and J.G.B. wrote the manuscript. All authors have read and agreed to the published version of the manuscript.

Funding: This research was funded by an EU-FP7 Marie Sklowdowska Curie IIF award to T.D. through his project Lyngbya-KENYA 29950 carried out at Newcastle University, United Kingdom (2012–2014) grant number Lyngbya-KENYA 29950; and by a fellowship to T.D. at the Helmholtz Institute for Pharmaceutical Research (HIPS), Saarland, Germany (2018–19) from the Organisation for the Prohibition of Chemical Weapons (OPCW) of the Hague, The Netherlands, grant number L/ICA/ICB/216416/18. The APC was funded by the Western Indian Ocean Marine Sciences Association (WIOMSA).

Institutional Review Board Statement: Not applicable.

Informed Consent Statement: Not applicable.

Acknowledgments: We acknowledge Rebecca Goss of the University of St Andrews, Scotland, UK, for the LCMS analyses, Rolf Mueller of HIPS for providing his lab and facilities to T.D and Brian Whitton of Durham University, UK for confirming the identity of *M. producens*' stalked diatoms.

Conflicts of Interest: The authors declare that there is no conflict of interest.

References

1. *WHO Report on Surveillance of Antibiotic Consumption 2016–2018 Early Implementation*; WHO: Geneva, Switzerland, 2018.
2. Demain, A.L.; Sanchez, S. Microbial drug discovery: 80 years of progress. *J. Antibiot.* **2009**, *62*, 5–16. [CrossRef] [PubMed]
3. Hutchings, M.I.; Truman, A.W.; Wilkinson, B. Antibiotics: Past, present and future. *Curr. Opin. Microbiol.* **2019**, *51*, 72–80. [CrossRef] [PubMed]
4. Ball, S.; Bessell, C.J.; Mortimer, A. The Production of Polyenic Antibiotics by Soil Streptomycetes. *J. Gen. Microbiol.* **1957**, *17*, 96–103. [CrossRef] [PubMed]
5. Matsuda, S.; Adachi, K.; Matsuo, Y.; Nukina, M.; Shizuri, Y. Salinisporamycin, a novel metabolite from *Salinispora arenicola*. *J. Antibiot.* **2009**, *62*, 519–526, Erratum in *J. Antibiot.* **2009**, *62*, 537. [CrossRef]
6. Jensen, P.R.; Moore, B.S.; Fenical, W. The marine actinomycete genus Salinispora: A model organism for secondary metabolite discovery. *Nat. Prod. Rep.* **2015**, *32*, 738–751. [CrossRef]
7. Takizawa, M.; Colwell, R.R.; Hill, R. Isolation and Diversity of Actinomycetes in the Chesapeake Bay. *Appl. Environ. Microbiol.* **1993**, *59*, 997–1002. [CrossRef]
8. Hoffmann, T.; Müller, S.; Nadmid, S.; Garcia, R.; Müller, R. Microsclerodermins from terrestrial myxobacteria: An intriguing biosynthesis likely connected to a sponge symbiont. *J. Am. Chem. Soc.* **2013**, *135*, 16904–16911. [CrossRef]
9. Gemperlein, K.; Zaburannyi, N.; Garcia, R.; La Clair, J.J.; Müller, R. Metabolic and Biosynthetic Diversity in Marine Myxobacteria. *Mar. Drugs* **2018**, *16*, 314. [CrossRef]
10. Nijland, R.; Hall, M.; Burgess, J.G. Dispersal of Biofilms by Secreted, Matrix Degrading, Bacterial DNase. *PLoS ONE* **2010**, *5*, e15668. [CrossRef]
11. Tomescu, A.M.; Honegger, R.; Rothwell, G.W. Earliest fossil record of bacterial-cyanobacterial mat consortia: The early Silurian Passage Creek biota (440 Ma, Virginia, USA). *Geobiology* **2008**, *6*, 120–124. [CrossRef]
12. Praveen Kumar, R.; Vijayan, D.; Leo Antony, M.; Muthu Kumar, C.; Thajuddin, N. Phylogenetic diversity of cultivable bacteria associated with filamentous non-hetrocystous marine cyanobacteria. *J. Algal Biomass Util.* **2009**, *1*, 86–101.

13. Engene, N.; Rottacker, E.C.; Kaštovský, J.; Byrum, T.; Choi, H.; Ellisman, M.H.; Komárek, J.; Gerwick, W.H. *Moorea producens* gen. nov., sp. nov. and *Moorea bouillonii* comb. nov., tropical marine cyanobacteria rich in bioactive secondary metabolites. *Int. J. Syst. Evol. Microbiol.* **2012**, *62*, 1171–1178. [CrossRef]
14. Omarova, E.O.; Zenova, G.M.; Orleanskii, V.K.; Lobakova, E.S. Experimental associations of cyanobacteria and actinomycetes. *Mosc. Univ. Biol. Sci. Bull.* **2007**, *62*, 1–6. [CrossRef]
15. Gil-Turnes, M.S. Antimicrobial Metabolites Produced by Epibiotic Bacteria: Their Role in Microbial Competition and Host Defense. Ph.D. Thesis, University of California at San Diego, San Diego, CA, USA, 1988.
16. Orjala, J.; Gerwick, W.H. Two quinoline alkaloids from the caribbean cyanobacterium *Lyngbya majuscula*. *Phytochemistry* **1997**, *45*, 1087–1090. [CrossRef]
17. Cummings, S.L.; Barbé, D.; Leao, T.F.; Korobeynikov, A.; Engene, N.; Glukhov, E.; Gerwick, W.H.; Gerwick, L. A novel uncultured heterotrophic bacterial associate of the cyanobacterium *Moorea producens* JHB. *BMC Microbiol.* **2016**, *16*, 198. [CrossRef]
18. Harr, K.E.; Szabo, N.J.; Cichra, M.; Phlips, E.J. Debromoaplysiatoxin in Lyngbya-dominated mats on manatees (*Trichechus manatus latirostris*) in the Florida King's Bay ecosystem. *Toxicon* **2008**, *52*, 385–388. [CrossRef]
19. Dzeha, T.; Nyiro, C.; Kardasopoulos, D.; Mburu, D.; Mwafaida, J.; Hall, M.J.; Burgess, J.G. UV Resistance of bacteria from the Kenyan Marine cyanobacterium *Moorea producens*. *MicrobiologyOpen* **2019**, *8*, e00697. [CrossRef]
20. Tronholm, A.; Engene, N. Moorena gen. nov., a valid name for "Moorea Engene & al." nom. inval. (Oscillatoriaceae, Cyanobacteria). *Not. Algarum* **2019**, *122*, 1–2.
21. Davies-Coleman, M.T.; Dzeha, T.M.; Gray, C.A.; Hess, S.; Pannell, L.K.; Hendricks, D.T.; Arendse, C.E. Isolation of Homodolastatin 16, a New Cyclic Depsipeptide from a Kenyan Collection of *Lyngbya majuscula*. *J. Nat. Prod.* **2003**, *66*, 712–715. [CrossRef]
22. Engene, N.; Gerwick, W.H. Intra-genomic 16S rRNA gene heterogeneity in cyanobacterial genomes. *Fottea* **2011**, *11*, 17–24. [CrossRef]
23. Engene, N.; Gunasekera, S.P.; Gerwick, W.H.; Paul, V.J. Phylogenetic inferences reveal a large extent of novel biodiversity in chemically rich tropical marine cyanobacteria. *Appl. Environ. Microbiol.* **2013**, *79*, 1882–1888. [CrossRef] [PubMed]
24. Jones, A.C.; Monroe, E.A.; Podell, S.; Hess, W.R.; Klages, S.; Esquenazi, E.; Niessen, S.; Hoover, H.; Rothmann, M.; Lasken, R.S.; et al. Genomic insights into the physiology and ecology of the marine filamentous cyanobacterium *Lyngbya majuscula*. *Proc. Natl. Acad. Sci. USA* **2011**, *108*, 8815–8820. [CrossRef] [PubMed]
25. Lasken, R.S. Single-cell genomic sequencing using Multiple Displacement Amplification. *Curr. Opin. Microbiol.* **2007**, *10*, 510–516. [CrossRef] [PubMed]
26. Vaara, T.; Vaara, M.; Niemela, S. Two improved methods for obtaining axenic cultures of cyanobacteria. *Appl. Environ. Microbiol.* **1979**, *38*, 1011–1014. [CrossRef]
27. Grass, G.; Rensing, C.; Solioz, M. Metallic Copper as an Antimicrobial Surface. *Appl. Environ. Microbiol.* **2011**, *77*, 1541–1547. [CrossRef]
28. Dollwet, H.H.A.; Sorenson, J.R.J. Historic uses of copper compounds in medicine. *Trace Elem. Med.* **1985**, *2*, 80–87.
29. Nubel, U.; Garcia-Pichel, F.; Muyzer, G. PCR primers to amplify 16S rRNA genes from cyanobacteria. *Appl. Environ. Microbiol.* **1997**, *63*, 3327–3332. [CrossRef]
30. Whitton, B.; Durham University, Durham, UK. Personal communication, 2013.
31. Rainey, F.A.; Ward-Rainey, N.; Kroppenstedt, R.M.; Stackebrandt, E. The genus Nocardiopsis represents a phylogenetically coherent taxon and a distinct actinomy-cete lineage: Proposal of *Nocardiopsaceae* fam. nov. *Int. J. Syst. Bacteriol.* **1996**, *46*, 1088–1092. [CrossRef]
32. Lechevalier, M.P.; De Bievre, C.; Lechevalier, H. Chemotaxonomy of aerobic Actinomycetes: Phospholipid composition. *Biochem. Syst. Ecol.* **1977**, *5*, 249–260. [CrossRef]
33. Harker, M.; Hirschberg, J.; Oren, A. *Paracoccus marcusii* sp. nov., an orange Gram-negative coccus. *Int. J. Syst. Bacteriol.* **1998**, *48*, 543–548. [CrossRef]
34. Su, T.L. Micrococcin, an antibacterial substance formed by a strain of Micrococcus. *Br. J. Exp. Pathol.* **1948**, *29*, 473–481.
35. Bycroft, B.W.; Gowland, M.S. The structures of the highly modified peptide antibiotics micrococcin P1 and P2. *J. Chem. Soc. Chem. Commun.* **1978**, *1978*, 256–258. [CrossRef]
36. Lefranc, D.; Ciufolini, M.A. Total Synthesis and Stereochemical Assignment of Micrococcin P1. *Angew. Chem. Int. Ed.* **2009**, *48*, 4198–4201. [CrossRef]
37. Walsh, C.T.; Acker, M.G.; Bowers, A.A. Thiazolyl peptide antibiotic biosynthesis: A cascade of post-translational modifications on ribosomal nascent proteins. *J. Biol. Chem.* **2010**, *285*, 27525–27531. [CrossRef]
38. Wang, W.; Park, K.-H.; Lee, J.; Oh, E.; Park, C.; Kang, E.; Lee, J.; Kang, H. A New Thiopeptide Antibiotic, micrococcin P3, from a marine-derived Strain of the bacterium *Bacillus stratosphericus*. *Molecules* **2020**, *25*, 4383. [CrossRef]
39. Kranjec, C.; Ovchinnikov, K.V.; Grønseth, T.; Ebineshan, K.; Srikantam, A.; Diep, D.B. A bacteriocin-based antimicrobial formulation to effectively disrupt the cell viability of methicillin-resistant *Staphylococcus aureus* (MRSA) biofilms. *NPJ Biofilms Microbiomes* **2020**, *6*, 1–13. [CrossRef]
40. Jansen, R.; Sood, S.; Huch, V.; Kunze, B.; Stadler, M.; Müller, R. Pyrronazols, Metabolites from the Myxobacteria *Nannocystis pusilla* and *N. exedens*, Are Unusual Chlorinated Pyrone-Oxazole-Pyrroles. *J. Nat. Prod.* **2014**, *77*, 320–326. [CrossRef]
41. Okanya, P.W.; Mohr, K.I.; Gerth, K.; Jansen, R.; Müller, R. Marinoquinolines A–F, Pyrroloquinolines from *Ohtaekwangia kribbensis* (Bacteroidetes). *J. Nat. Prod.* **2011**, *74*, 603–608. [CrossRef]

42. Bader, C.D.; Neuber, M.; Panter, F.; Krug, D.; Müller, R. Supercritical Fluid Extraction Enhances Discovery of Secondary Metabolites from Myxobacteria. *Anal. Chem.* **2020**, *92*, 15403–15411. [CrossRef]
43. Morin, N.; Vallaeys, T.; Hendrickx, L.; Natalie, L.; Wilmotte, A. An efficient DNA isolation protocol for filamentous cyanobacteria of the genus *Arthrospira*. *J. Microbiol. Methods* **2010**, *80*, 148–154. [CrossRef]
44. Sambrook, J.; Russell, D. *Molecular Cloning: A Laboratory Manual*, 3rd ed.; Cold Spring Harbor Laboratory Press: Cold Spring Harbor, NY, USA, 2001.
45. Kumar, S.; Stecher, G.; Li, M.; Knyaz, C.; Tamura, K. MEGA X: Molecular Evolutionary Genetics Analysis across Computing Platforms. *Mol. Biol. Evol.* **2018**, *35*, 1547–1549. [CrossRef]
46. Caulier, S.; Nannan, C.; Gillis, A.; Licciardi, F.; Bragard, C.; Mahillon, J. Overview of the Antimicrobial Compounds Produced by Members of the *Bacillus subtilis* Group. *Front. Microbiol.* **2019**, *10*, 302. [CrossRef]
47. Charousová, I.; Steinmetz, H.; Medo, J.; Javoreková, S.; Wink, J. Characterization of Antimycins—Producing Streptomycete Strain VY46 Isolated from Slovak Soil. *Braz. Arch. Biol. Technol.* **2016**, *59*, e16160274. [CrossRef]

marine drugs

Article

Chitin Degradation Machinery and Secondary Metabolite Profiles in the Marine Bacterium *Pseudoalteromonas rubra* S4059

Xiyan Wang, Thomas Isbrandt, Mikael Lenz Strube, Sara Skøtt Paulsen, Maike Wennekers Nielsen, Yannick Buijs, Erwin M. Schoof, Thomas Ostenfeld Larsen, Lone Gram and Sheng-Da Zhang *

Department of Bioengineering, Technical University of Denmark, DK-2800 Kgs Lyngby, Denmark; xwan@dtu.dk (X.W.); tispe@bio.dtu.dk (T.I.); milst@dtu.dk (M.L.S.); ssp@sbtinstruments.com (S.S.P.); mweni@dtu.dk (M.W.N.); yabu@dtu.dk (Y.B.); erws@dtu.dk (E.M.S.); tol@bio.dtu.dk (T.O.L.); gram@bio.dtu.dk (L.G.)
* Correspondence: shez@dtu.dk; Tel.: +45-5011-7765

Abstract: Genome mining of pigmented *Pseudoalteromonas* has revealed a large potential for the production of bioactive compounds and hydrolytic enzymes. The purpose of the present study was to explore this bioactivity potential in a potent antibiotic and enzyme producer, *Pseudoalteromonas rubra* strain S4059. Proteomic analyses (data are available via ProteomeXchange with identifier PXD023249) indicated that a highly efficient chitin degradation machinery was present in the red-pigmented *P. rubra* S4059 when grown on chitin. Four GH18 chitinases and two GH20 hexosaminidases were significantly upregulated under these conditions. GH19 chitinases, which are not common in bacteria, are consistently found in pigmented *Pseudoalteromonas*, and in S4059, GH19 was only detected when the bacterium was grown on chitin. To explore the possible role of GH19 in pigmented *Pseudoalteromonas*, we developed a protocol for genetic manipulation of S4059 and deleted the GH19 chitinase, and compared phenotypes of the mutant and wild type. However, none of the chitin degrading ability, secondary metabolite profile, or biofilm-forming capacity was affected by GH19 deletion. In conclusion, we developed a genetic manipulation protocol that can be used to unravel the bioactive potential of pigmented pseudoalteromonads. An efficient chitinolytic enzyme cocktail was identified in S4059, suggesting that this strain could be a candidate with industrial potential.

Keywords: chitin; chitinase; chitin degradation machinery; *Pseudoalteromonas*; secondary metabolites

Citation: Wang, X.; Isbrandt, T.; Strube, M.L.; Paulsen, S.S.; Nielsen, M.W.; Buijs, Y.; Schoof, E.M.; Larsen, T.O.; Gram, L.; Zhang, S.-D. Chitin Degradation Machinery and Secondary Metabolite Profiles in the Marine Bacterium *Pseudoalteromonas rubra* S4059. *Mar. Drugs* **2021**, *19*, 108. https://doi.org/10.3390/md19020108

Academic Editor: Hitoshi Sashiwa

Received: 22 December 2020
Accepted: 4 February 2021
Published: 12 February 2021

1. Introduction

Marine microorganisms have emerged as a promising source of novel antimicrobial compounds or hydrolytic enzymes [1,2]. In particular, the marine genus *Pseudoalteromonas* harbors a wide range of bioactive compounds with antimicrobial, antifouling, and algicidal activities [3–6]. Based on both phenotypes and genome-wide analyses, *Pseudoalteromonas* can be divided into two groups: pigmented and non-pigmented species [3]. The genomes of pigmented species contain a high number of biosynthetic gene clusters (BGCs) as compared to those of non-pigmented species [7]. Both groups carry the genetic potential to produce a wide range of glycosyl hydrolases, and the pigmented *Pseudoalteromonas* especially harbors a powerful chitin degrading machinery containing several chitinolytic enzymes [7].

Chitin is the most abundant carbon source in the marine environment [8], where it is present in three crystalline allomorphs: α-, β-, and γ-chitin. α-chitin has antiparallel chains, β-chitin has parallel chains, and γ-chitin has the mixture of both chains [9]. Chitin in nature is predominantly degraded by microorganisms [10], and chitin degradation depends on secreted extracellular chitinases (EC.3.2.1.14) and other chitinolytic enzymes/proteins, such as lytic polysaccharide monooxygenases (LPMOs) [11]. Chitinases are glycoside hydrolases (GHs) and are classified into GH18, GH19, and GH20 in the CAZy database [12,13]. The GH18 family chitinases are common in bacteria, whereas the GH19 chitinases are mostly found in plants and are believed to function as a defense mechanism against fungal pathogens [14,15]. Chitinases of both families catalyze the degradation of chitin polymers [12]. The GH 20 family β-N-acetylhexosaminidases hydrolyze amorphous chitin polymers [16], and the LPMOs are metalloenzymes that cleave glycosidic bonds in crystalline chitin and facilitate access of chitinase [17]. Paulsen et al. [7] found that pigmented and non-pigmented *Pseudoalteromonas* evolved divergent GH profiles in their genomic contents. Further, all pigmented *Pseudoalteromonas* species contain at least one GH19 chitinase, which is rarely reported in bacteria. However, only a very few non-pigmented *Pseudoalteromonase* species contain a GH19 chitinase [7]. A GH19 chitinase of the pigmented *Pseudoalteromonas tunicata* CCUG 44952T has been heterologously expressed in *Escherichia coli* and displayed antifungal activity [18]. However, whether this is the dominant role of GH19 in pigmented *Pseodoalteromonas* is yet to be investigated.

The secondary metabolome of several bacteria is influenced by carbon-source, and chitin may serve to enhance the production of secondary metabolites, as observed in strains of Vibrionaceae [19–21]. Likewise, the addition of chitin to *Streptomyces coelicolor* A3 (2) growing in autoclaved soil induced the expression of genes associated with secondary metabolites' production [22]. Due to the potent chitinolytic machinery in *Pseudoalteromonas* [7], we speculated that there could be a link between chitin degradation and secondary metabolism. Since *P. rubra* S4059 dedicates 15% of its genome to secondary metabolites [7] and as other pigmented pseudoalteromonads contain GH19 chitinases [7], we further explored the bioactivity of this prodigiosin-producing strain as a model organism. The purpose of this study was to explore the chitin degradation machinery and secondary metabolite profiles when grown on chitin and to investigate the possible function of GH19 chitinase in *P. rubra* S4059.

2. Results

2.1. *In Silico Analysis of Chitin Degrading Machinery and Bioactive Potential in P. rubra S4059*

The genome of S4059 consists of two circular chromosomes, of 4,595,233 bp and 1,348,119 bp, with an average G + C content of 47.71% and 46.93%. Fourteen putative chitinolytic enzymes were identified according to the prediction of the S4059 proteome in Uniprot (proteome ID UP000305729), including seven of the GH18 chitinase family, two of the GH19 chitinase family, and three of the GH20 hexosaminidase family, as well as two lytic polysaccharide monooxygenases (LPMOs) of the auxiliary activity (AA) family 10 (Table 1). All the chitinolytic enzymes contained a signal peptide at the N-terminal, except for one GH19 chitinase (A0A5S3UPT5).

Table 1. The chitinolytic machinery in *Pseudoalteromonas rubra* S4059 according to the prediction of the proteome from Uniprot (Proteome ID UP000305729). The signal peptide was predicted using amino acid sequence by SignalP-5.0 (http://www.cbs.dtu.dk/services/SignalP/ (accessed on 22 September 2018)).

Glycoside Hydrolase Type	Accession	Signal Peptide
GH18	A0A5S3USE2	Y
	A0A5S3V351	Y
	A0A5S3V6T3	Y
	A0A5S3V0U4	Y
	A0A5S3USH6	Y
	A0A5S3V3K3	Y
	A0A5S3V378	Y
GH19	A0A5S3UX38	Y
	A0A5S3UPT5	N
GH20	A0A5S3UX95	Y
	A0A5S3UV09	Y
	A0A5S3V1X9	Y
LPMO	A0A5S3UTD1	Y
	A0A5S3V4S2	Y

The genome of S4059 harbors nineteen predicted BGCs identified by antiSMASH 6.0, distributed with thirteen on chr I and six on chr II. BGC 2-5, 17, and 18 are non-ribosomal peptide synthetase clusters (NRPs), BGC 8, 13, and 16 are other unspecified ribosomally synthesized and post-translationally modified peptide products (RiPP) clusters, BGC 10, 11, and 15 are the hybrids of NRPs and Type I polyketide (PKs), BGC 7 is a hserlactone BGC, BGC 9 is prodigiosin BGC, and BGC 12, 13 belong to lanthipepride-class. Four of the BGCs located on chr I were predicted to produce indigoidine, kalimantacin A, amonabactin P 750, and prodigiosins (Table S1), however, only the prodigiosin gene cluster was predicted to be conserved to the known BGC with a similarity score of 70%, while the others were below 40% as shown in Table S1. The products of the rest of the BGCs are not known.

2.2. Global Proteome Profiles of P. rubra S4059 Grown on Chitin

The proteomes of *P. rubra* S4059 grown on different carbon sources were analyzed by liquid chromatography–tandem mass spectrometry (LC-MS/MS)-based label-free quantitative proteomics approach. The analyses were done on both cells and culture supernatant (excreted proteins) of S4059 grown in crystalline chitin or mannose containing medium. A total of 2813 proteins were identified in the global proteome of S4059, of which 738 and 142 proteins were up- and downregulated in S4059 culture supernatant when grown on crystalline chitin as compared to growth on mannose (Figure 1A). Simultaneously, 1861 and 141 proteins were up- and downregulated in S4059 cells when grown on crystalline chitin compared to on mannose (Figure 1B). Proteins involved in bacterial chemotaxis, cell division, flagellar assembly, and Type IV pilus assembly were upregulated when S4059 was grown on crystalline chitin (Table S3). Proteins associated with the core metabolism were also upregulated on chitin (Table S3). A protein involved in mannosidase from the GH92 family was upregulated when grown on mannose compared to when grown on crystalline chitin (Table S3).

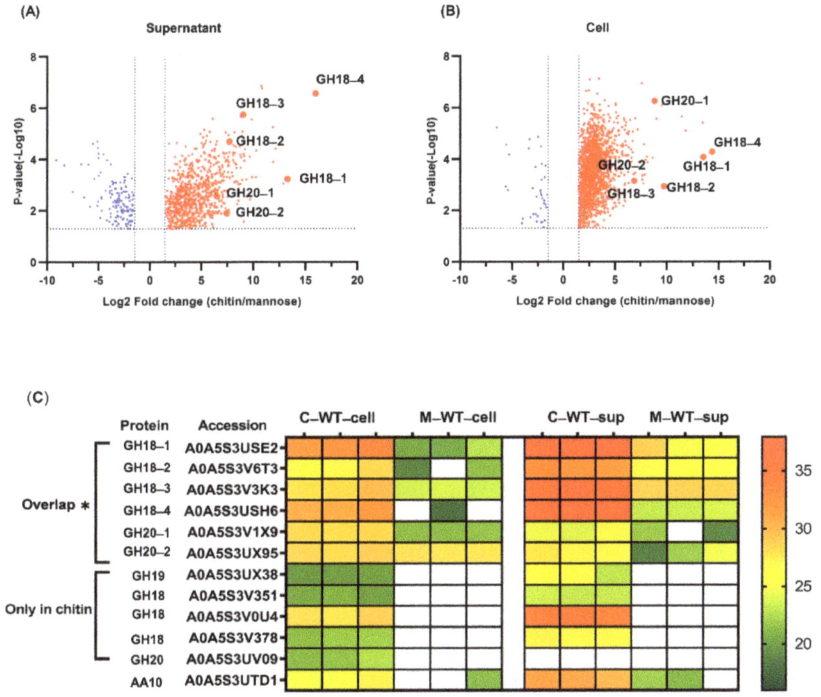

Figure 1. Comparison of identified proteins in the culture supernatant (**A**) and cells (**B**) of *Pseudoalteromonas rubra* S4059

when grown on chitin compared to on mannose. The dotted lines indicated that a threshold value for the cut off was a combination of p-value ≤ 0.05 and Log_2 fold-change ≥ 1.5. Red dots represent upregulated proteins, and blue dots represent downregulated proteins. Chitinolytic enzymes with significant fold changes are highlighted by enlarged dots with protein names in (**A**,**B**). Heat map comparison of identified chitinolytic enzymes in the supernatant and cells of *Pseudoalteromonas rubra* S4059 is color-coded by increasing abundance (**C**). C–WT–cell: cells of S4059 grown on chitin; M–WT–cell: cells of S4059 grown on mannose; C–WT–sup: culture supernatant of S4059 grown on chitin; M–WT–sup: culture supernatant of S4059 grown on mannose. White denotes proteins not detected under this condition. 'Overlap' indicates these proteins were detected in both chitin and mannose-grown samples, and an asterisk (*) highlights proteins significantly upregulated when grown on chitin compared to on mannose.

2.3. Comparative Analysis of the Expression of Chitinolytic Enzymes in P. rubra S4059

A total of twelve chitin utilization associated proteins, including seven GH18s, three GH20s, a GH19, and a LPMO, were identified with a confidence rate of 99% at the peptide and protein levels in the *P. rubra* S4059 global proteome, while a GH19 (A0A5S3UPT5) and an LPMO (A0A5S3V4S2) were not detected (Figure 1C).

All chitinolytic enzymes could be detected in both cells and culture supernatant of S4059, except the enzyme A0A5S3UV09 from the GH20 family, which was not detected in the culture supernatant (Figure 1C). The GH18 chitinase A0A5S3USH6, annotated as ChiC, was the most highly expressed chitinolytic enzyme in both cells and culture supernatant during growth on chitin. Four GH18s (A0A5S3USE2, A0A5S3V6T3 A0A5S3V3K3, and A0A5S3USH6) and two GH20s (A0A5S3V1X9 and A0A5S3UX95) enzymes were significantly upregulated when S4059 was grown on crystalline chitin compared to on mannose (Figure 1). Meanwhile, several chitin-utilization associated proteins were induced and could only be detected when grown on crystalline chitin, including a GH19 chitinase and three GH18 chitinases (A0A5S3V351, A0A5S3V0U4, and A0A5S3V378) (Figure 1C). In addition, an LPMO from the AA10 family was identified under both growth conditions, but with no significant expression difference (Figure 1C).

2.4. Influence of Chitin on the Metabolome of S4059

To investigate the potential link between chitin degradation and secondary metabolite production, the S4059 wild type was grown on mannose, crystalline chitin, colloidal chitin, or N-acetyl glucosamine (NAG) containing marine minimal medium (MMM) in stationary phase. Chemical analysis using high-performance liquid chromatography coupled to diode array detection and high-resolution mass spectrometry (HPLC-DAD-HRMS) showed that mannose and crystalline chitin resulted in largely the same chemical profiles, although two unknown tentative prodigiosin analogs were produced in higher amounts on mannose (Figure S1). NAG containing media resulted in an overall higher production of secondary metabolites compared to mannose, crystalline, and colloidal chitin, and NAG and colloidal chitin both led to increased production of two unknown non-prodigiosin derived (based on UV-Vis absorption) compounds (Figure S1). Prodigiosin, hexyl prodigiosin, and heptyl prodigiosin (Figure S1B–D) were produced in varying amounts on all media. The identity of prodigiosin was confirmed using an authentic standard in combination with our in-house MS/MS library, and the two analogs were identified based on similarities with MS/MS and UV-Vis absorption spectra. Additionally, using our in-house MS/MS library, combined with a compound list generated from all *Pseudoalteromonas*-derived secondary metabolites found in the Reaxys database, no other known secondary metabolites were identified in S4059.

2.5. The Deletion of GH19 Chitinase Does Not Affect Growth or Chitin Degradation

To explore the function of GH19 chitinase in pigmented *P. rubra* S4059 and investigate a possible link between chitin degradation and secondary metabolites production, an in-frame deletion of GH19 chitinase gene (the GH19 A0A5S3UX38 with a signal peptide) was generated in S4059 by homologous recombination (Figure 2A,B). Wild type S4059 and GH19 deletion mutant (Δ*GH19*) were grown in MMM supplemented with crystalline chitin, colloidal chitin, NAG, or mannose. The mutant grew similarly to the wild type in all substrates with the same growth rate and maximum cell density (Figure 2C,D and Figure S2). The maximum cell density reached 10^9 colony-forming unit (CFU)/mL in all substrates supplemented with casamino acid while only reaching 10^8 CFU/mL when the strains grew in chitin containing MMM without casamino acid. The generation time of wild type and the mutant was 43.80 ± 8.46 min in all substrates with casamino acid, while without casamino acid, the value was 91.27 ± 2.23 min in crystalline chitin and 74.87 ± 0.30 min in colloidal chitin contained MMM.

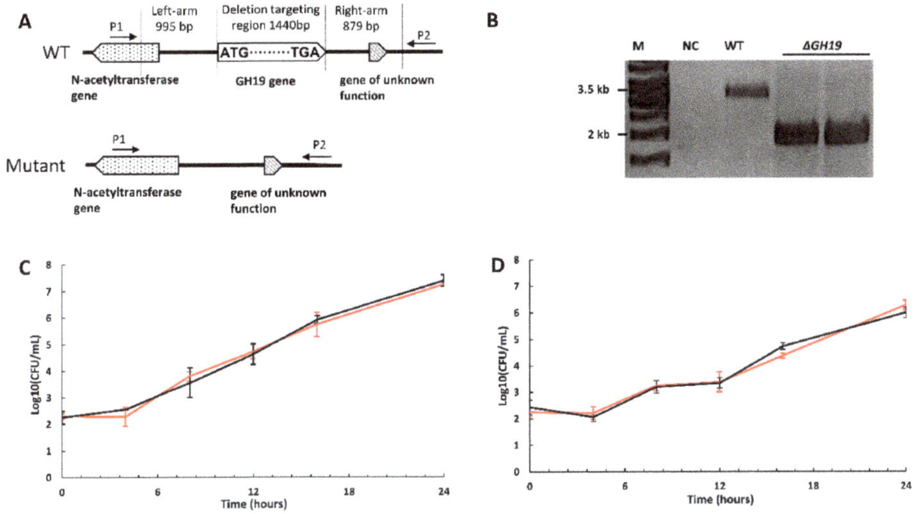

Figure 2. The in-frame deletion of the GH19 chitinase gene in *Pseudoalteromonas rubra* S4059 was verified by PCR with primers P1 and P2 that target the left and right homology arm of the GH19 chitinase gene (**A**). The PCR products were analyzed by electrophoresis (**B**). M: DNA ladder; NC: negative control with water as the PCR template; WT: PCR products with gDNA of wild type strain S4059 as a template; Δ*GH19*: PCR products with gDNA of Δ*GH19* as a template. Growth kinetics of *Pseudoalteromonas rubra* S4059 wild type (red lines) and Δ*GH19* (black lines) when grown in a marine minimal medium containing (**C**) colloidal chitin or (**D**) crystalline chitin (shrimp chitin) without casamino acids at 25 °C for 24 h, shaking at 200 rpm. Data were analyzed on three biological replicates, and the error bars represent the standard deviation.

The chitin degradation capacity of the *P. rubra* S4059 wild type and the GH19 mutant was also tested on chitin (crystalline and colloidal chitin) plates. As expected from the growth experiment, the mutant had the same chitinolytic ability (the size of clearing zone) as the wild type (Figure S2E–F). According to a previous study, the heterologously expressed GH19 chitinase in *E. coli* showed antifungal activity against *Aspergillus niger*. Therefore, the antifungal activity was also explored by co-cultivating both the strains with the fungus *Aspergillus niger* on marine agar (MA) plates, showing that the GH19 mutant displayed the same inhibitory effects as the wild type (data not shown).

2.6. Biofilm Formation and Chitin Surface Attachment of P. rubra S4059 Was Not Affected by Deletion of GH19 Chitinase Gene

Many *Pseudoalteromonas* species are good biofilm formers that are able to colonize crustaceans in marine environments [23], and since chitin colonization has been linked to biofilm formation in other bacteria [24], the biofilm formation of S4059 wild type and the mutant were compared in chitin containing media. The surface formed biofilm of the mutant and wild type was detected at the same level in all media (Figure S3).

The growth and attachment of the wild type and the mutant on natural chitin (shrimp shells) was assessed, and both strains grew from an initial density of 10^4 CFU/mL to a final cell density of 10^7 CFU/mL in the liquid surrounding the shells (Figure 3). Surface-attached bacteria were removed from shrimp shells by sonication resulting in an increase in cell density to 10^8 CFU/mL with similar levels reached by wild type and the mutant (Figure 3).

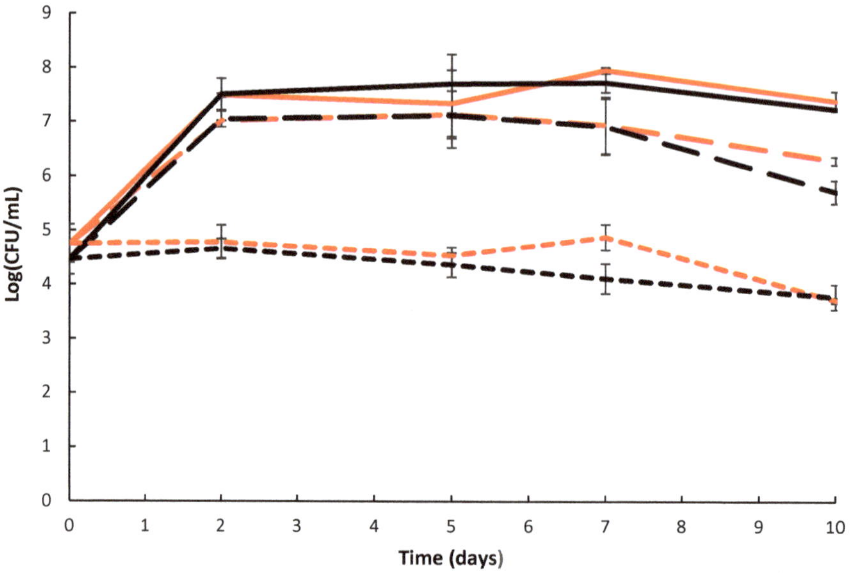

Figure 3. Growth and attachment of *Pseudoalteromonas rubra* S4059 wild type (red) and mutant Δ*GH19* (black) on Vannamei shrimp shells. Long dash lines: samples from liquid surrounding shrimp shells before sonication. Solid lines: samples from liquid surrounding shrimp shells after sonication. Short dash lines: samples from 3% Sigma sea salt without shrimp shells as a control. Data were analyzed on three biological replicates, and the error bars represent standard deviation.

2.7. Deletion of GH19 Chitinase Does Not Significantly Influence the Proteome of S4059

To investigate the impact of the GH19 chitinase deletion on the proteome of S4059, the GH19 mutant, and the wild type were grown on a chitin-based medium to stationary phase. Supernatant and cells were separated for proteome analysis. A total of 2512 proteins were identified, but no significant changes in any of the detected proteins were observed between wild type and GH19 mutant in either supernatant or cells when grown on crystalline chitin, except that GH19 chitinase could not be detected in the mutant cultures.

2.8. Similar Secondary Metabolome Pattern in Wild Type Strain and GH19 Mutant

Following the measurement of growth kinetics, the extracts of cultures grown in MMM were analyzed by HPLC-HRMS. Each strain was cultivated in three biological replicates in media containing one of the four carbon sources: mannose, NAG, colloidal chitin, or shrimp chitin. The wild type and the mutant had similar secondary metabolome profiles, as shown in Figure S1A. Screening for known natural products was also undertaken, revealing that only prodigiosin, as well as three of its analogs, could be identified (Figure S1B).

3. Discussion

Chitinolytic bacteria have been widely studied due to the possible use as antifungal agents in biocontrol [25]. In addition, the involvement of chitin in the ecology of *Vibrio cholerae* and its virulence regulation has been the focus of many studies [26–28]. Recently, a novel perspective on chitin degradation has been seen in some strains of *Vibrionaceae*, where growth on chitin as compared to on glucose leads to enhanced expression of several BGCs [19] along with enhanced antibacterial activity [20]. Chitin is the most abundant polymer in the ocean, and, hence, many marine bacteria are potent chitin degraders [10]. In silico analysis has demonstrated that pigmented species of the genus *Pseudoalteromonas* have elaborate chitinolytic machinery containing at least one of the otherwise rare GH19 chitinase in their genomes, and also, they devote up to 15% of their genome to BGCs with a vast potential for secondary metabolite production [7]. Here, we demonstrated that the pigmented bacterium *P. rubra* S4059 grew well using both purified chitin (crystalline and colloidal chitin) and natural shrimp shells as a sole source of nutrients. These results were further substantiated by proteome analyses that demonstrated that the strain S4059, indeed, produces an efficient chitinolytic enzyme cocktail, including GH18, GH19, LPMO, and GH20.

GH18 chitinases are the predominant chitinolytic enzymes in bacteria [29–31], and the strain S4059 harbored seven putative GH18 chitinases as determined by genome analysis, four of which were significantly upregulated when grown on chitin. Secretome analysis of the soil-derived and chitinolytic bacterium *Cellvibrio japonicus* indicated that many chitinolytic enzymes, including GH18 chitinases, and GH19 chitinases and LPMOs, were highly upregulated when grown on β-chitin as compared to α-chitin [29]. Out of fourteen putative chitinolytic enzymes in S4059, only the two putative enzymes, GH19 A0A5S3UPT5 and LPMO A0A5S3V4S2, were not detected when S4059 was grown on an α-chitin surface, suggesting that these two enzymes may have other functions. Proteome analysis of *P. rubra* S4059 culture supernatant confirmed the presence of all chitinolytic enzymes except for the two enzymes GH19 A0A5S3UPT5 and LPMO A0A5S3V4S2, and an even higher amount of the enzymes in culture supernatant than in cells (Figure 1C), implying that those detected proteins indeed are secreted enzymes able to degrade chitin. Secretome analysis of *Cellvibrio japonicus* showed that thousands of proteins were detected in the filtered culture supernatant. However, the authors mentioned that cell lysis can lead to overestimating the numbers of secreted proteins [29]. Further, they used the plate-based method that was developed by Bengtson et al. [32] to detect truly secreted proteins, and the result indicated that only 267 secreted proteins were detected in α-chitin containing medium [29]. In our study, due to the insoluble property of chitin, secreted chitinases may bind to small chitin particles, and, thus, the secreted chitinases cannot be passed through sterile filters leading to misestimating the expression of secreted chitinases. Thus, we did not filter the culture supernatant for retaining bound chitinases, which were on chitin particles. We found that 880 proteins were influenced by chitin in the culture supernatant of S4059, as compared to on mannose, and these high numbers of influenced proteins may be due to a combination factor of the unfiltered culture supernatant and cell lysis during centrifugation [33]. Further, the agar plate-based method probably can point out the true numbers of secreted proteins in S4059.

One of the two GH19 chitinases in *P. rubra* S4059 was highly expressed when the bacterium was grown on chitin, and while some GH19 chitinases have been linked to antifungal activity, their broader role in bacteria remains enigmatic [18,34,35]. The results suggesting antifungal activity have mainly relied on heterologous expression of GH19 in hosts such as *E. coli*, and this provides information about the enzyme per se, but not necessarily about the actual role in its native host. We, therefore, chose to delete the GH19 that was highly expressed on chitin to explore its possible role in S4059 further. Both the mutant and wild type displayed similar antifungal activity (data not shown). Despite the high expression of GH19 when S4059 was grown on chitin, the GH19 deficient mutant showed no difference in growth compared to the WT when grown on chitin (Figure 2 and Figure S2). Our results, therefore, indicate that GH19 chitinase is not the predominant chitin degrading enzyme in *P. rubra* S4059, given the wide array of other chitinolytic enzymes. Chitin utilization capacity has been investigated in a chitinolytic soil bacterium *Cellvibrio japonicus* [30]. Through a combination of secretome and genetic manipulation approaches, a highly expressed GH18 chitinase was identified as the enzyme essential for the degradation of chitin in the strain [30]. Proteome analyses in S4059 demonstrated that two GH18 chitinases A0A5S3USH6 and A0A5S3USE2 are the most highly expressed chitinases in both cells and culture supernatant according to protein abundance when S4059 was grown on chitin (Table S7), suggesting that the GH18 chitinases could be potentially essential enzymes for chitin degradation in S4059 under testing conditions.

In conclusion, the proteomic analysis showed that a highly efficient chitin degradation machinery was identified in pigmented *P. rubra* S4059, and four GH18 chitinases and two GH20 hexosaminidases in S4059 were significantly upregulated when grown on chitin. In contrast to different proteome profiles, the different growth conditions on chitin investigated here did not significantly alter the metabolite profile of S4059, in contrast to what has been reported in other *Vibrio* species and *Streptomyces coelicolor* A3 (2) [19–22]. Although the deletion of GH19 chitinase did not influence chitin degradation activity in S4059, we developed a conjugation-based approach allowing genetic manipulation in this bioactive bacterium S4059. Given the large potential for secondary metabolism as found by genome mining and from uncharacterized compounds produced on especially chitin derived substrates, the genetic approach developed here will allow exploration of the novel chemical space of this organism.

4. Materials and Methods

4.1. Bacterial Strains, Plasmids, and Growth Conditions

All bacterial strains and plasmids used in this study are listed in Table S5. *P. rubra* S4059 was isolated during the Galathea 3 expedition [36] and cultured in marine broth (MB, BD Difco 2216, Le Pont de Claix, France) or APY medium [37] at 25 °C, 200 rpm. *P. rubra* S4059 carrying a chromosomal-integrated suicide plasmid was cultured in MB containing 30 μg/mL chloramphenicol (Sigma, C0378, St. Louis, MO, USA) at 25 °C, 200 rpm. All chitin used in this study are α-chitin. *P. rubra* S4059 mutants and wild type were cultured in a marine minimal medium (MMM) [38] supplemented with four different carbon sources (0.2% mannose, 0.2% crystalline chitin, 0.2% colloidal chitin, or 0.2% NAG) and growth, biofilm formation, and secondary metabolome determined. To compare chitin degradation of mutants and wild type S4059, they were grown on plates containing 2% Sea Salt (Sigma, S9883, St. Louis, MO, USA), 1.5% agar, and 0.2% chitin (crystalline or colloidal). Colloidal chitin was prepared as described in a previous study [39].

All *Escherichia coli* strains were cultured in Luria Bertani (LB) Broth (BD Difco 244520, Le Pont de Claix, France) at 37 °C, 200 rpm. *E. coli* GB *dir-pir*116 [40] was used for constructing suicide plasmid. *E. coli* WM3064 was used as the donor strain in intergeneric conjugation experiments. *E. coli* WM3064 is a *dapA* mutant that requires exogenously supplied diaminopimelic acid (DAP, Sigma, D1377, St. Louis, MO, USA) with a final concentration of 0.3 μM for growth [41]. Plasmid pDM4 was used as the backbone of suicide vectors [42]. *E. coli* strains harboring pDM4, or its derivatives were grown in LB Broth with 10 μg/mL chloramphenicol or in LB agar with 15 μg/mL chloramphenicol.

4.2. Whole Genome Sequencing and Assembly of P. rubra S4059

Genomic DNA of *P. rubra* S4059 was extracted using the Genomic DNA buffer set (QIAGEN, 19060, Hilden, Germany) following the supplier's instructions. The closed genome of *P. rubra* S4059 was obtained by minION sequencing using the EXP-FLP002 flow cell priming kit, SQK-RAD004 rapid sequencing kit, FLO-MINSP6 flow cell, and the associated protocol (version RSE_9046_V1_revB-17Nov2017 and RSE_9046_V1_revB-14 AUG2019). Illumina reads, obtained from a previous study [7], were combined with the minION reads for hybrid assembly using the Unicycler package [43]. Before assembly, the minION reads were filtered using the Filtlong package, only keeping the top 500,000,000 bp. The genome was annotated using Prokka [44]. The genome is available at the National Center for Biotechnology Information (NCBI) under the accession number CP045429 and CP045430.

4.3. In Silico Analysis of Chitin Degrading Genes and Secondary Metabolites

The assembled genome was analyzed using the CLC Main Workbench 8.0.1 (CLC bio, Aarhus, Denmark) and the online platform MaGe MicroScope [45]. The chitinolytic enzymes and the prediction of the chitin degradation pathway in S4059 were annotated according to the prediction of the S4059 proteome in Uniprot (UniProt ID UP000305729). Amino acid sequences of the candidate chitinases were also submitted to the SignalP 5.0 Server [46] to identify the signal peptides. In addition, genomes were submitted to antiSMASH version 6.0 (https://antismash.secondarymetabolites.org/#!/start (accessed on 15 January 2021)) for the prediction of putative biosynthetic gene clusters involved in the production of secondary metabolites.

4.4. Growing Bacteria and Sample Preparation for Proteomic Analyses

The protein samples were prepared according to Chevallier et al. [47]. *P. rubra* S4059 wild type and GH19 mutant were grown in 20 mL MMM with crystalline chitin for 2 days at 25 °C, 200 rpm. All experiments were carried out in biological triplicates. A five milliliter culture was harvested (5000× *g*, 20 min), and then the culture supernatant was transferred into a new 15 mL Falcon tube, and ice-cold acetone (−20 °C) was added to the supernatant to a final concentration of 80%. Then the mixture was kept at −20 °C overnight and harvested at 2000× *g* for 20 min. Acetone was carefully removed. The harvested bacterial cells were washed twice with ice-cold phosphate-buffered saline (PBS), and the pellet was lysed using 20 µL of lysis buffer (consisting of 6 M Guanidinium Hydrochloride, 10 mM Tris (2-carboxyethyl) phosphine hydrochloride, 40 mM 2-chloroacetamide, 50 mM HEPES (4-(2-hydroxyethyl)-1-piperazineethanesulfonic acid) pH 8.5). Samples were inactivated at 95 °C for 5 min and were then sonicated on high 3 times for 10 s in a 4 °C Bioruptor sonication water bath (Diagenode). A Bradford assay (Sigma) was used to determine protein concentration, and 50 µg of each sample was used for digestion. Samples were diluted 1:3 with 10% Acetonitrile, 50 mM HEPES pH 8.5, LysC (MS grade, Wako, Japan) added in a 1:50 (enzyme to protein) ratio, and samples were incubated at 37 °C for 4 h. Samples were further diluted to 1:10 with 10% Acetonitrile, 50 mM HEPES pH 8.5, trypsin (MS grade, Promega) added in a 1:100 (enzyme to protein) ratio, and samples were incubated overnight at 37 °C. Enzyme activity was quenched by adding 2% trifluoroacetic acid (TFA) to a final concentration of 1%. Before mass spectrometry analysis, the peptides were desalted on SOLAu C18 plates (ThermoFisher Scientific, Roskilde, Denmark). After each solvent application, the plate was centrifuged for 1 min at 350× *g*. For each sample, the C18 material was activated with 200 µL of 100% Methanol (HPLC grade, Sigma), then 200 µL of 80% Acetonitrile, 0.1% formic acid. The C18 material was subsequently equilibrated 2 x with 200 µL of 1% TFA, 3% Acetonitrile, after which the samples were loaded. After washing the tips twice with 200 µL of 0.1% formic acid, the peptides were eluted using 40% Acetonitrile, 0.1% formic acid, and transferred into clean 500 µL Eppendorf tubes. The eluted peptides were concentrated in an Eppendorf Speedvac and reconstituted in 1% TFA, 2% Acetonitrile for Mass Spectrometry (MS, Merck, Darmstadt, Germany) analysis.

4.5. Proteomic Data Acquisition

The proteomic data acquisition approach was modified from Haddad Momeni et al. [48]. Briefly, peptides were loaded onto a 2 cm C18 trap column (ThermoFisher 164705), connected in-line to a 15 cm C18 reverse-phase analytical column (Thermo EasySpray ES803) using 100% Buffer A (0.1% Formic acid in water) at 750 bar, using the Thermo EasyLC 1200 HPLC system (ThermoFisher, Roskilde, Denmark), and the column oven operating at 30 °C. Peptides were eluted over a 140 min gradient ranging from 10 to 60% of 80% acetonitrile, 0.1% formic acid at 250 nL/min, and a Q-Exactive instrument (ThermoFisher Scientific, Roskilde, Denmark) was run in a DD-MS2 top 10 method. Full MS spectra were collected at a resolution of 70,000, with an automatic gain control (AGC) target of 3×10^6 or maximum injection time of 20 ms and a scan range of 300 to 1750 m/z. The MS2 spectra were obtained at a resolution of 17,500, with an AGC target value of 1×10^6 or maximum injection time of 60 ms, a normalized collision energy of 25, and an intensity threshold of 1.7 × 10^4. Dynamic exclusion was set to 60 s, and ions with a charge state <2 or unknown were excluded. MS performance was verified for consistency by running complex cell lysate quality control standards, and chromatography was monitored to check for reproducibility. The mass spectrometry data have been deposited to the ProteomeXchange Consortium (http://proteomecentral.proteomexchange.org (accessed on 21 December 2020)) via the PRIDE partner repository with the dataset identifier PXD 023249. The reviewer account details: Username: reviewer_pxd023249@ebi.ac.uk; Password: xteOmcDd. The raw files were analyzed using Proteome Discoverer 2.4. Label-free quantitation (LFQ) was enabled in the processing and consensus steps, and spectra were matched against the *P. rubra* S4059 database obtained from Uniprot (UniProt ID: UP000305729). Dynamic modifications were set as Oxidation (M), Deamidation (N, Q), and Acetyl on the protein N-termini. Cysteine carbamidomethyl was set as a static modification.

The methods of proteomic analyses were modified from Beyene et al. [49]. Briefly, all the statistical analyses were performed using Perseus software (version 1.6.14.0, Max-Planck Institute of Biochemistry, Martinsried, Germany), https://maxquant.net/perseus/ (accessed on 20 September 2020)), and all results were filtered to a 1% false discovery rate (FDR). The normalized abundance values for each protein were $\log_2$ transformed, and at least two valid values were required in the bio-triplicates for quantitation. When the original signals were zero, they were imputed with random numbers from a normal distribution, in which the mean and standard deviation were chosen from low abundance values below the noise level (Width = 0.3; shift = 1.8) [49,50]. To identify proteins with significantly different abundances when S4059 were grown on chitin compared to on mannose, the FDR were estimated using Benjamini–Hochberg method, and a two-tailed unpaired *t*-test was used with a combination of p-value ≤ 0.05 and Log_2 fold-change ≥ 1.5 [51]. The resulting significant proteins were exported from Perseus and visualized in GraphPad Prism 8 (Graphpad Software, San Diego, CA, USA, https://www.graphpad.com/scientific-software/prism/ (accessed 5 October 2020)) using volcano plots.

4.6. DNA Manipulation

Genomic DNA of *P. rubra* S4059 was extracted using the Genomic DNA buffer set (QIAGEN, 19060, Hilden, Germany), as mentioned above. All primers used in this study are listed in Table S6. All purified DNA fragments were amplified using PrimeSTAR® Max Premix (TaKaRa, catalog number: R045A, Kusatsu, Japan). Blue TEMPase Hot Start Master Mix K (catalog number: 733-2584, Haasrode, Belgium) was used for homologous recombination event checking by PCR. All primers and plasmids were designed in A Plasmid Editor-ApE. The specificity of primers was checked by BLAST against the *P. rubra* S4059 genome. All primers were ordered from Integrated DNA technologies (Leuven, Belgium).

4.7. Construction of Suicide Plasmids for in-Frame Deletion of GH19 Chitinase in P. rubra S4059

The suicide plasmid was constructed by the direct cloning method using pDM4 as the backbone [40,42]. The pDM4 plasmid contains an R6K replicon origin, *mob* genes and *oir*T for conjugation, and a chloramphenicol resistance gene *cat* and a *sacB* gene for counter selection [42]. An approximately 1-kb upstream and downstream region flanking of GH19 gene was amplified with primer pairs GH19-L-F/GH19-L-R, GH19-R-F/GH19-R-R (Table S6). The amplified recombining arms were fused with overlap extension PCR to form the recombining arm segments, which were cloned into pJET1.2 subcloning vector using a CloneJET PCR Cloning Kit (ThermoFisher Scientific, K1231, Vilnius, Lithuania) for sequencing. Subsequently, the homologous segment was amplified from sequencing-confirmed pJET1.2-dGH19 arms using primers GH19-pJET1.2-F and GH19-pJET1.2-R. The linear backbone was amplified from the pDM4 suicide vector using primers (GH19-pDM4-F/GH19-pDM4-R). After gel purification, the linear vector and the homologous fragment were co-electroporated into *E. coli* GB *dir-pir116* and ligated by the RecET direct cloning system [40]. The restriction cloning method was also attempted several times to construct this plasmid. However, it was unsuccessful. All plasmids were extracted using a QIAprep Spin Miniprep Kit (QIAGEN, 27106, Hilden, Germany).

4.8. Conjugation of *P. rubra S4059*

The conjugation protocol was modified from Yu et al. and Wang et al. [52,53]. *E. coli* WM3064 harboring the suicide plasmid were used as the donor and *P. rubra* S4059 as the recipient. Overnight cultures of donor and recipient were prepared as pre-cultures one day before the conjugation. During conjugation, both strains were diluted 100 times and grown to $OD_{600} \approx 0.6$. One-mL donor cells were harvested at 6000× *g* for 1 min. The pellets were resuspended and washed once using 1 mL LB + DAP. Then, 1 mL recipient was added to the *E. coli* WM3064 pellet and centrifuged at 6000× *g* for 1 min. One-mL MB + DAP was added to wash the mixture by pipetting and centrifuging at 6000× *g* for 1 min. The supernatant was removed until 20–30 µL liquid remained. The mixture of cells was resuspended and placed on a 0.2-µm pore-size membrane (MF-Millipore, GSWP02500) that was placed on an APY + DAP agar plate. The mating plates were incubated at 20 °C for 24 h. The cells were suspended in 1 mL MB and incubated with shaking at 750 rpm in an Eppendorf® thermomixer comfort, 25 °C for 1 h. After recovery, cells were spread on MA plates with 30 µg/mL chloramphinical (Table S4) and incubated at 25 °C for 24–48 h.

4.9. Confirmation of the First Crossing over Mutants and Deletion Mutants

Colonies from the first crossover selective plates were picked and cultured in 5 mL MB containing 30 µg/mL chloramphenicol overnight. Genomic DNA extraction from pre-cultures using NucleoSpin® Tissue kit (Macherey–Nagel, Düren, Germany, 740952.250). To determine whether the plasmid integrated into target regions, the genomic DNA was used as the template for PCR checking with primers (Cm^r-F/Cm^r-R, GH19-p 1/GH19-p 4, and GH19-p 2/GH19-p 3). Colonies carrying the integrated plasmid were cultured in MB with 30 µg/mL chloramphenicol at 25 °C overnight as pre-culture. The pre-culture was diluted 100 times and inoculated in 5 mL fresh MB without antibiotics until $OD_{600} \approx 0.6$. The culture was 10-fold diluted and spread on the counter selection plates (half nutrients of MA) containing 10% sucrose. These counter selection plates were incubated at 20 °C until colonies were visible. Confirmation of the in-frame deletion mutants was carried out by PCR application and sequencing. Primers (GH19-p1/GH19-p2) were designed to amplify the mutation region, and the PCR produced was purified and sent for DNA sequencing.

4.10. Growth Curves of Wild Type and Mutant

Growth kinetics of *P. rubra* S4059 WT (wild type) and Δ*GH19* (GH19 chitinase mutant) were established in MMM with or without 0.3% casamino acids and supplemented with 0.2% colloidal chitin, 0.2% crab chitin (C9752, Sigma, St. Louis, MO, USA), 0.2% mannose (63580, Sigma, St. Louis, MO, USA), or 0.2% NAG (A3286, Sigma, St. Louis, MO, USA), respectively, as carbon source. Pre-cultures of *P. rubra* WT and mutants were grown in MB overnight at 25 °C. The cultures were diluted to a starting concentration of 10^3 CFU/mL in MMM. Samples were taken every 4 h for estimation of cell density by plate counting. All experiments were done in three biological replicates.

4.11. Growth and Attachment on Shrimp Shells

Six millimeter diameter circular disks were prepared from the exoskeleton of Vannamei shrimps (description in Supplementary Material). Bacterial cultures (WT and mutants) were grown in 5 mL MB in 50 mL flasks at 25 °C, 200 rpm overnight. The cultures were diluted to 10^4 CFU/mL in artificial seawater (3% sea salt, Sigma, S9883) and incubated with or without shrimp shells in 1.5 mL Eppendorf tubes. Samples of the suspension were taken after 0, 2, 5, 7, 10 days incubation and plated after serial dilution. The tubes were sonicated five minutes at 50/60 Hz in an ultrasonic bath (Emmi D20 Q, EMAG, Mörfelden-Walldorf, Germany) and vortexed 10 s to remove bacteria attached to the shrimp shells [54]. A suspension of cells with known cell counts was subjected to the same sonication and cell counts done after sonication, demonstrating that this procedure did not reduce cell counts. Then serial dilutions and colony counts were done to determine cell densities. The experiment was done in biological duplicate.

4.12. Extraction of Metabolites for Chemical Analysis

Bacterial cultures were grown in MMM with different carbon sources, and samples were taken for chemical analyses after 72 h incubation. Ten milliliters of the sample were extracted with an equal volume of high-performance liquid chromatography (HPLC)-grade Ethyl acetate in 50 mL Falcon tubes. The organic phase was transferred to a new vial and evaporated under nitrogen. The dried extract was re-dissolved in 500 µL methanol and stored at −20 °C. Chemical analysis was performed in biological triplicate.

4.13. Chemical Analysis by UHPLC-HRMS

The chemical analysis approach was modified from Holm et al. [55]. Chemical analysis was performed on a Bruker maXis 3G orthogonal acceleration quadrupole time-of-flight mass spectrometer (Bruker Daltonics, Billlerica, MA, USA) equipped with an electrospray ionization (ESI) source and connected to an Ultimate 3000 UHPLC system (Dionex, Sunnyvale, CA, USA). The column used was a reverse-phase Kinetex 1.7 µm C18, 100 mm × 2.1 mm (Phenomenex). The column temperature was kept at 40 °C throughout the analysis. A linear gradient of LC-MS grade water and acetonitrile both buffered with formic acid was used, starting at 10% (*v/v*) acetonitrile and increased to 100% in 10 min, maintaining this rate for 3 min before returning to the starting conditions in 0.1 min and staying there for 2.4 min before the following run. A flow rate of 0.40 mL/min was used. Time-of-flight mass spectrometry (TOFMS) was performed in ESI+ with a data acquisition range of 10 scans per second at *m/z* 75–1250. The TOFMS was calibrated using the Bruker Daltonics high precision calibration algorithm by means of the internal standard sodium formate, which was automatically infused before each run. This provided a mass accuracy of better than 1.5 ppm in MS mode. UV-visible spectra were collected at wavelengths from 200 to 700 nm. Data processing was performed using DataAnalysis 4.0 (Bruker Daltonics, Billerica, MA, USA) and Target Analysis 1.2 software (Bruker Daltonics). Tandem MS spectra were acquired on an Agilent 6545 QTOF-MS using the method described in Isbrandt et al. (2020) [56].

Supplementary Materials: The following are available online at https://www.mdpi.com/1660-3397/19/2/108/s1, Table S1. The predicted biosynthetic gene clusters (BGCs) of Pseudoalteromonas rubra S4059 by antiSMASH 6.0. Table S2. The fold change of six significantly upregulated chitinolytic enzymes in cell or supernatant samples. Table S3. Significantly up-and downregulated proteins in Pseudoalteromonas rubra S4059 proteome when grown on chitin compared to on mannose. Table S4. Antibiotic sensitivity of Pseudoalteromonas rubra S4059 growth on an MB agar plate. Table S5. Bacteria and plasmids used in this study. Table S6. Primers used in this study. Table S7. The normalized protein abundance of chitinolytic enzymes in S4059. Figure S1. (A) Base peak chromatograms of Pseudoalteromonas rubra S4059 wild type (WT) and ΔGH19 mutant when cultivated on a marine minimal medium using mannose, crystalline chitin, colloidal chitin, or N-acetyl glucosamine (NAG) as the carbon source. The red pigment prodigiosin and two of its analogs (hexyl prodigiosin and heptyl prodigiosin) could be identified in the extract and confirmed based on MS/MS experiments and the acquired absorption spectra. Experiments were done in biological triplicates, and a reference chromatogram of the sterile growth medium was included to show media components also present in the experiments. (B) Tandem MS spectra recorded for (1) prodigiosin, (2) hexyl-prodigiosin, and (3) heptyl-prodigiosin. The prodigiosin MS/MS spectra matched our in-house MS/MS library, and the characteristic fragment m/z 252.11 and loss of CH3 (m/z 15.02) additionally matched those previously reported for prodigiosin and analogs [57]. (C) Recorded UV-Vis absorption spectrum of prodigiosin. All proposed prodigiosins share identical absorption spectra. The spectrum is in agreement with previously reported literature [58]. Figure S2. (A–D) Growth kinetics of Pseudoalteromonas rubra S4059 wild type (WT) and ΔGH19 mutant in mannose (A), colloidal chitin (B), crystalline chitin (crab chitin) (C), and NAG (chitin monomer) (D) containing a marine minimal medium (MMM) with casamino acids. (E,F) WT and ΔGH19 growth in crystalline chitin (E) or colloidal chitin containing MMM without casamino acid. Square: WT; Triangle: ΔGH19. The points are bio-replicates, and error bars are standard deviation. (G,H) Chitin degradation activities of wild type and the mutant on colloidal chitin plate (G) and crystalline chitin plate (H). Figure S3. Biofilm formation on the microtiter-well plastic surface of Pseudoalteromonas rubra S4059 wild type and ΔGH19 mutant in four different sole carbon contained medium as determined by the O'Toole and Kolter crystal violet assay. (A) in mannose; (B) in NAG (chitin monomer); (C) in colloidal chitin; (D) in crab chitin. All experiments were in bio-triplicates, and error bars are standard deviation.

Author Contributions: X.W., S.S.P., S.-D.Z., and L.G. conceived and design the experiments; X.W. performed the experiments; T.I. and T.O.L. performed the chemical analysis; E.M.S. and M.W.N. performed the proteomic analyses. M.L.S. assembled the genome of *P. rubra* S4059 and supervised the statistical analysis. Y.B. assisted in approving that GH19 was expressed in *P. rubra* S4059 when grown on chitin. X.W. wrote the first manuscript draft; S.-D.Z. and L.G. supervised the edited and finalized the manuscript. All authors have read and agreed to the published version of the manuscript.

Funding: This research was supported by the Chinese Scholarship Council (CSC scholarship No. 201706170066), the Danish National Research Foundation (DNRF137) for the Center for Microbial Secondary Metabolites, the Independent Research Fund Denmark (grant DFF–7017-00003), and the European Union's Horizon 2020 research and Innovation Programme under the Marie Sklodowska-Curie grant agreement no. 713683 (COFUND fellows DTU) via the H. C. Ørsted fellowship program.

Data Availability Statement: Proteomic data are available via ProteomeXchange with identifier PXD023249 (http://www.proteomexchange.org/) and the genome of *Pseudoalteromonas rubra* S4059 is available at the National Center for Biotechnology Information (NCBI) under the accession number CP045429 (https://www.ncbi.nlm.nih.gov/nuccore/CP045429.1/ (accessed on 23 November 2020)) and CP045430 (https://www.ncbi.nlm.nih.gov/nuccore/CP045430.1/ (accessed on 23 November 2020)). Further inquiries can be directed to the corresponding author/s.

Acknowledgments: We gratefully acknowledge Youming Zhang and Zhen Li from the Shandong University for kindly providing the RecET direct cloning strains and vectors.

Conflicts of Interest: The authors declare no conflict of interest. The funders had no role in the design of the study; in the collection, analyses, or interpretation of data; in the writing of the manuscript, or in the decision to publish the results.

References

1. Romano, G.; Costantini, M.; Sansone, C.; Lauritano, C.; Ruocco, N.; Ianora, A. Marine microorganisms as a promising and sustainable source of bioactive molecules. *Mar. Environ. Res.* **2017**, *128*, 58–69. [CrossRef]
2. Parte, S.; Sirisha, V.L.; D'Souza, J.S. Biotechnological applications of marine enzymes from algae, bacteria, fungi, and sponges. *Adv. Food Nutr. Res.* **2017**, *80*, 75–106. [CrossRef] [PubMed]
3. Bowman, J.P. Bioactive compound synthetic capacity and ecological significance of marine bacterial genus *Pseudoalteromonas*. *Mar. Drugs* **2007**, *5*, 220–241. [CrossRef]
4. Offret, C.; Desriac, F.; Le Chevalier, P.; Mounier, J.; Jégou, C.; Fleury, Y. Spotlight on antimicrobial metabolites from the marine bacteria *Pseudoalteromonas*: Chemodiversity and ecological significance. *Mar. Drugs* **2016**, *14*, 129. [CrossRef] [PubMed]
5. Tang, B.L.; Yang, J.; Chen, X.L.; Wang, P.; Zhao, H.L.; Su, H.N.; Li, C.Y.; Yu, Y.; Zhong, S.; Wang, L.; et al. A predator-prey interaction between a marine *Pseudoalteromonas* sp. and Gram-positive bacteria. *Nat. Commun.* **2020**, *11*, 285. [CrossRef] [PubMed]
6. Zhao, H.L.; Chen, X.L.; Xie, B.B.; Zhou, M.Y.; Gao, X.; Zhang, X.Y.; Zhou, B.C.; Weiss, A.S.; Zhang, Y.Z. Elastolytic mechanism of a novel M23 metalloprotease pseudoalterin from deep-sea *Pseudoalteromonas* sp. CF6-2: Cleaving not only glycyl bonds in the hydrophobic regions but also peptide bonds in the hydrophilic regions involved in cross-linking. *J. Biol. Chem.* **2012**, *287*, 39710–39720. [CrossRef]
7. Paulsen, S.S.; Strube, M.L.; Bech, P.K.; Gram, L.; Sonnenschein, E.C. Marine chitinolytic *Pseudoalteromonas* represents an untapped reservoir of bioactive potential. *Msystems* **2019**, *4*, 1–12. [CrossRef] [PubMed]
8. Rinaudo, M. Chitin and chitosan: Properties and applications. *Prog. Polym. Sci.* **2006**, *31*, 603–632. [CrossRef]
9. Rudall, K.M.; Kenchington, W. The chitin system. *Biol. Rev.* **1973**, *49*, 597–636. [CrossRef]
10. Beier, S.; Bertilsson, S. Bacterial chitin degradation-mechanisms and ecophysiological strategies. *Front. Microbiol.* **2013**, *4*, 149. [CrossRef] [PubMed]
11. Vaaje-Kolstad, G.; Horn, S.J.; Sørlie, M.; Eijsink, V.G.H. The chitinolytic machinery of *Serratia marcescens*—A model system for enzymatic degradation of recalcitrant polysaccharides. *FEBS J.* **2013**, *280*, 3028–3049. [CrossRef] [PubMed]
12. Oyeleye, A.; Normi, Y.M. Chitinase: Diversity, limitations, and trends in engineering for suitable applications. *Biosci. Rep.* **2018**, *38*, 1–21. [CrossRef] [PubMed]

13. Gooday, G.W. The ecology of chitin degradation. *Adv. Microb. Ecol.* **1990**, 387–430. [CrossRef]
14. Bai, Y.; Eijsink, V.G.H.; Kielak, A.M.; van Veen, J.A.; de Boer, W. Genomic comparison of chitinolytic enzyme systems from terrestrial and aquatic bacteria. *Environ. Microbiol.* **2016**, *18*, 38–49. [CrossRef] [PubMed]
15. Udaya Prakash, N.A.; Jayanthi, M.; Sabarinathan, R.; Kangueane, P.; Mathew, L.; Sekar, K. Evolution, homology conservation, and identification of unique sequence signatures in GH19 family chitinases. *J. Mol. Evol.* **2010**, *70*, 466–478. [CrossRef]
16. Konno, N.; Takahashi, H.; Nakajima, M.; Takeda, T.; Sakamoto, Y. Characterization of β-N-acetylhexosaminidase (LeHex20A), a member of glycoside hydrolase family 20, from *Lentinula edodes* (shiitake mushroom). *AMB Express* **2012**, *2*, 1–7. [CrossRef] [PubMed]
17. Vaaje-Kolstad, G.; Westereng, B.; Horn, S.J.; Liu, Z.; Zhai, H.; Sørlie, M.; Eijsink, V.G.H. An oxidative enzyme boosting the enzymatic conversion of recalcitrant polysaccharides. *Science* **2010**, *330*, 219–222. [CrossRef] [PubMed]
18. García-Fraga, B.; da Silva, A.F.; López-Seijas, J.; Sieiro, C. A novel family 19 chitinase from the marine-derived *Pseudoalteromonas tunicata* CCUG 44952T: Heterologous expression, characterization and antifungal activity. *Biochem. Eng. J.* **2015**, *93*, 84–93. [CrossRef]
19. Giubergia, S.; Phippen, C.; Gotfredsen, C.H.; Nielsen, K.F.; Gram, L. Influence of niche-specific nutrients on secondary metabolism in *Vibrionaceae*. *Appl. Environ. Microbiol.* **2016**, *82*, 4035–4044. [CrossRef] [PubMed]
20. Giubergia, S.; Phippen, C.; Nielsen, K.F.; Gram, L. Growth on chitin impacts the transcriptome and metabolite profiles of antibiotic-producing *Vibrio coralliilyticus* S2052 and *Photobacterium galatheae* S2753. *Msystems* **2017**, *2*, 1–12. [CrossRef] [PubMed]
21. Wietz, M.; Duncan, K.; Patin, N.V.; Jensen, P.R. Antagonistic interactions mediated by marine bacteria: The role of small molecules. *J. Chem. Ecol.* **2013**, *39*, 879–891. [CrossRef]
22. Nazari, B.; Kobayashi, M.; Saito, A.; Hassaninasab, A.; Miyashita, K.; Fujiia, T. Chitin-induced gene expression in secondary metabolic pathways of *Streptomyces coelicolor* A3(2) grown in soil. *Appl. Environ. Microbiol.* **2013**, *79*, 707–713. [CrossRef]
23. Saravanan, P.; Nancharaiah, Y.V.; Venugopalan, V.P.; Rao, T.S.; Jayachandran, S. Biofilm formation by *Pseudoalteromonas ruthenica* and its removal by chlorine. *Biofouling* **2006**, *22*, 371–381. [CrossRef] [PubMed]
24. Margolis, J.J.; El-Etr, S.; Joubert, L.M.; Moore, E.; Robison, R.; Rasley, A.; Spormann, A.M.; Monack, D.M. Contributions of *Francisella tularensis* subsp. *novicida* chitinases and Sec secretion system to biofilm formation on chitin. *Appl. Environ. Microbiol.* **2010**, *76*, 596–608. [CrossRef] [PubMed]
25. Veliz, E.A.; Martínez-Hidalgo, P.; Hirsch, A.M. Chitinase-producing bacteria and their role in biocontrol. *AIMS Microbiol.* **2017**, *3*, 689–705. [CrossRef] [PubMed]
26. Reguera, G.; Kolter, R. Virulence and the environment: A novel role for *Vibrio cholerae* toxin-coregulated pili in biofilm formation on chitin. *J. Bacteriol.* **2005**, *187*, 3551–3555. [CrossRef] [PubMed]
27. Sun, S.; Tay, Q.X.M.; Kjelleberg, S.; Rice, S.A.; McDougald, D. Quorum sensing-regulated chitin metabolism provides grazing resistance to *Vibrio cholerae* biofilms. *ISME J.* **2015**, *9*, 1812–1820. [CrossRef]
28. Pruzzo, C.; Vezzulli, L.; Colwell, R.R. Global impact of *Vibrio cholerae* interactions with chitin. *Environ. Microbiol.* **2008**, *10*, 1400–1410. [CrossRef] [PubMed]
29. Tuveng, T.R.; Arntzen, M.Ø.; Bengtsson, O.; Gardner, J.G.; Vaaje-Kolstad, G.; Eijsink, V.G.H. Proteomic investigation of the secretome of *Cellvibrio japonicus* during growth on chitin. *Proteomics* **2016**, *16*, 1904–1914. [CrossRef]
30. Monge, E.C.; Tuveng, T.R.; Vaaje-Kolstad, G.; Eijsink, V.G.H.; Gardner, J.G. Systems analysis of the glycoside hydrolase family 18 enzymes from *Cellvibrio japonicus* characterizes essential chitin degradation functions. *J. Biol. Chem.* **2018**, *293*, 3849–3859. [CrossRef]
31. Hayes, C.A.; Dalia, T.N.; Dalia, A.B. Systematic genetic dissection of chitin degradation and uptake in *Vibrio cholerae*. *Environ. Microbiol.* **2017**, *19*, 4154–4163. [CrossRef]
32. Bengtsson, O.; Arntzen, M.; Mathiesen, G.; Skaugen, M.; Eijsink, V.G.H. A novel proteomics sample preparation method for secretome analysis of *Hypocrea jecorina* growing on insoluble substrates. *J. Proteom.* **2016**, *131*, 104–112. [CrossRef] [PubMed]
33. Peterson, B.W.; Sharma, P.K.; van der Mei, H.C.; Busscher, H.J. Bacterial cell surface damage due to centrifugal compaction. *Appl. Environ. Microbiol.* **2012**, *78*, 120–125. [CrossRef] [PubMed]
34. Martínez-Caballero, S.; Cano-Sánchez, P.; Mares-Mejía, I.; Díaz-Sánchez, A.G.; Macías-Rubalcava, M.L.; Hermoso, J.A.; Rodríguez-Romero, A. Comparative study of two GH19 chitinase-like proteins from *Hevea brasiliensis*, one exhibiting a novel carbohydrate-binding domain. *FEBS J.* **2014**, *281*, 4535–4554. [CrossRef] [PubMed]
35. Ohno, T.; Armand, S.; Hata, T.; Nikaidou, N.; Henrissat, B.; Mitsutomi, M.; Watanabe, T. A modular family 19 chitinase found in the prokaryotic organism *Streptomyces griseus* HUT 6037. *J. Bacteriol.* **1996**, *178*, 5065–5070. [CrossRef] [PubMed]
36. Gram, L.; Melchiorsen, J.; Bruhn, J.B. Antibacterial activity of marine culturable bacteria collected from a global sampling of ocean surface waters and surface swabs of marine organisms. *Mar. Biotechnol.* **2010**, *12*, 439–451. [CrossRef] [PubMed]
37. Zhang, S.D.; Santini, C.L.; Zhang, W.J.; Barbe, V.; Mangenot, S.; Guyomar, C.; Garel, M.; Chen, H.T.; Li, X.G.; Yin, Q.J.; et al. Genomic and physiological analysis reveals versatile metabolic capacity of deep-sea *Photobacterium phosphoreum* ANT-2200. *Extremophiles* **2016**, *20*, 301–310. [CrossRef] [PubMed]
38. Östling, J.; Goodman, A.; Kjelleberg, S. Behaviour of IncP-1 plasmids and a miniMu transposon in a marine *Vibrio* sp.: Isolation of starvation inducible *lac* operon fusions. *FEMS Microbiol. Lett.* **1991**, *86*, 83–94. [CrossRef]
39. Paulsen, S.S.; Andersen, B.; Gram, L.; MacHado, H. Biological potential of chitinolytic marine bacteria. *Mar. Drugs* **2016**, *14*, 230. [CrossRef] [PubMed]

40. Wang, H.; Li, Z.; Jia, R.; Hou, Y.; Yin, J.; Bian, X.; Li, A.; Müller, R.; Stewart, A.F.; Fu, J.; et al. RecET direct cloning and Redαβ recombineering of biosynthetic gene clusters, large operons or single genes for heterologous expression. *Nat. Protoc.* **2016**, *11*, 1175–1190. [CrossRef] [PubMed]
41. Dehio, C.; Meyer, M. Maintenance of broad-host-range incompatibility group P and group Q plasmids and transposition of Tn5 in *Bartonella henselae* following conjugal plasmid transfer from *Eescherichia coli*. *J. Bacteriol.* **1997**, *179*, 538–540. [CrossRef] [PubMed]
42. Milton, D.L.; O'Toole, R.; Hörstedt, P.; Wolf-Watz, H. Flagellin A is essential for the virulence of *Vibrio anguillarum*. *J. Bacteriol.* **1996**, *178*, 1310–1319. [CrossRef]
43. Wick, R.R.; Judd, L.M.; Gorrie, C.L.; Holt, K.E. Unicycler: Resolving bacterial genome assemblies from short and long sequencing reads. *PLoS Comput. Biol.* **2017**, *13*, e1005595. [CrossRef] [PubMed]
44. Seemann, T. Prokka: Rapid prokaryotic genome annotation. *Bioinformatics* **2014**, *30*, 2068–2069. [CrossRef]
45. Vallenet, D.; Calteau, A.; Dubois, M.; Amours, P.; Bazin, A.; Beuvin, M.; Burlot, L.; Bussell, X.; Fouteau, S.; Gautreau, G.; et al. MicroScope: An integrated platform for the annotation and exploration of microbial gene functions through genomic, pangenomic and metabolic comparative analysis. *Nucleic Acids Res.* **2019**. [CrossRef] [PubMed]
46. Almagro Armenteros, J.J.; Tsirigos, K.D.; Sønderby, C.K.; Petersen, T.N.; Winther, O.; Brunak, S.; von Heijne, G.; Nielsen, H. SignalP 5.0 improves signal peptide predictions using deep neural networks. *Nat. Biotechnol.* **2019**, *37*, 420–423. [CrossRef] [PubMed]
47. Chevallier, V.; Schoof, E.M.; Malphettes, L.; Andersen, M.R.; Workman, C.T. Characterization of glutathione proteome in CHO cells and its relationship with productivity and cholesterol synthesis. *Biotechnol. Bioeng.* **2020**, *117*, 3448–3458. [CrossRef] [PubMed]
48. Haddad Momeni, M.; Leth, M.L.; Sternberg, C.; Schoof, E.; Nielsen, M.W.; Holck, J.; Workman, C.T.; Hoof, J.B.; Abou Hachem, M. Loss of AA13 LPMOs impairs degradation of resistant starch and reduces the growth of *Aspergillus nidulans*. *Biotechnol. Biofuels* **2020**, *13*, 1–13. [CrossRef] [PubMed]
49. Beyene, G.T.; Kalayou, S.; Riaz, T.; Tonjum, T. Comparative proteomic analysis of *Neisseria meningitidis* wildtype and dprA null mutant strains links DNA processing to pilus biogenesis. *BMC Microbiol.* **2017**, *17*, 1–18. [CrossRef] [PubMed]
50. Yimer, S.A.; Birhanu, A.G.; Kalayou, S.; Riaz, T.; Zegeye, E.D.; Beyene, G.T.; Holm-Hansen, C.; Norheim, G.; Abebe, M.; Aseffa, A.; et al. Comparative proteomic analysis of *Mycobacterium tuberculosis* lineage 7 and lineage 4 strains reveals differentially abundant proteins linked to slow growth and virulence. *Front. Microbiol.* **2017**, *8*, 795. [CrossRef] [PubMed]
51. Dunn, J.; Ferluga, S.; Sharma, V.; Futschik, M.; Hilton, D.A.; Adams, C.L.; Lasonder, E.; Hanemann, C.O. Proteomic analysis discovers the differential expression of novel proteins and phosphoproteins in meningioma including NEK9, HK2 and SET and deregulation of RNA metabolism. *EBioMedicine* **2019**, *40*, 77–91. [CrossRef]
52. Yu, Z.C.; Zhao, D.L.; Ran, L.Y.; Mi, Z.H.; Wu, Z.Y.; Pang, X.; Zhang, X.Y.; Su, H.N.; Shi, M.; Song, X.Y.; et al. Development of a genetic system for the deep-sea psychrophilic bacterium *Pseudoalteromonas* sp. SM9913. *Microb. Cell Fact.* **2014**, *13*, 1–9. [CrossRef]
53. Wang, P.; Yu, Z.; Li, B.; Cai, X.; Zeng, Z.; Chen, X.; Wang, X. Development of an efficient conjugation-based genetic manipulation system for Pseudoalteromonas. *Microb. Cell Fact.* **2015**, *14*, 1–11. [CrossRef]
54. Kim, E.; Kinney, W.H.; Ovrutsky, A.R.; Vo, D.; Bai, X.; Honda, J.R.; Marx, G.; Peck, E.; Lindberg, L.; Falkinham, J.O.; et al. A surface with a biomimetic micropattern reduces colonization of *Mycobacterium abscessus*. *FEMS Microbiol. Lett.* **2014**, *360*, 17–22. [CrossRef] [PubMed]
55. Holm, D.K.; Petersen, L.M.; Klitgaard, A.; Knudsen, P.B.; Jarczynska, Z.D.; Nielsen, K.F.; Gotfredsen, C.H.; Larsen, T.O.; Mortensen, U.H. Molecular and chemical characterization of the biosynthesis of the 6-MSA-derived meroterpenoid yanuthone D in *Aspergillus niger*. *Chem. Biol.* **2014**, *21*, 519–529. [CrossRef] [PubMed]
56. Isbrandt, T.; Tolborg, G.; Ødum, A.; Workman, M.; Larsen, T.O. Atrorosins: A new subgroup of *Monascus* pigments from *Talaromyces atroroseus*. *Appl. Microbiol. Biotechnol.* **2020**, *104*, 615–622. [CrossRef] [PubMed]
57. Lee, J.S.; Kim, Y.S.; Park, S.; Kim, J.; Kang, S.J.; Lee, M.H.; Ryu, S.; Choi, J.M.; Oh, T.K.; Yoon, J.H. Exceptional production of both prodigiosin and cycloprodigiosin as major metabolic constituents by a novel marine bacterium, *Zooshikella rubidus* S1-1. *Appl. Environ. Microbiol.* **2011**, *77*, 4967–4973. [CrossRef] [PubMed]
58. Couturier, M.; Bhalara, H.D.; Chawrai, S.R.; Monson, R.; Williamson, N.R.; Salmond, G.P.C.; Leeper, F.J. Substrate flexibility of the flavin-dependent dihydropyrrole oxidases Pigb and Hapb involved in antibiotic prodigiosin biosynthesis. *ChemBioChem* **2020**, *21*, 523–530. [CrossRef]

marine drugs

MDPI

Article

An Integrative Bioinformatic Analysis for Keratinase Detection in Marine-Derived *Streptomyces*

Ricardo Valencia [1,†,‡], Valentina González [1,†], Agustina Undabarrena [1], Leonardo Zamora-Leiva [1], Juan A. Ugalde [2] and Beatriz Cámara [1,*]

1 Laboratory of Molecular Microbiology and Environmental Biotechnology, Department of Chemistry and Center for Biotechnology Daniel Alkalay Lowitt, Federico Santa María Technical University, Valparaíso 2340000, Chile; ricardo.valenciaa@alumnos.usm.cl (R.V.); valentina.gonzalez@alumnos.usm.cl (V.G.); agustina.undabarrena@usm.cl (A.U.); leonardo.zamoral@sansano.usm.cl (L.Z.-L.)
2 Millennium Initiative for Collaborative Research on Bacterial Resistance (MICROB-R), Santiago 8320000, Chile; juan@ecogenomica.cl
* Correspondence: beatriz.camara@usm.cl; Tel.: +56-32-2654732
† These authors have contributed equally to this work.
‡ Current address: Institute of Quantitative Biology, Biochemistry and Biotechnology, School of Biological Sciences, The University of Edinburgh, King's Buildings, Edinburgh EH9 3BF, UK.

Abstract: Keratinases present promising biotechnological applications, due to their ability to degrade keratin. *Streptomyces* appears as one of the main sources of these enzymes, but complete genome sequences of keratinolytic bacteria are still limited. This article reports the complete genomes of three marine-derived streptomycetes that show different levels of feather keratin degradation, with high (strain G11C), low (strain CHD11), and no (strain Vc74B-19) keratinolytic activity. A multi-step bioinformatics approach is described to explore genes encoding putative keratinases in these genomes. Despite their differential keratinolytic activity, multiplatform annotation reveals similar quantities of ORFs encoding putative proteases in strains G11C, CHD11, and Vc74B-19. Comparative genomics classified these putative proteases into 140 orthologous groups and 17 unassigned orthogroup peptidases belonging to strain G11C. Similarity network analysis revealed three network communities of putative peptidases related to known keratinases of the peptidase families S01, S08, and M04. When combined with the prediction of cellular localization and phylogenetic reconstruction, seven putative keratinases from the highly keratinolytic strain *Streptomyces* sp. G11C are identified. To our knowledge, this is the first multi-step bioinformatics analysis that complements comparative genomics with phylogeny and cellular localization prediction, for the prediction of genes encoding putative keratinases in streptomycetes.

Keywords: keratinases; keratinolytic proteases; marine-derived *Streptomyces*; genomic comparison

Citation: Valencia, R.; González, V.; Undabarrena, A.; Zamora-Leiva, L.; Ugalde, J.A.; Cámara, B. An Integrative Bioinformatic Analysis for Keratinase Detection in Marine-Derived *Streptomyces*. *Mar. Drugs* **2021**, *19*, 286. https://doi.org/10.3390/md19060286

Academic Editor: Max Crüsemann

Received: 14 April 2021
Accepted: 18 May 2021
Published: 21 May 2021

1. Introduction

Keratin is a fibrous and recalcitrant protein belonging to a large family of structural proteins that constitute hair, wool, feathers, nails, bristles, and horns of several animals [1]. This protein is densely packed in α-helix or β-sheet structures (α/β-keratin, respectively) and their high degree of cross-linkages by disulfide and hydrogen bonds confers high mechanical stability and resistance to common proteolytic enzymes such as pepsin, trypsin, and papain [2]. Its recalcitrant structure is a significant challenge for degradation, a process that naturally can take as long as many years [3]. Indeed, there are many known examples of preserved hair, skin, and feathers on archeological materials [4–6]. Its accumulation can be a major problem, especially for poultry processing farms, where feather keratin is a by-product of industrial activities. Therefore, finding microorganisms that present the ability to degrade this protein will become an eco-friendly alternative to improve the management of their waste resources. So far, several microorganisms have been reported to produce keratinases, including Fungi [7,8] and Bacteria, such as *Bacillus* [9–11] and *Streptomyces* [12–16].

Keratinases (EC 3.4.21/24/99.11) are a particular class of proteases that possess keratinolytic activity, being able to degrade several insoluble keratin substrates [3]. They are primarily extracellular; however, cell-bound [17] and intracellular [18] enzymes have also been reported. Most of the keratinases known to date are serine proteases [14,16,19], while a few have been classified as metalloproteases [20]. Nevertheless, it remains unclear which features are required for keratin degradation [21]. Most studies are focused on the purification and characterization of a unique keratinase or protease with keratinolytic activity [16,22–26]. However, purified keratinases known to date cannot completely solubilize native keratin, which confirms that one enzyme alone cannot fully decompose its recalcitrant structure [3,27]. For this reason, it has been hypothesized that a pool of proteases is needed to penetrate and break down keratin structure, instead of a single enzyme. Indeed, in natural environments, this degradation could result from the combined action of enzymes from various organisms, such as Fungi and Bacteria [3]. Moreover, due to the high cysteine content in keratin, and therefore, their respective disulfide bonds, it is believed that other enzymes, such as disulfide reductases, are likely to be involved in this process, acting in addition to keratinolytic proteases [28]. Although there are many publications describing keratinase characterization, the molecular mechanism of microbial keratinolysis is not yet completely elucidated.

Genomic analysis of keratinolytic bacteria is seldom reported [29–34]. *Streptomyces* species are one of the main producers of keratinases [35], but so far, there is only one recently reported genome of keratinolytic-degrading *Streptomyces* [36]. Moreover, according to our knowledge, there are no comparative studies between keratinolytic and non-keratinolytic bacteria, which may unveil the underlying genetic factors contributing to its degradative capacity. Recently, our Chilean marine actinobacterial culture collection [37–39] was screened for extracellular enzyme activities analyzing 75 strains [40], providing evidence of promising keratinolytic activity. To see whether we could bioinformatically predict the genes encoding putative keratinases, in this study, we sequenced the genome of three of these streptomycetes, selected for showing varying levels of keratin degradation: Strains G11C, CHD11, and Vc74B-19, with high, low, and no keratinolytic activity, respectively. We present an integrative comparative analysis between the universe of putative proteases belonging to these strains, complementing information from orthogroups of proteases, peptidase families, cell location prediction, and phylogeny, to finally deliver a bioinformatic prediction consisting of a set of genes considered to encode potential keratinases. Efforts addressing a thorough *in silico* investigation of putative proteases and peptidases, to obtain those likely to be involved in feather degradation, have been accomplished for the first time. Interestingly, 18 of 24 proteases predicted by this pipeline (6 of seven potential keratinases (predicted by phylogenetic analysis), and 12 of 17 unique genes of the G11C genome ("unassigned p-orthogroup" peptidases)) and thought to be involved in keratinolytic activity were validated in our previous study by being present in the secretome of strain G11C [40]. This study provides a not so far described bioinformatic multi-step pipeline, that helps decipher potential genetic factors that enable some strains to have higher efficiency in keratin degradation.

2. Results

2.1. Genome Features of Streptomyces Strains with Differential Keratinolytic Activity

Three strains (Table S1) from our Chilean marine actinobacterial culture collection [37–39] were selected for genome sequencing, based on a previous feather degradation screening [40]: *Streptomyces* sp. G11C, presented the highest level of keratinolytic activity, exhibiting complete feather degradation in liquid culture; *Streptomyces* sp. Vc74B-19, evidenced no keratinolytic activity, leaving the feather structure unaltered, and *Streptomyces* sp. CHD11 presented a low level of degradation, showing the partial dissolution of the fibers of the feathers [40]. To obtain insights into the genetic determinants involved in feather degradation, genomes were sequenced using the Illumina NextSeq platform with a 150 bp × 2 configuration. Final assembly statistics, including quality metrics, for each genome, are displayed in Table 1. CHD11 and Vc74B-19 genomes, of approximately 7.5 Mbp, are larger in size than the G11C genome (nearly 6.9 Mbp), although the GC content is similar for all three strains and is comparable with percentages found in actinobacterial strains [41].

Table 1. Assembly statistics of analyzed *Streptomyces* genomes.

Statistical Data	*Streptomyces* sp. G11C	*Streptomyces* sp. CHD11	*Streptomyces* sp. Vc74B-19
Total number of paired reads	7,253,694	9,168,658	8,356,602
Total raw reads bases (Gbp)	187.73	232.83	213.71
Assembly size (bp) (≥500 bp contigs)	6,873,298	7,469,836	7,625,040
Number of contigs (≥500 bp)	167	91	197
Contigs (N50) (kb)	204,147	98,291	76,195
G + C content (%)	73.15	71.67	72.33
Predicted CDS	5953	6661	6835
CheckM completeness (%)	99.53	100	99.24
L50 statistics	24	12	31

Previous taxonomic classification using the 16S rRNA gene indicated that these marine strains belong to the *Streptomyces* genus [37]. To obtain a precise taxonomic placement, we performed a phylogenomic analysis (Figure 1, Table S2) and calculated average nucleotide identity (ANI) (Figure S1, Table S3). In the case of the phylogenomic tree, the inference was made with Orthofinder [42] using 634 single-copy orthogroups. These analyses indicate that both streptomycete strains presenting either low and no keratinolytic activity, strains CHD11 and Vc74B-19, respectively, are phylogenetically close, grouping in the same sub-clade with the closest neighbor *Streptomyces emeiensis* CGMCC 4.3504^T [43]. This is consistent with ANI values obtained between strains Vc74B-19 and CHD11 (88.2%) and with *S. emeiensis* type strain—87.5% for strain CHD11 and 87.4% for strain Vc74B-19. On the other hand, strain G11C, with high keratinolytic activity, groups with *Streptomyces albidoflavus* NRRL B-1271^T [44], consistent with an ANIm of 96.1% that indicates strain G11C could be considered as part of the *albidoflavus* species [45]. A strain belonging to the *albidoflavus* species has been described in the literature to possess keratinolytic activity, secreting at least six extracellular proteases when cultured on a feather meal-based medium [14]. Altogether, these findings motivated us to study the minor differences between our genomes and examine a possible bioinformatic explanation for the observed differential keratinolytic activities.

2.2. Comparative Genomics of Differential Keratinolytic Streptomycete Strains

To identify potential genes encoding keratinases that could be involved in keratin hydrolysis and the observed differences in *Streptomyces* strains G11C, CHD11, and Vc74B-19, a comparison of the diversity and quantity of peptidases present in all three strains was accomplished using the following approaches: Genome annotation using the Prokka, PANNZER2, and eggNOG servers, classification by MEROPS database and identification of orthologous groups. In addition, to compare these protein sequences with functionally characterized keratinases obtained from literature, a similarity network was developed.

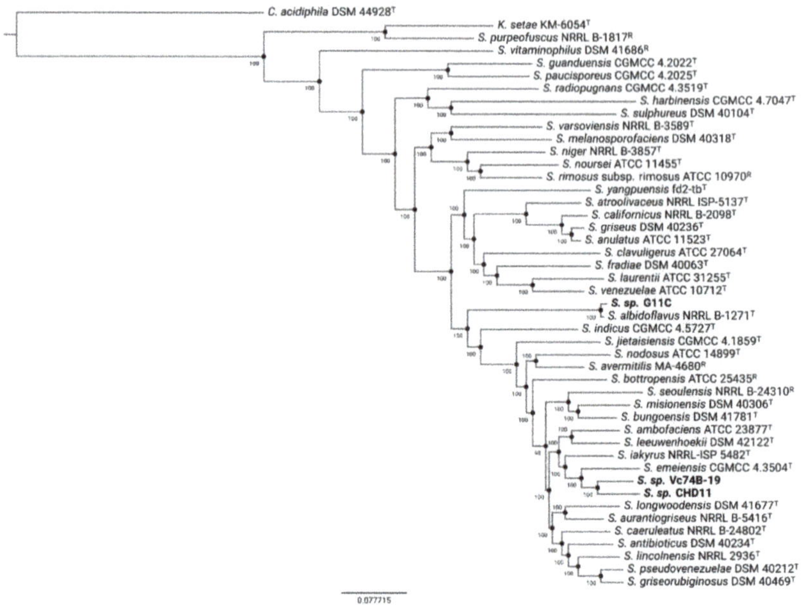

Figure 1. Phylogenomic tree of selected *Streptomyces* strains using 634 identified single-copy orthogroups via Orthofinder and subsequent Fasttree inference. Genomes of type (T) and reference (R) strains belonging to the *Streptomyces* genus were retrieved from the PATRIC database. *Catenulispora acidiphila* DSM44928 and *Kitasatospora setae* KM-6054 were used as outgroups, rooting the tree at the *Catenulispora* node. Bootstrap support values (b = 1000) are depicted for each branch. Strains sequenced in this study are displayed in bold font. The following abbreviations apply: *S.*, *Streptomyces*; *K.*, *Kitasatospora*; *C.*, *Catenulispora*.

2.2.1. Protease Search

Multiplatform annotation revealed that all three *Streptomyces* strains presented a similar abundance of genes encoding for putative peptidases, corresponding to 3% of their genomic content (Table 2, Table S4). According to MEROPS classification, approximately 85% of their putative peptidases were classified into a protease family (Table S5), where strains G11C, CHD11, and Vc74B-19 presented 46, 48, and 49 peptidase families, respectively. In general, the most substantial fraction of peptidases for all three strains belongs to the serine (47–48.6%) and metallo- super-families (36.7–41.1%), whereas the minor fraction consists of cysteine (6.6–11.4%), aspartic (1.1–1.3%), threonine (1.1–1.3%) and mixed (1.1–1.3%) super-families (Figure S2). This result is consistent with previous studies, where serine, metallo-, and cysteine peptidases are the dominant proteolytic enzymes (>90%) of Bacteria, and aspartic and threonine peptidases contribute to a minor extent [46,47]. Interestingly, *Streptomyces* sp. G11C presents two putative peptidases belonging to two unique families (C02 and S53) that are not present in strains CHD11 and Vc74B-19. C02 belongs to the cysteine peptidases of the calpain family, although its biological role in bacteria is unclear, and there are not many studies that clarify its properties [48]. On the other hand, serine S53 family peptidases belong to the sedolisin family, which has been strongly correlated with an acidophilic lifestyle [46]. In contrast, strains CHD11 and Vc74B-19 share five peptidase families (C14, C15, C40, C56, and M103) between them that are absent in strain G11C. Similarly, strain G11C only shares a peptidase family (M17) with the non-keratinolytic strain Vc74B-19, which is not present in strain CHD11. The similarities shared with the non-keratinolytic strain Vc74B-19 could indicate that such peptidases may not contribute to the degradative ability of the keratinolytic strains G11C and CHD11.

Table 2. Characteristics of putative proteases genes in *Streptomyces* strains G11C, CHD11, and Vc74B-19.

Number of:	*Streptomyces* sp. G11C	*Streptomyces* sp. CHD11	*Streptomyces* sp. Vc74B-19
ORFs encoding putative proteases	179	198	207
Putative proteases classified into a peptidase family	151	166	177
p-orthogroups in each strain	113	132	137
"unassigned p-orthogroup" peptidases	17	8	3

Subsequently, putative peptidases (584 sequences) of the three strains were classified into 140 protease orthologous groups (p-orthogroups) using Orthofinder [42]. As expected, putative peptidases from the same p-orthogroup belong to a single peptidase family (Table S6). In fact, 102 p-orthogroups are shared by all three strains (Figure 2), confirming the similarity of the protease space between these streptomycete genomes. As for strain G11C, three p-orthogroups are exclusively shared with strain CHD11, and eight p-orthogroups with Vc74B-19, that are not present in the other strain. Particularly, the three p-orthogroups 121, 122, and 134 (Table S6), shared between the keratinolytic strain G11C and the low-keratinolytic strain CHD11, belonging to the M50, S12, and S01 peptidase families, can be considered good candidates for potential keratinolytic proteases, assuming both strains could have similar degradation mechanisms. By contrast, the eight p-orthogroups shared between the keratinolytic strain G11C and the non-keratinolytic strain Vc74B-19 can be potentially discarded as keratinolytic peptidase candidates.

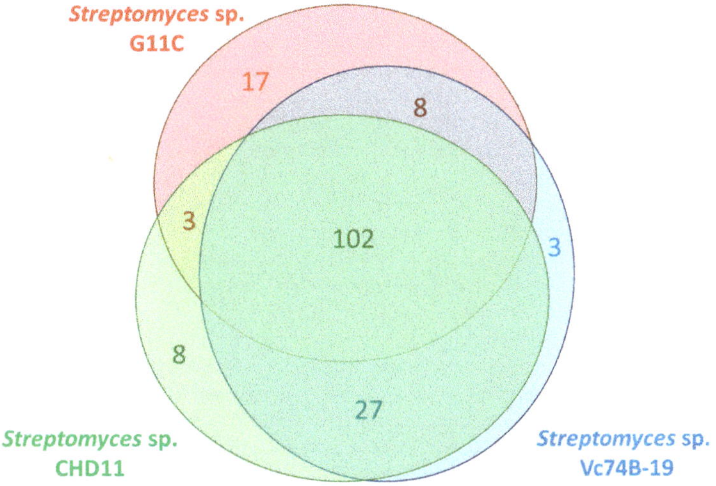

Figure 2. Venn diagram of common p-orthogroup representatives between streptomycete strains G11C, CHD11, and Vc74B-19. Numbers indicate the number of p-orthogroups found for each strain or between strains.

Most of the shared p-orthogroups belong to the serine (n = 37) and metallo- (n = 40) super-families, while the cysteine, aspartic, threonine, and mixed super-families are found in a smaller proportion (n = 2–5), which agrees with our previous MEROPS results. On the other hand, some peptidases are not classified into any p-orthogroup. Further exploration of these "unassigned p-orthogroup" peptidases could give an insight into the differences observed in terms of keratinolytic activity between the strains, considering that strain G11C presents comparatively the greatest keratin degradative capacity under the conditions analyzed [40]. Among the 17 putative peptidases unique for strain G11C, there are five serine peptidases (families S01, S16, S15, S53, and S51), three metallo-peptidases (families

M86, M50, and M56), two cysteine peptidases (families C82 and C02), and seven unassigned peptidases to any family.

Putative proteases belonging to families, S01, S08, and M04, where most known bacterial keratinases are found (Table S7), can serve as indicators to search for putative keratinolytic proteases. Two sequences of *Streptomyces* sp. G11C belonging to the S01 family draw our attention, which are absent in orthogroups shared with the non-keratinolytic strain Vc74B-19: An unassigned p-orthogroup peptidase (G11C_00267) and a peptidase (G11C_00756) belonging to one of the three p-orthogroups shared between the keratin degrading strains G11C and CHD11. Additionally, *Streptomyces* sp. G11C presents 8, 12, and 3 putative peptidases belonging to the families S08, S01, and M04, respectively, that may be of interest for the search for putative keratinases, despite belonging to orthogroups shared between the three strains. The detail of the promising sequences of *Streptomyces* sp. G11C (i.e., "unassigned p-orthogroup" peptidases, peptidases shared between the strains G11C and CHD11, and peptidases belonging to the peptidase families S01, S08, and M04) are summarized in Table S8.

2.2.2. Network Analysis

To complement the previous analysis, and identify those sequences related to families of known keratinases, a similarity network was constructed using an all-vs-all local alignment. For this analysis, 584 putative proteases of the three strains (hereinafter named "three-strain dataset"), 61 functional keratinases (mainly from Gram-positive bacteria) collected from NCBI (Table S7), and 50 selected trypsin, papain, and pepsin sequences, representing our hypothetical non-keratinase database (Table S9), were compared. Nodes in the network depict each protease, and an edge represents a hit in the resulting alignment (Figure 3; Table S10). Our protease similarity network graphically depicts the p-orthogroup distribution and identifies p-orthogroups that are related to functionally described keratinases. In total, 123 network communities composed of at least two or more nodes were detected by the Louvain algorithm.

Three network communities (N° 1, 4, and 41) possess sequences linked with functional keratinases with an E-value threshold of 1×10^{-40} (Table S11). The largest one, community N° 1 (Figure 3B), is related to sequences belonging to the peptidase family S08, constituted by most of the functional keratinases (n = 51 sequences) harboring 3, 5, and 6 sequences from strains G11C, CHD11, and Vc74B-19, respectively (p-orthogroups 0 and 11). Community N° 4 (Figure 3C) is composed of putative peptidases belonging to the family S01, where strains G11C, CHD11, and Vc74B-19 contribute with 5, 6, and 6 sequences, respectively (p-orthogroups 8, 17, and 116). This cluster presents six functional keratinases from *Actinomadura*, *Streptomyces*, and *Nocardiopsis*. Curiously, two putative non-keratinase sequences, annotated as trypsin-like serine protease (family S01) from other *Streptomyces* strains, also cluster together. This observation suggests that these two specific peptidases could have keratinolytic activity, although it has not been experimentally tested yet. Finally, in the smaller community N° 41 (Figure 3D), sequences belonging to the peptidase family M04 can be observed, consisting of 3, 2, and 5 sequences from strains G11C, CHD11, and Vc74B-19, respectively (p-orthogroups 16 and 64), clustering together with a functional keratinase from a *Geobacillus* strain (AJD77429.1). Scattered in the network, we found three keratinases from *Lactobacillus* and *Bifidobacterium* that do not group with any sequence from our three-strain dataset. In general, putative non-keratinase sequences are depicted as unconnected nodes or communities, except for specific cases such as communities N° 4 (mentioned above) and N° 47, both belonging to the peptidase family S01 (Table S10).

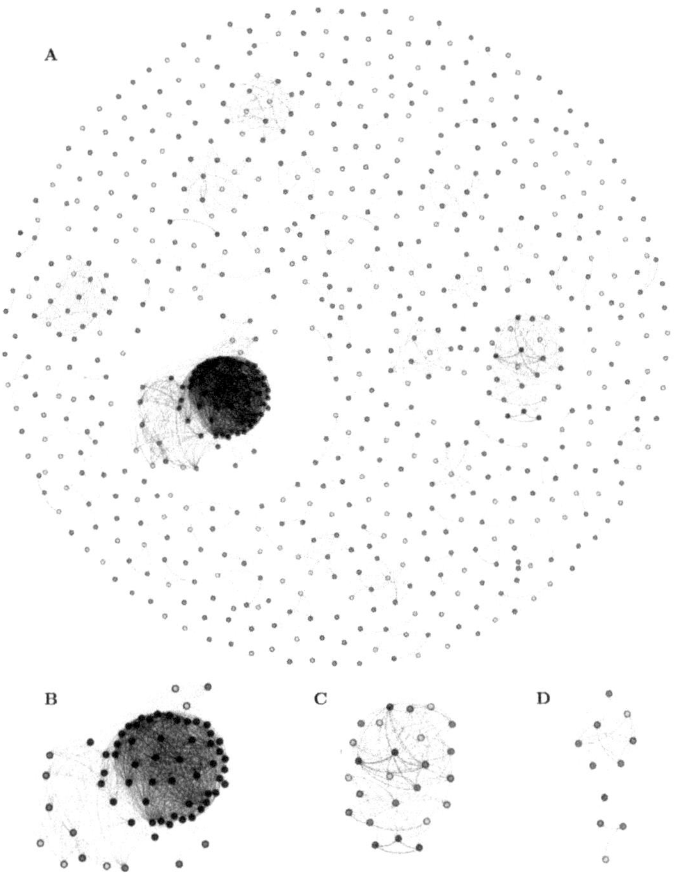

Figure 3. Protease similarity network, including the three-strain (584 sequences), keratinase (61 sequences), and non-keratinase (50 sequences) datasets. The E-value threshold of the blast alignment for the network is 1×10^{-40} Each node represents an identified putative protease, and the color fill indicates the origin of the sequence: Red, strain G11C; green, strain CHD11; blue, strain Vc74B-19; black, functionally known keratinases; yellow, putative non-keratinases. Edge transparency was adjusted to represent E-value difference: Darker edges correspond to smaller E-values. (**A**) entire network, (**B–D**) zoom into particular network clusters possessing known keratinases: Community 1, 4, and 41, respectively.

In summary, there are 11, 13, and 16 putative proteases linked to functional keratinases from *Streptomyces* strains G11C, CHD11, and Vc74B-19, respectively. Although the number of genes is less for keratinolytic-strain G11C, the percentage of identity when compared with some functional keratinase sequences is higher with this strain (Table S11). For instance, the first hit for all three strains is a keratinase synthesized by *Streptomyces albidoflavus* TBG-S13A5 (AYM48028.1), which presented a 96.4% amino acid identity with a predicted protein from strain G11C (G11C_01512), 72.8% identity for strain CHD11 (CHD11_02603) and 72.2% for strain Vc74B-19 (Vc74B-19_03690). The sequence found in G11C, belonging to peptidase family S01, p-orthogroup 8, and community N° 4, can be considered a putative keratinase, considering the high amino acid similarity with the known keratinase from *Streptomyces albidoflavus* TBG-S13A5, which can also be explained by the phylogenomic closeness between both strains.

2.3. Filtering by Cellular Localization Scores

Cellular localization data and phylogeny were employed to narrow the list of candidate keratinases that could potentially make a difference in keratin degradation for strain G11C. Proteases secreted into the extracellular medium are expected to play an important role in keratin degradation [2]. Thus, to identify those sequences predicted as extracellular, all previously mentioned datasets (three-strain set, functional keratinases, and putative non-keratinases) were inputted into three localization prediction software: PSORTb, CELLO, and SignalP (Table S12). To add informative categories and therefore, facilitate interpretation of results in the following steps, we separated the three-strain set into: (i) Keratinase-linked proteases (40 sequences), which are sequences linked to functional keratinases according to the network, (ii) "unassigned p-orthogroup" sequences (28 sequences) according to protease orthogroup classification, and (iii) the remaining into the three-strain category (516 sequences). Principal component analysis (PCA) and t-distributed stochastic neighbor embedding (t-SNE) were employed to embed sequences into a bidimensional space through the numerical scores retrieved from each tool (Figure 4). Two semi-defined clusters are visualized in the PCA plot (Figure 4A), representing intracellular (lower left corner) and extracellular (lower right corner) proteases. As expected, most of the keratinase-linked proteases from the three-strain dataset group together with known keratinases are represented as extracellular proteases. On the other hand, most of "unassigned p-orthogroup" sequences, including the peptidases unique of *Streptomyces* sp. G11C, are predicted as cytoplasmic and membrane-associated proteases. Non-keratinases were distributed in sparse coordinates, where seven sequences can be considered putative extracellular proteases.

Sequences were further clustered in the t-SNE bidimensional space using the DBSCAN algorithm [49], revealing a clear separation of the sequences into groups (Figure 4B, Figure S3). This clustering also guides the comparison of the sequence space representation between the PCA and the t-SNE. From Figure 4B, three DBSCAN clusters related to extracellular localization characteristics can be visualized. These were named t-SNE group 0, 1, and 2, each one with 68, 91, and 32 total sequences, respectively, where a considerable number of functional keratinases is present (Table 3; Table S13). Therefore, these groups are of great interest as they may contain promising sequences to encode potential extracellular keratinases. In all the identified groups, there are more sequences predicted as extracellular belonging to strains Vc74B-19, and CHD11 than from strain G11C. Possibly, differences in keratinolytic activity could be due to specific characteristics at the amino acid sequence level. To deepen our analysis, we complemented this study with a phylogenetic analysis of the sequences identified in the t-SNE groups.

Table 3. Peptidase sequence distribution in t-SNE groups.

	Number of Peptidases Present in:		
Category	**t-SNE Group 0**	**t-SNE Group 1**	**t-SNE Group 2**
Functional keratinase	40	5	10
Keratinase-linked sequence—strain G11C	1	9	1
Keratinase-linked sequence—strain CHD11	4	8	1
Keratinase-linked sequence—strain Vc74B-19	4	11	1
three-strain category—strain G11C	5	13	6
three-strain category—strain CHD11	4	18	5
three-strain category—strain Vc74B-19	8	24	7
Putative non-keratinase	2	3	1

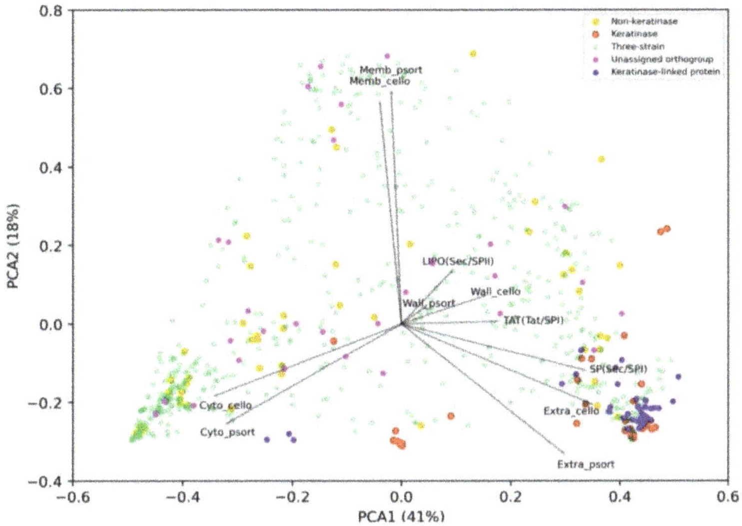

(A)

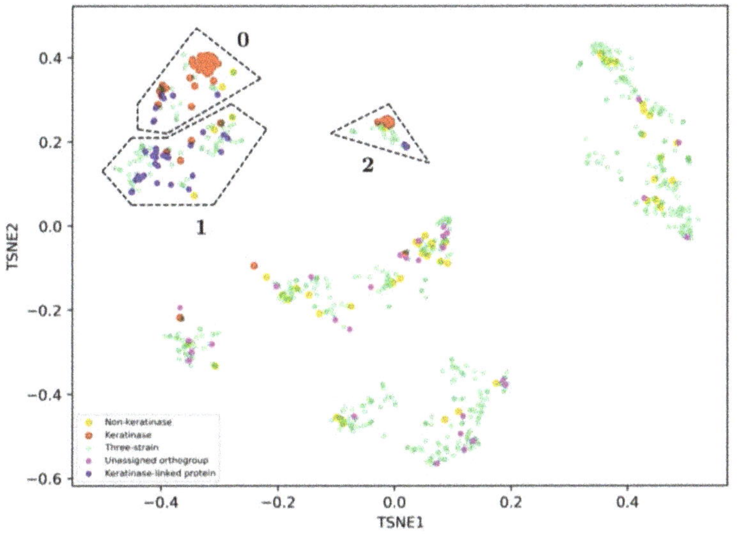

(B)

Figure 4. (**A**) Two-dimensional PCA using localization features for proteases. Protease sequences were retrieved from genomes of strain G11C, Vc74B-19, and CHD11. The x- and y-axis explain 41% and 18% of the observed variance of the data, respectively. Functional keratinases are depicted in red, putative non-keratinases in yellow, sequences from our three streptomycete genomes (i.e., three-strain category) in green, sequences without assigned p-orthogroup in magenta and keratinase-linked proteins, according to the network, are depicted in blue. Loadings represent the cellular localization features: Wall, membrane, cytoplasmic, and extracellular of the software CELLO and PSORTb, in addition to putative signal peptides: LIPO(Sec/SPII), SP(Sec/SPI), TAT(Tat/SPI) predicted with SignalP. (**B**) Two-dimensional t-SNE using localization features for the same group of proteases. Defined t-SNE group 0, 1, and 2 are enclosed by dashed polygons.

2.4. Phylogeny on t-SNE Groups

To identify extracellular peptidases of *Streptomyces* sp. G11C that are phylogenetically related to functional keratinases, multiple sequence alignments (MSA), and phylogenetic analysis were performed on the t-SNE groups 0, 1, and 2 (containing sequences predicted as extracellular). The average occupancy (average number of residues per position in the alignment) [50] of the three t-SNE groups MSAs was rather low as highly divergent sequences hinder phylogenetic tree construction: group 0—35.8%, group 1—19.3%, and group 2—35.7%. For this reason, we filtered positions with occupancy below 70% to generate more compact MSAs, and the new average occupancy for these compact alignments was t-SNE group 0—87.4%, group 1—85.1%, and group 2—90.3% (Figure S4). Then, we constructed bootstrapped maximum likelihood trees with these compact MSAs (Figure 5). Due to the high divergence observed for the sequences in each t-SNE group, an additional tool was applied, ancestral state reconstruction, to aid the interpretation of the trees.

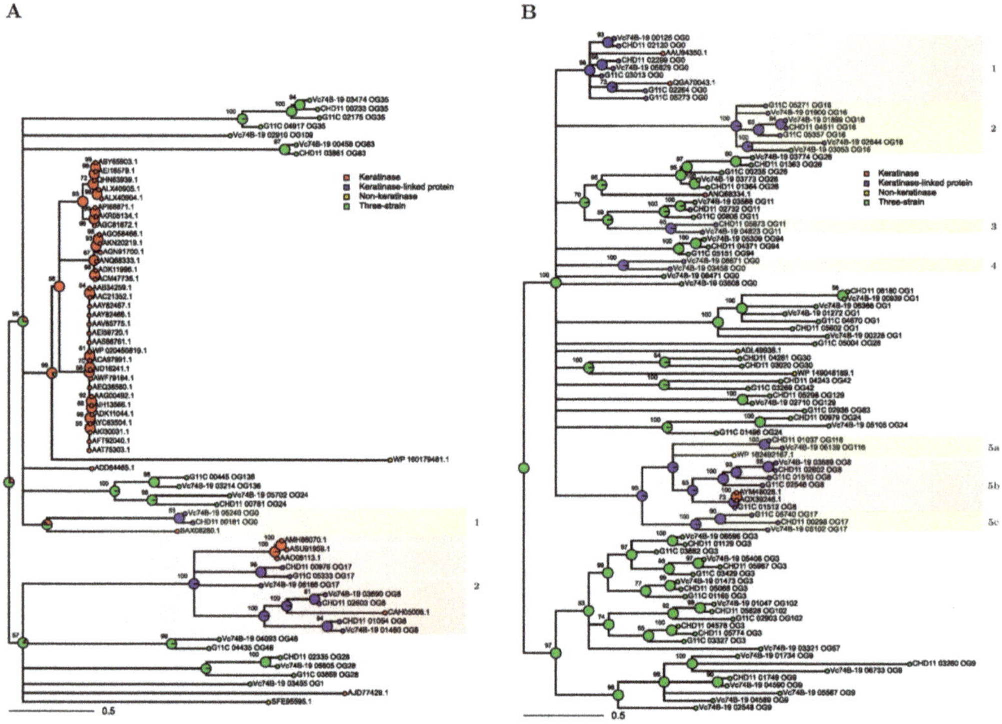

Figure 5. Maximum likelihood trees from filtered MSA of t-SNE group 0 (**A**) and t-SNE group 1 (**B**) sequences. Ancestral state probabilities inferred in internal nodes for each category (functional keratinase, keratinase-linked protein, three-strain, and non-keratinase) are depicted as pie charts, with a total of 1 for each pie chart. Support values based on bootstrapping are indicated for each node. Selected clades under stipulated criteria are enclosed by light red boxes, while discarded clades are enclosed by light yellow boxes.

The same discrete categories used in the PCA and t-SNE plots (i.e., functional keratinase, keratinase-linked protein, three-strain category, and non-keratinase) were used for the ancestral state reconstruction analysis. With this tool, a probability distribution is assigned to each ancestor node within the tree, indicating the likeliness of the ancestor to belong to one of these categories. This provides a visual interface to study which branches could potentially be related to proteases with keratinolytic activity, as the ancestral state depends on both branch length (i.e., sequence similarity) and tree topology [51,52]. We applied three filters to select clades for a more detailed description. First, we analyzed branches that presented >50% probability of belonging to the functional keratinase or keratinase-linked categories. Second, we selected clades that possess at least one functional keratinase. And third, we focused only on clades where at least one sequence from strain G11C is present. These criteria reduced the subsequent analysis to clade 2 in the t-SNE group 0 (Figure 5A, Box 2) and clades 1 and 5b from t-SNE group 1 (Figure 5A, Box 1 and 5b). Clades of the t-SNE group 2 did not meet these requirements, and therefore, were not analyzed (Figure S5).

Clade 2 of t-SNE group 0 (Figure 5A, Box 2) harbors seven proteases from the three-strain set, annotated as serine proteases belonging to the S01 family, community 4, three from the p-orthogroup 17, and four from the p-orthogroup 8. Within this clade, there are four keratinases, belonging to *Actinomadura* (ASU91959.1, AMH86070.1), *Nocardiopsis* (AAO06113.1), and *Streptomyces* (CAH05008.1) strains. Interestingly, a sequence of the keratinolytic strain G11C (G11C_05333) and low-keratinolytic strain CHD11 (CHD11_00976) are phylogenetically close, compared to the non-keratinolytic strain Vc74B-19. It is possible that specific motifs or amino acids within these sequences, not present in strain Vc74B-19, enhance the activity of the codified enzymes, and should be considered as candidates for putative keratinases. In addition, a subclade that presents Vc74B-19 and CHD11 sequences related to the known *Streptomyces fradiae* K11 keratinase CAH05008.1 was observed. In this case, branch lengths indicate significant sequence divergence, and therefore, no evidence of putative keratinolytic activity can be assigned to the three-strain genes of this subclade.

In the case of the t-SNE group 1 tree, clade 1 (Figure 5B, Box 1) groups seven three-strain proteases belonging to the p-orthogroup 0, community 1: Three from strain G11C (G11C_02264, G11C_03013, G11C_05273), two from strain CHD11 (CHD11_02120, CHD11_02299), and two from strain Vc74B-19 (Vc74B-19_00125, Vc74B-19_05629). All these sequences are annotated as serine proteases of the S08 family. There are only two sequences of functional keratinases within this clade, one is a partial sequence from *Streptomyces* sp. OWU 1633 (AAU94350.1) and the other is from *Amycolatopsis* sp. BJA-103 (QGA70043.1), both belonging to the family S08. In this clade, the sequences of CHD11 and Vc74B-19 strains are phylogenetically closer, compared to strain G11C.

Clade 5b (Figure 5B, Box 5b) comprises five three-strain sequences of the p-orthogroup 8, community 4: Three from strain G11C (G11C_01510, G11C_01512, G11C_02546), one from strain CHD11 (CHD11_02602) and one from strain Vc74B-19 (Vc74B-19_03689), annotated as streptogrisins A, B, and D. This clade has a branch that contains two keratinases from *Streptomyces albidoflavus*, strains Fea-10 (AQX39246.1) and TBG-S13A5 (AYM48028.1). In this branch, only one sequence of strain G11C is present (G11C_01512), and given its high similarity with the mentioned keratinases (96.4% amino acid identity), it is probably a potential keratinase, which could explain, to a certain extent, the differences in keratinolytic activity between our strains. All these sequences belong to the peptidase S01 family.

Focusing on *Streptomyces* sp. G11C, which evidenced the greater level of keratin degradation, we identified seven putative proteases of interest, that are phylogenetically close to known keratinases, and that could contribute to explaining the observed differential keratinolytic activities. These sequences are the following: G11C_05333, G11C_02264, G11C_03013, G11C_05273, G11C_01510, G11C_01512, and G11C_02546. They belong to p-orthogroups 0, 8, and 17, communities 1 and 4, which are related to peptidase families S01 and S08, therefore, supporting this prediction.

2.5. Summary of the Main Results of the Bioinformatic Pipeline

To determine the genetic determinants potentially involved in the keratinolytic capacity of marine *Streptomyces*, a comparative genomic analysis was carried out between three streptomycetes with different keratinolytic activities, strains G11C, CHD11, and Vc74B-19 with high, medium, and null activity, respectively (Figure 6). Initially, a search for proteases was performed by genomic annotation using three servers: Prokka, PANNZER2, and eggNOG. These proteases were manually cured using Blastp and classified into peptidase families according to the MEROPS database. Subsequently, a comparative genomic analysis between the universe of proteases of the three strains allowed the identification of protease orthogroups shared between the three streptomycete genomes, highlighting proteases unique to each strain. From this analysis, genes of interest were exclusively related to keratinolytic strains, where 17 genes unique to strain G11C and three peptidases belonging to orthogroups shared between strains CHD11 and G11C are found. Additionally, a similarity network analysis of all the proteases of the three strains together with two databases of functional keratinases and hypothetical non-keratinases, allowed the identification of three communities related to functional keratinases belonging to peptidase families S01, S08, and M04. 11 proteases from *Streptomyces* sp. G11C emerge from this analysis. Subsequently, to identify extracellular proteases related to keratinases, the information from the similarity networks and p-orthogroup analysis was integrated with a cell localization analysis through t-SNE based clustering. This analysis allowed the identification of three groups containing extracellular proteases, named groups t-SNE 0, 1, and 2. In this analysis, most of the unique peptidases of the strain G11C (unassigned p-orthogroup peptidases) and the peptidases shared between the keratinolytic strains CHD11 and G11C were predicted to be intracellular. However, given their exclusive relationship with the keratinolytic strains, they are still considered interesting because their presence may possibly explain the differences in keratinolytic activity between the three strains. On the other hand, the peptidases predicted to be extracellular present in the t-SNE groups were subjected to a phylogenetic analysis incorporating the tool: Ancestral state reconstruction, which assigns a probability distribution to each ancestor node within the tree, of belonging to the categories: Functional keratinase, keratinase-linked protein, three-strain category, and non-keratinase. Finally, after applying selection criteria for the analysis of the clades of the phylogenetic trees (presence of a functional keratinase, presence of a G11C sequence, and 50% probability in the ancestor node of being keratinase or keratinase-linked sequence), seven coding sequences for potential extracellular keratinases were identified in *Streptomyces* sp. G11C.

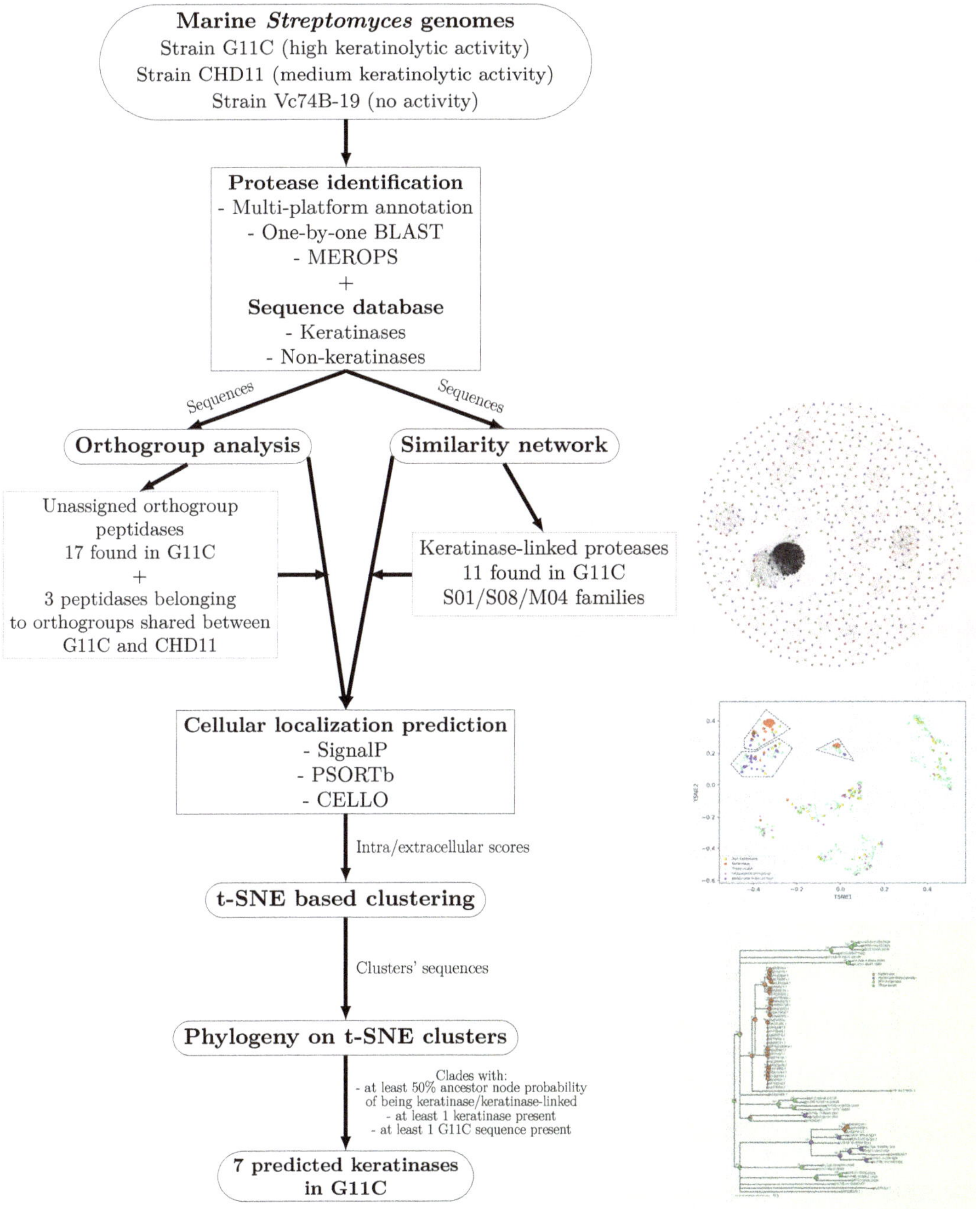

Figure 6. Bioinformatic pipeline to predict potential keratinases in *Streptomyces* sp. G11C. This analysis integrates a series of steps, including comparative genomics with network similarities, cellular localization prediction, and phylogeny to provide a set of genes considered to encode putative keratinases.

In this analysis, sequences codifying for (1) proteases related exclusively to keratinolytic strains and (2) proteases predicted to be extracellular and related to functional keratinases are considered as interesting candidates that could explain the differences in keratinolytic activity between the three strains.

3. Discussion

In this study, a multi-step bioinformatic pipeline, applying several comparative genomics tools, was developed to predict a set of genes that encode putative keratinases in a marine *Streptomyces* strain with keratinolytic activity. To see if genetic features related to these activities could be identified, three strains with differential keratinolytic activity were selected, *Streptomyces* sp. G11C presented a rather high percentage of feather degradation, reaching approximately 80% and with a relative keratinase activity of 60%, after five days of incubation, whereas *Streptomyces* sp. CHD11 presented lower relative keratinase activity (less than 10%) [40]. In contrast, *Streptomyces* sp. Vc74B-19 presented no keratinolytic activity, even after 10 days of incubation [40].

Genome comparison showed approximately 3% of the total gene count encoded putative peptidases, revealing an unexpected similar abundance and diversity in all three strains. Previous reports described that among bacterial species, the percentage of peptidases encoded in the genomes ranges from 1.5% to 4% [53]. A similar diversity of peptidase families was found in all three strains, with serine, metallo- and cysteine super-families being more abundant in all three genomes. Peptidase diversity may reflect their adaptation to environmental conditions [46]. Considering the marine origin of the *Streptomyces* analyzed, the diversity of peptidases could be related to environmental characteristics such as the pH of the ocean, which varies from slightly neutral to alkaline [54]. Serine, cysteine, and metallo-peptidases are generally active under these conditions [55,56] and may contribute to their ecologic success, and possibly, their degradative abilities. In general, strains CHD11 and Vc74B-19 showed to be more similar to each other, sharing a large number of peptidase families and p-orthogroups that are absent in strain G11C, in agreement with their close phylogenomic relatedness. By contrast, strain G11C presented more "unassigned p-orthogroup" peptidases (17 unique peptidases) compared to the other two strains CHD11 and Vc74B-19 (8 and 3, respectively), of which 12 were actively involved in keratin degradation, whose presence was confirmed in our previous secretome analysis in keratinolytic strain G11C [40], highlighting them as interesting candidates. According to the subcellular localization analysis, most of these sequences are predicted as cytoplasmic and membrane-associated proteases. Although most of the keratinolytic proteases known to date are predominantly extracellular, some cell-bound and intracellular keratinolytic proteases have also been described [57]. Therefore, the participation of the unique proteases of the strain G11C in the keratinolytic activity cannot be ruled out.

Most of the keratinases known to date, have been classified as serine proteases [14,16,19,58,59], and a few as metalloproteases [20,60,61]. The latter mainly come from Gram-negative bacteria and fungi [62]. To compare and identify promising sequences related to known keratinases, we constructed a functional keratinase database, mainly from Gram-positive bacteria (Table S7), retrieving data from the NCBI. An analysis based on the MEROPS classification indicates that keratinases from *Bacillus* belong to the peptidase S08 family, and keratinases from *Actinobacteria*, such as *Nocardiopsis*, *Actinomadura*, and *Streptomyces*, belong mostly to the S01 family. There is scarce information about the metalloprotease family associated with keratinases. In our database, only one of the keratinases, from a *Geobacillus* strain (AJD77429.1), belongs to the metalloprotease super-family, specifically to the family M04. A protease similarity network, using these functionally characterized keratinases together with our three streptomycete genomes and non-keratinases databases, highlighted three communities of nodes containing keratinase-linked peptidases belonging to the S1, S8 (serine proteases), and M4 (metalloprotease) families, allowing the identification of 11 promising sequences of the keratinolytic strain G11C. It is worth mentioning that community 41 (family M04) presented the least number of grouped sequences, which is possibly related to the presence of only one functional keratinase, as mentioned above. Furthermore, the three strains show few peptidases belonging to this family, for example, *Streptomyces* sp. G11C only presents three M04 metallopeptidases that were subsequently discarded because they did not meet the pipeline criteria (being extracellular and phylogenetically close to functional keratinases). On the other hand, the promising sequences, including the unique peptidases of the strain G11C (unassigned p-orthogroup peptidases), and the peptidases belonging to p-orthogroups shared between the keratinolytic strains CHD11 and G11C, did not group in any community of the network, since most belong to other protease families, being divergent from the known keratinase families. In these groups, there are only two serine proteases of the family S01, although they did not group in community 4 (family S01). In addition, it can be mentioned that one of these unique sequences of strain G11C (G11C_00267) presented high abundance in the secretome analysis carried out previously [40], indicating a relevant role in the degradation of keratin.

To narrow the search for potential keratinases, we complemented this information with the subcellular localization data and phylogeny. In the t-SNE clustering analysis, we identified those putative peptidases that are predicted as extracellular (including the keratinase-linked sequences mentioned above). In this analysis, we reasoned that cellular localization prediction is intimately related to a putative keratinolytic function. This is in line with previous reports, that have shown that the macromolecular characteristics of keratin prevent its direct absorption by microbial cells [2]. Thus, the utilization of keratin as a nutrient source usually requires the production of extracellular keratinases. Therefore, to finely separate and select potential extracellular keratinase sequences, we included a phylogenetic analysis of the clusters, which also provides a way to integrate the similarity network data into our selection process. The latter is one of the main challenges addressed in this work, since network sequence data has been mainly used as a standalone tool for functional inference [63], partly due to its graphics that are not completely compatible with tabular or structural sequence data. Finally, from this analysis, we identified seven gene sequences encoding potential keratinases (belonging to families S01 and S08) together with 17 unique genes encoding unassigned p-orthogroup peptidases in *Streptomyces* sp. G11C could explain the differences observed, in terms of keratinolytic activity, between the three strains. Apparently, the degradation of recalcitrant keratin wastes requires the cooperation of several keratinolytic proteases, as evidenced in some bacterial [36,64–67] and fungi species [7,68]. Recently, a work reported by Huang et al. [65], evidenced the presence of five proteases in the culture of *Bacillus* sp. 8A6 with keratin-rich substrates, belonging to four protease families M12, S01A, S8A, and T3. In fungi, the participation of a set of proteases in keratin degradation has also been reported. Pathogenic fungi mainly secrete endoproteases, including proteases from families A1, S8A, M36, and M35 [68]. The non-pathogenic fungus *Onygena corvina* secretes proteases belonging to three protease families: S08, M28, and M03, when cultivated with pig bristles [7]. However, we have not found proteases belonging to these families in our analysis with streptomycete genomes, except for some putative peptidases belonging to the M28 family, suggesting that the mechanisms of keratin degradation vary between fungi and bacteria. For most keratinolytic studies involving *Streptomyces*, the approach has been focused on purifying and characterizing the main keratinolytic enzyme. For example, in work reported by Bressollier et al. [14], at least six extracellular proteases were identified in the culture of *Streptomyces albidoflavus* grown on feather meal-based medium, but only the most abundant keratinolytic serine protease was further characterized. Recently, through a transcriptomic analysis performed by Li et al. in 2020, it was possible to elucidate a set of factors involved in the keratin degradation mechanism mediated by *Streptomyces* sp. SCUT-3 [36]. In this analysis, 19 genes codifying potential extracellular proteases, along with 10 genes codifying potential intracellular proteases belonging to serine-type, cysteine-type, and metalloproteases, were up-regulated during growth in medium containing feathers. In addition, two genes involved in mycothiol synthesis, and some genes related to sulfite production were also up-regulated, indicating a cooperative action of reducing agents in the breaking of feather disulfide bonds. According to this evidence, it is conceivable to propose a set of enzymes acting together in keratin degradation by a single bacterium. The literature mentioned above is solely based on the functional exploration of keratin degradation, and no systematic bioinformatics analysis has been approached. The advantage of our pipeline is it considers whole genomes instead of single sequences, which has not been previously addressed with keratinases. With the advances in genome sequencing and the improvement of the number of genome-scale studies, our pipeline could be enriched and further bioinformatic predictions tested.

To go further on this argument, in our recent work [40], we confirmed the presence of these predicted enzymes in the *Streptomyces* sp. G11C secretome: Six of seven keratinolytic proteases (predicted by phylogenetic analysis), and 12 of 17 unique genes of the G11C genome ("unassigned p-orthogroup" peptidases), were detected under the culture conditions with feathers as the sole carbon source, indicating that a set of enzymes may act synergistically during keratin degradation. Interestingly, one of the unique genes of the G11C strain (G11C_00267) presented one of the highest protein abundances in the proteomic analysis [40], suggesting an important role for this enzyme in the keratin degradation mechanism. These findings are consistent with our bioinformatic predictions. The coordination of all these extracellular and intracellular enzymes, including the unique peptidases of *Streptomyces* sp. G11C could be potentiating its keratinolytic activity, leading to an advantage over the other *Streptomyces* analyzed strains CHD11 and Vc74B-19. Genes encoding disulfide reductases and genes related to sulfite export were similar in the three strains (data not shown), suggesting that disulfide bond reduction is not related to the observed functional differences, at least not the common mechanisms described in the literature [35]. Additional efforts to discover the reasons for such functional differences between these strains are part of our ongoing investigation. Our novel bioinformatic pipeline, together with the increased sequencing of keratinolytic strains genomes, could serve as the basis for future predictions of keratinolytic proteases, facilitating the selection of potential keratinolytic bacteria. To our knowledge, this is the first comprehensive bioinformatics analysis that complements comparative genomics with phylogeny, network similarities, and cellular localization prediction to provide a set of candidate genes considered to encode putative keratinases.

4. Materials and Methods

4.1. Bacterial Strains

Previously, bacterial strains belonging to our Chilean marine actinobacterial culture collection, isolated from marine sediments, sponges, and sea urchins collected from the coast of Chile [37–39], were analyzed for keratinolytic activity through a simple feather degradation test on agar plates and culture tubes [40]. Based on these results, three *Streptomyces* were chosen to perform a genomic comparison according to their keratinolytic activity. *Streptomyces* sp. G11C isolated from marine sediments derived from Penas Gulf, with high keratinolytic activity, *Streptomyces* sp. CHD11, isolated from a marine sponge from Chañaral de Aceituno Island, with low keratinolytic activity and *Streptomyces* sp. Vc74B-19, isolated from marine sediments from Valparaíso Bay, with no keratinolytic activity (Table S1).

4.2. Genomic DNA Extraction

Strains were grown on ISP2 media for 24–48 h, and cells were collected by centrifugation (13,000× *g*, 2 min), resuspended in 50 mM EDTA, and then mechanically separated with a shank. For cell rupture, disaggregated cells were treated with Lysozyme 10 mg/mL, Lysostaphin 10 mg/mL, and Proteinase K 1 mg/mL for 1 h at 37 °C. Then, for DNA purification, the Promega Wizard DNA extraction kit was used, according to the manufacturer's description. Finally, an alcohol treatment was used for DNA precipitation and cleaning, with 100% isopropanol for DNA precipitation, followed by 70% ethanol to wash the DNA pellet. The sample was rehydrated and stored according to the Promega Wizard DNA Extraction Kit instructions.

4.3. Genome Sequencing, Assembly, and Annotation

Sequencing was performed using the Illumina NextSeq platform with a 150 bp × 2 configuration. Raw reads were examined for coverage and trimmed for a minimum quality of 20 using Sickle v.1.33 [69]. Genome assembly was performed using SPAdes v.3.13.1 with default parameters [70,71] and Unicycler in normal mode [72] (internally using SPAdes v.3.11.1. The SPAdes assembly pipeline contains a final step of scaffolding using SSPACE [73]. Assembly quality was measured using QUAST v.5.0.2 [74], and genome completeness and contamination were evaluated using CheckM v1.0.18 [75]. A unique working assembly for each strain was selected based on the one with a smaller number of contigs, largest contigs (N50, L50 evaluation), and the lowest contamination metrics. Assembled genomes were annotated using Prokka v.1.13.4 [76], PANNZER2 [77], and eggNOG 5.0 [78] web servers.

4.4. Phylogenomic Tree Inference

Streptomyces genomes were selected from the tree described in Nouioui et al. [79], spanning over subclades. The selection criteria used was genome quality (fewer contigs and higher completeness based on CheckM), and type strains were preferred for the analysis. Assembly metrics were obtained using QUAST v.5.0.2 and CheckM v.1.0.18. The genomes of strains that closely resembled our strains by 16S rRNA identity [37] were also added: *Streptomyces albidoflavus* NBRC 13010 (=NRRL B-1271) and *Streptomyces aurantiogriseus* NRRL B-5416. *S. albogriseoleus* genome was not included, since assemblies presented anomalies, according to NCBI Genbank. The genomes of a *Catenulispora* strain (DSM 44928) and a *Kitasatospora* strain (KM-6054) were used as outgroups. Selected genomes and the outgroup genomes were retrieved from the Pathosystems Resource Integration Center (PATRIC) database and are described in Table S2. Phylogenomic reconstruction was performed using Orthofinder v.2.3.11 [42], with FastTree v.2.1.10 [80], in multiple sequence alignment mode (-M msa option), employing the default parameters for the orthogroup definition. Complementary to the phylogenomic analysis, average nucleotide identity calculation was performed using all of the selected genomes (Table S3), with the Python PyANI package [81] and depicted using the seaborn package in Python.

4.5. Putative Protease Identification

Annotations obtained from Prokka, PANNZER2, and eggNOG were consolidated in Table S4. Putative proteases were identified by matching annotations with the following keywords: Peptidase, protease, proteinase, sortase, caspase, penicillin-binding protein, insulinase, snapalysin, and mycosin. Each coding sequence that presented a keyword in at least one of the predictions was manually checked using BLASTp v.2. against the NR database, to confirm the proteolytic nature of the enzyme. In this work, the terms "protease" and "peptidase" have been used indistinctly [82].

4.6. Classification of Protease Families and Identification of Protease Orthogroups

For the classification into protease families, a reciprocal best hit search (E-value threshold, 1×10^{-20} of the three-strain dataset was performed against MEROPS, the peptidase database, release 11, using the HMMER-based web-server utility [83]. This database classifies peptidases into seven superfamilies based on the catalytic residue (Aspartic (A), Cysteine (C), Glutamic (G), Metallo (M), Asparagine (N), Serine (S), Threonine (T)) along with two superfamilies of Mixed (P) and Unknown (U) catalytic types, and further divides these superfamilies into 255 proteolytic families based on similarities in amino acid sequences [84]. Additionally, the curated list of proteases for the three strains was grouped into orthogroups using Orthofinder [42] with the default E-value 1×10^{-40} These were named protease orthogroup or p-orthogroup. Venn diagram visualization of common p-orthogroups between strains was done using the package eulerr in R [85].

4.7. Creation of Custom Databases: Functional Keratinases and Putative Non-Keratinases

To identify putative keratinases in the genomes, two custom databases with sequences of functional keratinases and putative non-keratinases were constructed by retrieving sequences from the NCBI NR database (query date: March 2020). The functional keratinase database was built according to literature and contains 61 sequences from *Actinomadura, Amycolatopsis, Bacillus, Bifidobacterium, Brevibacillus, Deinococcus, Geobacillus, Lactobacillus, Meiothermus, Nocardiopsis, Streptomyces*, and *Thermus* (Table S7). In addition, to differentiate and discard those sequences that do not encode possible keratinolytic proteases, a putative non-keratinase database was created. Several reports indicate that keratin has high stability against common proteases, such as pepsin, papain, and trypsin [1,2]. Based on this information, a hypothetical non-keratinase database was constructed (Table S9). This database contains 50 protein sequences belonging either to the trypsin, papain, or pepsin families. All sequences are derived from Gram-positive bacteria belonging to the genera *Bacillus, Bifidobacterium, Brevibacterium, Chloroflexi, Clostridium, Corynebacterium, Enterococcus, Lactobacillus, Listeria, Staphylococcus, Streptococcus*, and *Streptomyces*.

4.8. Similarity Network

For the similarity network of the three-strain dataset, a blastp all-vs-all output was processed in Python using the networkX package [86]. Both functional keratinase and non-keratinase databases were added to the three-strain dataset for network construction. In the network, nodes correspond to each protease and edges to a hit in the resulting alignment. The E-value cutoff for the display of the edge weights was set to 1×10^{-5} 1×10^{-20}, 1×10^{-40}, and 1×10^{-80}, being 1×10^{-40} the value chosen for the analysis, since it is a typical value (order of magnitude) employed in sequence similarity networks [87], and subsequent steps in the pipeline have small sensitivity to using stricter cutoffs (Figure S6). Community detection was performed using a weighted Louvain algorithm with a default resolution parameter of 1 [88]. A depiction of the network was obtained using Gephi v.0.9.2 [89] with a combination of Fruchtermann-Reingold [90] and Yifan Hu [91] layout algorithms.

4.9. Cellular Localization and Dimension Reduction

Prediction of subcellular localization for proteases was performed using CELLO v2.5 [92] and PSORTb v3.0.2 [93]. Putative signal peptides were predicted with SignalP 5.0 [94]. All predictions are consolidated and shown in Table S12. Numerical cellular localization data per sequence were used as features for dimension reduction techniques. This list includes wall, membrane, extracellular and intracellular scores from PSORTb (four features) and CELLO (four features), and also export pathway scores SP(Sec/SPI), TAT(Tat/SPI), LIPO(Sec/SPII), OTHER, intracellular and signal peptide possibility from SignalP (six features). The resulting matrix consisted of n sequences by 14 features. The set of sequences of size n includes the functional keratinase dataset, the putative non-keratinase dataset, and the three-strain dataset. The raw data matrix was standard-normalized, and dimensional reduction analysis was performed using Principal Component Analysis (PCA) and t-Distributed Stochastic Neighbor Embedding (t-SNE) (perplexity 30, 1000 iterations, fixed seed) [95]. Output coordinates for both methods were normalized using a min-max range. For the PCA, loadings for each feature were calculated from eigenvectors and depicted using arrows. The whole procedure was done using the Scikit-learn v.0.22.2 Python package [96].

4.10. Clustering and Phylogeny of t-SNE Groups

t-SNE points, i.e., coordinates by sequence, were clustered into groups, called "t-SNE groups", using the DBSCAN algorithm [49] implemented in Scikit-learn v.0.22.2. Multiple sequence alignment (MSA) for each t-SNE group was performed using MAFFT v7.455 [97] with options G-ins and -maxiter 1000. Average occupancy (average number of residues per position in the alignment) and MSA filtering by occupancy were obtained using the Prody Python package [50]. Positions with occupancy below 70% were removed from original MSAs to generate more compact MSAs. A substitution model was fitted to each MSAs using ProtTest 3 [98], considering all distributions plus I and G models, and then a multithread maximum likelihood tree was obtained using RaxML v.8.2.12 [99] with the best parameters calculated by ProtTest and the rapid bootstrapping configuration (-f a option, 1000 bootstraps). Because no outgroup sequence was provided, the trees were midpoint rooted. Ancestral state reconstruction on trees [100] over the discrete categories: Keratinase, non-keratinase, three-strain, and keratinase-linked protein was performed using the package Phytools in R [101]. The set up was defined in 1000 iterations and an "ER" model, which means that equal rates for all permitted transitions.

5. Conclusions

Our robust comparative genomic analysis between three *Streptomyces* strains with varying keratinolytic activities permitted the identification of a set of putative proteases that could potentially be involved in the keratinolytic capacity of *Streptomyces* sp. G11C. According to peptidase family classification and orthogroup identification, we consider as promising candidates: (1) Unique putative peptidases in the keratinolytic strain G11C (17 unassigned p-orthogroup peptidases), including those belonging to the peptidase families C02 and S53; and (2) three peptidases present in the orthologous groups shared between strains G11C and CHD11, but not present in the non-keratinolytic strain Vc74B-19. Additionally, similarity network analysis identified three communities of keratinases-linked peptidases belonging to families S01, S08, and M04. Complementing this information with sub-cellular localization data and phylogenetic analysis, we identified seven promising genes likely to encode potential keratinases from *Streptomyces* sp. G11C, belonging to peptidase families S01 and S08. These findings provide genetic information for the proteomic analysis in the keratinolytic strain G11C, described in related work [40], which functionally validates the predictions accomplished in this study. This is the first comprehensive bioinformatics analysis that complements comparative genomics with phylogeny, network similarities, and cellular localization prediction to provide a set of genes considered to encode putative keratinases. This semi-supervised pipeline, involving t-SNE clustering on cellular localization data, is a novel approach in the keratinase literature, and we consider it as a significant advance that will help build more sophisticated pipelines in the future. In addition, it can be useful for various other hydrolytic enzyme families, such as lipases, glycosidases, esterases, among others.

Supplementary Materials: The following are available online at https://www.mdpi.com/article/10.3390/md19060286/s1, Figure S1: ANIm matrix of genomes employed for the phylogeny, Figure S2: Classification of putative peptidases from *Streptomyces* strains G11C, CHD11, and Vc74B-19 using MEROPS database, Figure S3: Clustering of t-SNE points by the DBSCAN algorithm, Figure S4: Occupancy plots, Figure S5: Maximum likelihood tree from the filtered MSA of t-SNE group 2 sequences, Figure S6: Protease similarity network using E-value threshold 1×10^{-80} and Maximum likelihood trees from filtered MSA of t-SNE group 0 and t-SNE group 1 sequences, Table S1: List of strains utilized in this study, isolation sources, and 16S rRNA identification, Table S2: Assembly metrics of genomes incorporated in the phylogenomic tree, Table S3: ANIm matrix, Table S4: Annotation and selection of proteases, Table S5: Classification of peptidases by MEROPS database, Table S6: Orthogroup classification of proteases, Table S7: Functional keratinases from databases, Table S8: Promising genes of *Streptomyces* sp. G11C, Table S9: Putative non-keratinases from databases, Tabla S10: Nodes and edges of the network, Table S11: Edges of nodes connected with a functional keratinase, Table S12: Consolidated table of subcellular localization data for each protein sequence, Table S13: t-SNE group tables.

Author Contributions: R.V., V.G. and B.C. contributed to the conception and design of the experiments. V.G. performed the experiments of keratin degradation. L.Z.-L. and A.U. extracted the genomic DNA. V.G. and R.V. analyzed the data and prepared figures and tables. J.A.U. and B.C.

supervised bioinformatic analyses. R.V., V.G., A.U. and B.C. wrote and edited the manuscript. All authors contributed to manuscript revision, read and approved the submitted version. All authors have read and agreed to the published version of the manuscript.

Funding: Financial support was provided by CONICYT FONDECYT N°1171555 and CONICYT PIA GAMBIO Project N° ACT172128 (to BC). VG was funded by Conicyt PhD fellowship and Conicyt Gastos Operacionales N° 21161188, and PIIC program (UTFSM). AU was funded by 'CONICYT FONDECYT POSTDOCTORADO N° 3180399'. LZ was supported by Conicyt PhD fellowship N° 21180908. JAU was supported by the ANID Millennium Science Initiative/Millenium Initiative for Collaborative Research on Bacterial Resistance, MICROB-R, NCN17_081. The funders had no role in study design, data collection and analysis, decision to publish, or preparation of the manuscript.

Institutional Review Board Statement: Not applicable.

Informed Consent Statement: Not applicable.

Data Availability Statement: Complete genome sequences of *Streptomyces* sp. G11C, CHD11, and Vc74B-19 are available in NCBI Genbank under WGS accession numbers JABTTT000000000, JABTTS000000000, and JABTTR000000000, respectively. Prokka annotations of the genomes of *Streptomyces* sp. G11C, CHD11, Vc74B-19 are available via Figshare through the following link https://doi.org/10.6084/m9.figshare.13133270.v1 (accessed on 28 October 2020). Fasta headers are consistent with reported sequence labels in this work.

Acknowledgments: We thank Brigitte Böckle for her initial guidance and Danilo Pérez-Pantoja for facilitating computational access to perform the necessary analyses.

Conflicts of Interest: The authors declare no conflict of interest.

References

1. Korniłłowicz-Kowalska, T.; Bohacz, J. Biodegradation of keratin waste: Theory and practical aspects. *Waste Manag.* **2011**, *31*, 1689–1701. [CrossRef] [PubMed]
2. Brandelli, A. Bacterial keratinases: Useful enzymes for bioprocessing agroindustrial wastes and beyond. *Food Bioprocess Technol.* **2008**, *1*, 105–116. [CrossRef]
3. Lange, L.; Huang, Y.; Busk, P.K. Microbial decomposition of keratin in nature—A new hypothesis of industrial relevance. *Appl. Microbiol. Biotechnol.* **2016**, *100*, 2083–2096. [CrossRef] [PubMed]
4. Schweitzer, M.H.; Zheng, W.; Moyer, A.E.; Sjövall, P.; Lindgren, J. Preservation potential of keratin in deep time. *PLoS ONE* **2018**, *13*, e0206569. [CrossRef] [PubMed]
5. Moyer, A.E.; Zheng, W.; Schweitzer, M.H. Keratin durability has implications for the fossil record: Results from a 10 year feather degradation experiment. *PLoS ONE* **2016**, *11*, e0157699. [CrossRef] [PubMed]
6. De Souza Carvalho, I.; Novas, F.E.; Agnolín, F.L.; Isasi, M.P.; Freitas, F.I.; Andrade, J.A. A Mesozoic bird from Gondwana preserving feathers. *Nat. Commun.* **2015**, *6*, 1–5. [CrossRef] [PubMed]
7. Huang, Y.; Busk, P.K.; Herbst, F.A.; Lange, L. Genome and secretome analyses provide insights into keratin decomposition by novel proteases from the non-pathogenic fungus *Onygena corvina*. *Appl. Microbiol. Biotechnol.* **2015**, *99*, 9635–9649. [CrossRef] [PubMed]
8. Mazotto, A.M.; Couri, S.; Damaso, M.C.T.; Vermelho, A.B. Degradation of feather waste by *Aspergillus niger* keratinases: Comparison of submerged and solid-state fermentation. *Int. Biodeterior. Biodegrad.* **2013**, *85*, 189–195. [CrossRef]
9. Balaji, S.; Senthil Kumar, M.; Karthikeyan, R.; Kumar, R.; Kirubanandan, S.; Sridhar, R.; Sehgal, P.K. Purification and characterization of an extracellular keratinase from a hornmeal-degrading *Bacillus subtilis* MTCC (9102). *World J. Microbiol. Biotechnol.* **2008**, *24*, 2741–2745. [CrossRef]
10. Cheng, S.W.; Hu, H.M.; Shen, S.W.; Takagi, H.; Asano, M.; Tsai, Y.C. Production and characterization of keratinase of a feather-degrading *Bacillus licheniformis* PWD-1. *Biosci. Biotechnol. Biochem.* **1995**, *59*, 2239–2243. [CrossRef]
11. Cedrola, S.M.L.; de Melo, A.C.N.; Mazotto, A.M.; Lins, U.; Zingali, R.B.; Rosado, A.S.; Peixoto, R.S.; Vermelho, A.B. Keratinases and sulfide from *Bacillus subtilis* SLC to recycle feather waste. *World J. Microbiol. Biotechnol.* **2012**, *28*, 1259–1269. [CrossRef] [PubMed]
12. Jaouadi, B.; Abdelmalek, B.; Fodil, D.; Ferradji, F.Z.; Rekik, H.; Zaraî, N.; Bejar, S. Purification and characterization of a thermostable keratinolytic serine alkaline proteinase from *Streptomyces* sp. strain AB1 with high stability in organic solvents. *Bioresour. Technol.* **2010**, *101*, 8361–8369. [CrossRef]
13. Mabrouk, M.E.M. Feather degradation by a new keratinolytic *Streptomyces* sp. MS-2. *World J. Microbiol. Biotechnol.* **2008**, *24*, 2331–2338. [CrossRef]

14. Bressollier, P.; Letourneau, F.; Urdaci, M.; Verneuil, B. Purification and characterization of a keratinolytic serine proteinase from *Streptomyces albidoflavus*. *Appl. Environ. Microbiol.* **1999**, *65*, 2570–2576. [CrossRef]
15. Chitte, R.R.; Nalawade, V.K.; Dey, S. Keratinolytic activity from the broth of a feather-degrading thermophilic *Streptomyces thermoviolaceus* strain SD8. *Lett. Appl. Microbiol.* **1999**, *28*, 131–136. [CrossRef]
16. Böckle, B.; Galunsky, B.; Muller, R. Characterization of a Keratinolytic Serine Proteinase from *Streptomyces Pactum* DSM 40530. *Appl. Environ. Microbiol.* **1995**, *61*, 3705–3710. [CrossRef]
17. Nam, G.W.; Lee, D.W.; Lee, H.S.; Lee, N.J.; Kim, B.C.; Choe, E.A.; Hwang, J.K.; Suhartono, M.T.; Pyun, Y.R. Native-feather degradation by *Fervidobacterium islandicum* AW-1, a newly isolated keratinase-producing thermophilic anaerobe. *Arch. Microbiol.* **2002**, *178*, 538–547. [CrossRef]
18. El-Naghy, M.A.; El-Ktatny, M.S.; Fadl-Allah, E.M.; Nazeer, W.W. Degradation of chicken feathers by *Chrysosporium georgiae*. *Mycopathologia* **1998**, *143*, 77–84. [CrossRef]
19. Macedo, A.J.; Gava, R.; Driemeier, D.; Termignoni, C. Novel Keratinase from *Bacillus subtilis* S14 Exhibiting Remarkable Dehairing Capabilities. *Appl. Environ. Microbiol.* **2005**, *71*, 594–596. [CrossRef]
20. Thys, R.C.S.; Brandelli, A. Purification and properties of a keratinolytic metalloprotease from *Microbacterium* sp. *J. Appl. Microbiol.* **2006**, *101*, 1259–1268. [CrossRef]
21. Wu, W.L.; Chen, M.Y.; Tu, I.F.; Lin, Y.C.; Eswarkumar, N.; Chen, M.Y.; Ho, M.C.; Wu, S.H. The discovery of novel heat-stable keratinases from *Meiothermus taiwanensis* WR-220 and other extremophiles. *Sci. Rep.* **2017**, *7*, 1–12. [CrossRef] [PubMed]
22. Barman, N.C.; Zohora, F.T.; Das, K.C.; Mowla, M.G.; Banu, N.A.; Salimullah, M.; Hashem, A. Production, partial optimization and characterization of keratinase enzyme by *Arthrobacter* sp. NFH5 isolated from soil samples. *AMB Express* **2017**, *7*, 1–8. [CrossRef] [PubMed]
23. Habbeche, A.; Saoudi, B.; Jaouadi, B.; Haberra, S.; Kerouaz, B.; Boudelaa, M.; Badis, A.; Ladjama, A. Purification and biochemical characterization of a detergent-stable keratinase from a newly thermophilic actinomycete *Actinomadura keratinilytica* strain Cpt29 isolated from poultry compost. *J. Biosci. Bioeng.* **2014**, *117*, 413–421. [CrossRef] [PubMed]
24. Jaouadi, N.Z.; Rekik, H.; Badis, A.; Trabelsi, S.; Belhoul, M.; Yahiaoui, A.B.; Aicha, H.B.; Toumi, A.; Bejar, S.; Jaouadi, B. Biochemical and Molecular Characterization of a Serine Keratinase from *Brevibacillus brevis* US575 with Promising Keratin-Biodegradation and Hide-Dehairing Activities. *PLoS ONE* **2013**, *8*, e76722. [CrossRef]
25. Syed, D.G.; Lee, J.C.; Li, W.J.; Kim, C.J.; Agasar, D. Production, characterization and application of keratinase from *Streptomyces gulbargensis*. *Bioresour. Technol.* **2009**, *100*, 1868–1871. [CrossRef]
26. Mitsuiki, S.; Ichikawa, M.; Oka, T.; Sakai, M.; Moriyama, Y.; Sameshima, Y.; Goto, M.; Furukawa, K. Molecular characterization of a keratinolytic enzyme from an alkaliphilic *Nocardiopsis* sp. TOA-1. *Enzyme Microb. Technol.* **2004**, *34*, 482–489. [CrossRef]
27. Gupta, R.; Ramnani, P. Microbial keratinases and their prospective applications: An overview. *Appl. Microbiol. Biotechnol.* **2006**, *70*, 21–33. [CrossRef]
28. Daroit, D.J.; Brandelli, A. A current assessment on the production of bacterial keratinases. *Crit. Rev. Biotechnol.* **2014**, *34*, 372–384. [CrossRef]
29. Inada, S.; Watanabe, K. Draft genome sequence of *Meiothermus ruber* H328, which degrades chicken feathers, and identification of proteases and peptidases responsible for degradation. *Genome Announc.* **2013**, *1*, 3–4. [CrossRef]
30. Yong, B.; Yang, B.; Zhao, C.; Feng, H. Draft Genome Sequence of *Bacillus subtilis* Strain S1-4, Which Degrades Feathers Efficiently. *Genome Announc.* **2013**, *1*, 13–14. [CrossRef]
31. Park, G.-S.; Hong, S.-J.; Lee, C.-H.; Khan, A.R.; Ullah, I.; Jung, B.K.; Choi, J.; Kwak, Y.; Back, C.-G.; Jung, H.-Y.; et al. Draft Genome Sequence of *Chryseobacterium* sp. Strain P1-3, a Keratinolytic Bacterium Isolated from Poultry Waste. *Genome Announc.* **2014**, *2*, 10–11. [CrossRef]
32. Pereira, J.Q.; Ambrosini, A.; Sant'Anna, F.H.; Tadra-Sfeir, M.; Faoro, H.; Pedrosa, F.O.; Souza, E.M.; Brandelli, A.; Passaglia, L.M.P. Whole-genome shotgun sequence of the keratinolytic bacterium *Lysobacter* sp. A03, isolated from the Antarctic environment. *Genome Announc.* **2015**, *3*, 1–2. [CrossRef]
33. Kim, E.-M.; Hwang, K.H.; Park, J.-S. Complete Genome Sequence of *Chryseobacterium camelliae* Dolsongi-HT1, a Green Tea Isolate with Keratinolytic Activity. *Genome Announc.* **2018**, *6*, 1–2. [CrossRef]
34. Li, B.; Liu, F.; Ren, Y.; Ding, Y.; Li, Y.; Tang, X.-F.; Tang, B. Complete Genome Sequence of *Thermoactinomyces vulgaris* Strain CDF, a Thermophilic Bacterium Capable of Degrading Chicken Feathers. *Genome Announc.* **2019**, *8*, 1–2. [CrossRef]
35. Peng, Z.; Zhang, J.; Du, G.; Chen, J. Keratin Waste Recycling Based on Microbial Degradation: Mechanisms and Prospects. *ACS Sustain. Chem. Eng.* **2019**, *7*, 9727–9736. [CrossRef]
36. Li, Z.W.; Liang, S.; Ke, Y.; Deng, J.J.; Zhang, M.S.; Lu, D.L.; Li, J.Z.; Luo, X.C. The feather degradation mechanisms of a new *Streptomyces* sp. isolate SCUT-3. *Commun. Biol.* **2020**, *3*, 1–13. [CrossRef]
37. Cumsille, A.; Undabarrena, A.; González, V.; Claverías, F.; Rojas, C.; Cámara, B. Biodiversity of actinobacteria from the South Pacific and the assessment of *Streptomyces* chemical diversity with metabolic profiling. *Mar. Drugs* **2017**, *15*, 286. [CrossRef]
38. Undabarrena, A.; Beltrametti, F.; Claverías, F.P.; González, M.; Moore, E.R.; Seeger, M.; Cámara, B. Exploring the diversity and antimicrobial potential of marine actinobacteria from the comau fjord in Northern Patagonia, Chile. *Front. Microbiol.* **2016**, *7*, 1–16. [CrossRef]

39. Claverías, F.P.; Undabarrena, A.; Gonzalez, M.; Seeger, M.; Camara, B. Culturable diversity and antimicrobial activity of Actinobacteria from marine sediments in Valparaíso bay, Chile. *Front. Microbiol.* **2015**, *6*, 1–11. [CrossRef]
40. González, V.; Vargas-Straube, M.J.; Beys-da-Silva, W.O.; Santi, L.; Valencia, P.; Beltrametti, F.; Cámara, B. Enzyme Bioprospection of Marine-Derived Actinobacteria from the Chilean Coast and New Insight in the Mechanism of Keratin Degradation in *Streptomyces* sp. G11C. *Mar. Drugs* **2020**, *18*, 537. [CrossRef]
41. Ventura, M.; Canchaya, C.; Tauch, A.; Chandra, G.; Fitzgerald, G.F.; Chater, K.F.; van Sinderen, D. Genomics of Actinobacteria: Tracing the evolutionary history of an ancient phylum. *Microbiol. Mol. Biol. Rev.* **2007**, *71*, 495–548. [CrossRef] [PubMed]
42. Emms, D.M.; Kelly, S. OrthoFinder: Phylogenetic orthology inference for comparative genomics. *Genome Biol.* **2019**, *20*, 1–14. [CrossRef] [PubMed]
43. Sun, W.; Huang, Y.; Zhang, Y.Q.; Liu, Z.H. *Streptomyces emeiensis* sp. nov., a novel streptomycete from soil in China. *Int. J. Syst. Evol. Microbiol.* **2007**, *57*, 1635–1639. [CrossRef] [PubMed]
44. Hain, T.; Ward-Rainey, N.; Kroppenstedt, R.M.; Stackebrandt, E.; Rainey, F.A. Discrimination of *Streptomyces albidoflavus* strains based on the size and number of 16S-23S ribosomal DNA intergenic spacers. *Int. J. Syst. Bacteriol.* **1997**, *47*, 202–206. [CrossRef]
45. Jain, C.; Rodriguez-R., L.M.; Phillippy, A.M.; Konstantinidis, K.T.; Aluru, S. High throughput ANI analysis of 90K prokaryotic genomes reveals clear species boundaries. *Nat. Commun.* **2018**, *9*, 1–8. [CrossRef]
46. Nguyen, T.T.H.; Myrold, D.D.; Mueller, R.S. Distributions of extracellular peptidases across prokaryotic genomes reflect phylogeny and habitat. *Front. Microbiol.* **2019**, *10*, 1–14. [CrossRef]
47. Page, M.J.; Di Cera, E. Evolution of peptidase diversity. *J. Biol. Chem.* **2008**, *283*, 30010–30014. [CrossRef] [PubMed]
48. Rawlings, N.D. Bacterial calpains and the evolution of the calpain (C2) family of peptidases. *Biol. Direct* **2015**, *10*, 1–12. [CrossRef]
49. Hahsler, M.; Piekenbrock, M.; Doran, D. Dbscan: Fast density-based clustering with R. *J. Stat. Softw.* **2019**, *91*, 1–30. [CrossRef]
50. Bakan, A.; Meireles, L.M.; Bahar, I. ProDy: Protein dynamics inferred from theory and experiments. *Bioinformatics* **2011**, *27*, 1575–1577. [CrossRef]
51. Mooers, A. Effects of tree shape on the accuracy of maximum likelihood-based ancestor reconstructions. *Syst. Biol.* **2004**, *53*, 809–814. [CrossRef] [PubMed]
52. Litsios, G.; Salamin, N. Effects of phylogenetic signal on ancestral state reconstruction. *Syst. Biol.* **2012**, *61*, 533–538. [CrossRef] [PubMed]
53. Potempa, J.; Pike, R.N. Bacterial peptidases. *Contrib. Microbiol.* **2005**, *12*, 132–180. [CrossRef] [PubMed]
54. Jiang, L.Q.; Carter, B.R.; Feely, R.A.; Lauvset, S.K.; Olsen, A. Surface ocean pH and buffer capacity: Past, present and future. *Sci. Rep.* **2019**, *9*, 1–11. [CrossRef]
55. Rao, M.B.; Tanksale, A.M.; Ghatge, M.S.; Deshpande, V.V. Molecular and biotechnological aspects of microbial proteases. *Microbiol. Mol. Biol. Rev.* **1998**, *62*, 597–635. [CrossRef]
56. Rawlings, N.D. Peptidase specificity from the substrate cleavage collection in the MEROPS database and a tool to measure cleavage site conservation. *Biochimie* **2016**, *122*, 5–30. [CrossRef]
57. Brandelli, A.; Daroit, D.J.; Riffel, A. Biochemical features of microbial keratinases and their production and applications. *Appl. Microbiol. Biotechnol.* **2010**, *85*, 1735–1750. [CrossRef]
58. Williams, C.M.; Richter, C.S.; Mackenzie, J.M.; Shih, J.C.H. Isolation, Identification, and Characterization of a Feather-Degrading Bacterium. *Appl. Environ. Microbiol.* **1990**, *56*, 1509–1515. [CrossRef]
59. Mitsuiki, S.; Sakai, M.; Moriyama, Y.; Goto, M.; Furukawa, K. Purification and Some Properties of a Keratinolytic Enzyme from an Alkaliphilic *Nocardiopsis* sp. TOA-1. *Biosci. Biotechnol. Biochem.* **2002**, *66*, 164–167. [CrossRef]
60. Riffel, A.; Lucas, F.; Heeb, P.; Brandelli, A. Characterization of a new keratinolytic bacterium that completely degrades native feather keratin. *Arch. Microbiol.* **2003**, *179*, 258–265. [CrossRef]
61. Tatineni, R.; Doddapaneni, K.K.; Potumarthi, R.C.; Vellanki, R.N.; Kandathil, M.T.; Kolli, N.; Mangamoori, L.N. Purification and characterization of an alkaline keratinase from *Streptomyces* sp. *Bioresour. Technol.* **2008**, *99*, 1596–1602. [CrossRef]
62. Qiu, J.; Wilkens, C.; Barrett, K.; Meyer, A.S. Microbial enzymes catalyzing keratin degradation: Classification, structure, function. *Biotechnol. Adv.* **2020**, *44*, 1–22. [CrossRef]
63. Gerlt, J.A. Genomic Enzymology: Web Tools for Leveraging Protein Family Sequence-Function Space and Genome Context to Discover Novel Functions. *Biochemistry* **2017**, *56*, 4293–4308. [CrossRef]
64. Yamamura, S.; Morita, Y.; Hasan, Q.; Yokoyama, K.; Tamiya, E. Keratin degradation: A cooperative action of two enzymes from *Stenotrophomonas* sp. *Biochem. Biophys. Res. Commun.* **2002**, *294*, 1138–1143. [CrossRef]
65. Huang, Y.; Łężyk, M.; Herbst, F.A.; Busk, P.K.; Lange, L. Novel keratinolytic enzymes, discovered from a talented and efficient bacterial keratin degrader. *Sci. Rep.* **2020**, *10*, 1–11. [CrossRef]
66. Wang, S.L.; Hsu, W.T.; Liang, T.W.; Yen, Y.H.; Wang, C.L. Purification and characterization of three novel keratinolytic metalloproteases produced by *Chryseobacterium indologenes* TKU014 in a shrimp shell powder medium. *Bioresour. Technol.* **2008**, *99*, 5679–5686. [CrossRef]
67. Liu, Q.; Zhang, T.; Song, N.; Li, Q.; Wang, Z.; Zhang, X.; Lu, X.; Fang, J.; Chen, J. Purification and characterization of four key enzymes from a feather-degrading *Bacillus subtilis* from the gut of tarantula *Chilobrachys guangxiensis*. *Int. Biodeterior. Biodegrad.* **2014**, *96*, 26–32. [CrossRef]

68. Monod, M.; Capoccia, S.; Léchenne, B.; Zaugg, C.; Holdom, M.; Jousson, O. Secreted proteases from pathogenic fungi. *Int. J. Med. Microbiol.* **2002**, *292*, 405–419. [CrossRef]
69. Joshi, N.A.; Fass, J.N. Sickle: A Sliding-Window, Adaptive, Quality-Based Trimming Tool for FastQ Files—Version 1.33. 2011. Available online: https://github.com/najoshi/sickle (accessed on 8 June 2020).
70. Bankevich, A.; Nurk, S.; Antipov, D.; Gurevich, A.A.; Dvorkin, M.; Kulikov, A.S.; Lesin, V.M.; Nikolenko, S.I.; Pham, S.; Prjibelski, A.D.; et al. SPAdes: A new genome assembly algorithm and its applications to single-cell sequencing. *J. Comput. Biol.* **2012**, *19*, 455–477. [CrossRef] [PubMed]
71. Nurk, S.; Bankevich, A.; Antipov, D.; Gurevich, A.A.; Korobeynikov, A.; Lapidus, A.; Prjibelski, A.D.; Pyshkin, A.; Sirotkin, A.; Sirotkin, Y.; et al. Assembling single-cell genomes and mini-metagenomes from chimeric MDA products. *J. Comput. Biol.* **2013**, *20*, 714–737. [CrossRef]
72. Wick, R.R.; Judd, L.M.; Gorrie, C.L.; Holt, K.E. Unicycler: Resolving bacterial genome assemblies from short and long sequencing reads. *PLoS Comput. Biol.* **2017**, *13*, e1005595. [CrossRef] [PubMed]
73. Boetzer, M.; Henkel, C.V.; Jansen, H.J.; Butler, D.; Pirovano, W. Scaffolding pre-assembled contigs using SSPACE. *Bioinformatics* **2011**, *27*, 578–579. [CrossRef] [PubMed]
74. Gurevich, A.; Saveliev, V.; Vyahhi, N.; Tesler, G. QUAST: Quality assessment tool for genome assemblies. *Bioinformatics* **2013**, *29*, 1072–1075. [CrossRef] [PubMed]
75. Parks, D.H.; Imelfort, M.; Skennerton, C.T.; Hugenholtz, P.; Tyson, G.W. CheckM: Assessing the quality of microbial genomes recovered from isolates, single cells, and metagenomes. *Genome Res.* **2015**, *25*, 1043–1055. [CrossRef]
76. Seemann, T. Prokka: Rapid prokaryotic genome annotation. *Bioinformatics* **2014**, *30*, 2068–2069. [CrossRef]
77. Törönen, P.; Medlar, A.; Holm, L. PANNZER2: A rapid functional annotation web server. *Nucleic Acids Res.* **2018**, *46*, W84–W88. [CrossRef]
78. Huerta-Cepas, J.; Szklarczyk, D.; Heller, D.; Hernández-Plaza, A.; Forslund, S.K.; Cook, H.; Mende, D.R.; Letunic, I.; Rattei, T.; Jensen, L.J.; et al. EggNOG 5.0: A hierarchical, functionally and phylogenetically annotated orthology resource based on 5090 organisms and 2502 viruses. *Nucleic Acids Res.* **2019**, *47*, D309–D314. [CrossRef]
79. Nouioui, I.; Carro, L.; García-López, M.; Meier-Kolthoff, J.P.; Woyke, T.; Kyrpides, N.C.; Pukall, R.; Klenk, H.P.; Goodfellow, M.; Göker, M. Genome-based taxonomic classification of the *phylum* Actinobacteria. *Front. Microbiol.* **2018**, *9*, 1–119. [CrossRef] [PubMed]
80. Price, M.N.; Dehal, P.S.; Arkin, A.P. FastTree 2—Approximately maximum-likelihood trees for large alignments. *PLoS ONE* **2010**, *5*, e9490. [CrossRef] [PubMed]
81. Pritchard, L.; Glover, R.H.; Humphris, S.; Elphinstone, J.G.; Toth, I.K. Genomics and taxonomy in diagnostics for food security: Soft-rotting enterobacterial plant pathogens. *Anal. Methods* **2016**, *8*, 12–24. [CrossRef]
82. Barrett, A.J.; McDonald, J.K. Nomenclature: Protease, proteinase and peptidase. *Biochem. J.* **1986**, *237*, 935. [CrossRef]
83. HMMER-Based MEROPS Web-Server. Available online: https://www.ebi.ac.uk/merops/submit_searches.shtml. (accessed on 14 April 2020).
84. Rawlings, N.D.; Barrett, A.J.; Thomas, P.D.; Huang, X.; Bateman, A.; Finn, R.D. The MEROPS database of proteolytic enzymes, their substrates and inhibitors in 2017 and a comparison with peptidases in the PANTHER database. *Nucleic Acids Res.* **2018**, *46*, D624–D632. [CrossRef]
85. Larsson, J. eulerr: Area-Proportional Euler and Venn Diagrams with Ellipses. R package version 6.1.0. 2020. Available online: https://cran.r-project.org/package=eulerr (accessed on 18 March 2021).
86. Hagberg, A.A.; Schult, D.A.; Swart, P.J. Exploring network structure, dynamics, and function using NetworkX. In Proceedings of the 7th Python in Science Conference (SciPy 2008), Pasadena, CA, USA, 19–24 August 2008; pp. 11–15.
87. Atkinson, H.J.; Morris, J.H.; Ferrin, T.E.; Babbitt, P.C. Using sequence similarity networks for visualization of relationships across diverse protein superfamilies. *PLoS ONE* **2009**, *4*, e4345. [CrossRef]
88. Blondel, V.D.; Guillaume, J.L.; Lambiotte, R.; Lefebvre, E. Fast unfolding of communities in large networks. *J. Stat. Mech. Theory Exp.* **2008**, P10008. [CrossRef]
89. Bastian, M.; Heymann, S.; Jacomy, M. Gephi: An open source software for exploring and manipulating networks. In Proceedings of the Third International AAAI Conference on Weblogs and Social Media, San Jose, CA, USA, 17–20 May 2009; pp. 361–362.
90. Hu, Y. Efficient and High Quality Force-Directed Graph. *Math. J.* **2005**, *10*, 37–71.
91. Fruchterman, T.M.J.; Reingold, E.M. Graph drawing by force-directed placement. *Softw. Pract. Exp.* **1991**, *21*, 1129–1164. [CrossRef]
92. Sanchez, G.; Yu, C.-S.; Chen, Y.-C.; Lu, C.-H.; Hwang, J.-K. Prediction of Protein Subcellular Localization. *PROTEINS Struct. Funct. Bioinform.* **2006**, *64*, 643–651. [CrossRef]
93. Yu, N.Y.; Wagner, J.R.; Laird, M.R.; Melli, G.; Rey, S.; Lo, R.; Dao, P.; Cenk Sahinalp, S.; Ester, M.; Foster, L.J.; et al. PSORTb 3.0: Improved protein subcellular localization prediction with refined localization subcategories and predictive capabilities for all prokaryotes. *Bioinformatics* **2010**, *26*, 1608–1615. [CrossRef]
94. Almagro Armenteros, J.J.; Tsirigos, K.D.; Sønderby, C.K.; Petersen, T.N.; Winther, O.; Brunak, S.; von Heijne, G.; Nielsen, H. SignalP 5.0 improves signal peptide predictions using deep neural networks. *Nat. Biotechnol.* **2019**, *37*, 420–423. [CrossRef]

95. Van Der Maaten, L.; Hinton, G. Visualizing data using t-SNE. *J. Mach. Learn. Res.* **2008**, *9*, 2579–2625.
96. Pedregosa, F.; Varoquaux, G.; Gramfort, A.; Michel, V.; Thirion, B.; Grisel, O.; Blondel, M.; Prettenhofer, P.; Weiss, R.; Dubourg, V.; et al. Scikit-learn: Machine learning in Python. *J. Mach. Learn. Res.* **2011**, *12*, 2825–2830.
97. Katoh, K.; Misawa, K.; Kuma, K.I.; Miyata, T. MAFFT: A novel method for rapid multiple sequence alignment based on fast Fourier transform. *Nucleic Acids Res.* **2002**, *30*, 3059–3066. [CrossRef] [PubMed]
98. Darriba, D.; Taboada, G.L.; Doallo, R.; Posada, D. ProtTest 3: Fast selection of best-fit models of protein evolution. *Bioinformatics* **2011**, *27*, 1164–1165. [CrossRef] [PubMed]
99. Stamatakis, A. RAxML version 8: A tool for phylogenetic analysis and post-analysis of large phylogenies. *Bioinformatics* **2014**, *30*, 1312–1313. [CrossRef]
100. Bollback, J.P. SIMMAP: Stochastic character mapping of discrete traits on phylogenies. *BMC Bioinform.* **2006**, *7*, 1–7. [CrossRef]
101. Revell, L.J. phytools: An R package for phylogenetic comparative biology (and other things). *Methods Ecol. Evol.* **2012**, *3*, 217–223. [CrossRef]

MDPI
St. Alban-Anlage 66
4052 Basel
Switzerland
Tel. +41 61 683 77 34
Fax +41 61 302 89 18
www.mdpi.com

Marine Drugs Editorial Office
E-mail: marinedrugs@mdpi.com
www.mdpi.com/journal/marinedrugs

www.ingramcontent.com/pod-product-compliance
Lightning Source LLC
LaVergne TN
LVHW070433100526
838202LV00014B/1590
* 9 7 8 3 0 3 6 5 3 2 9 9 8 *

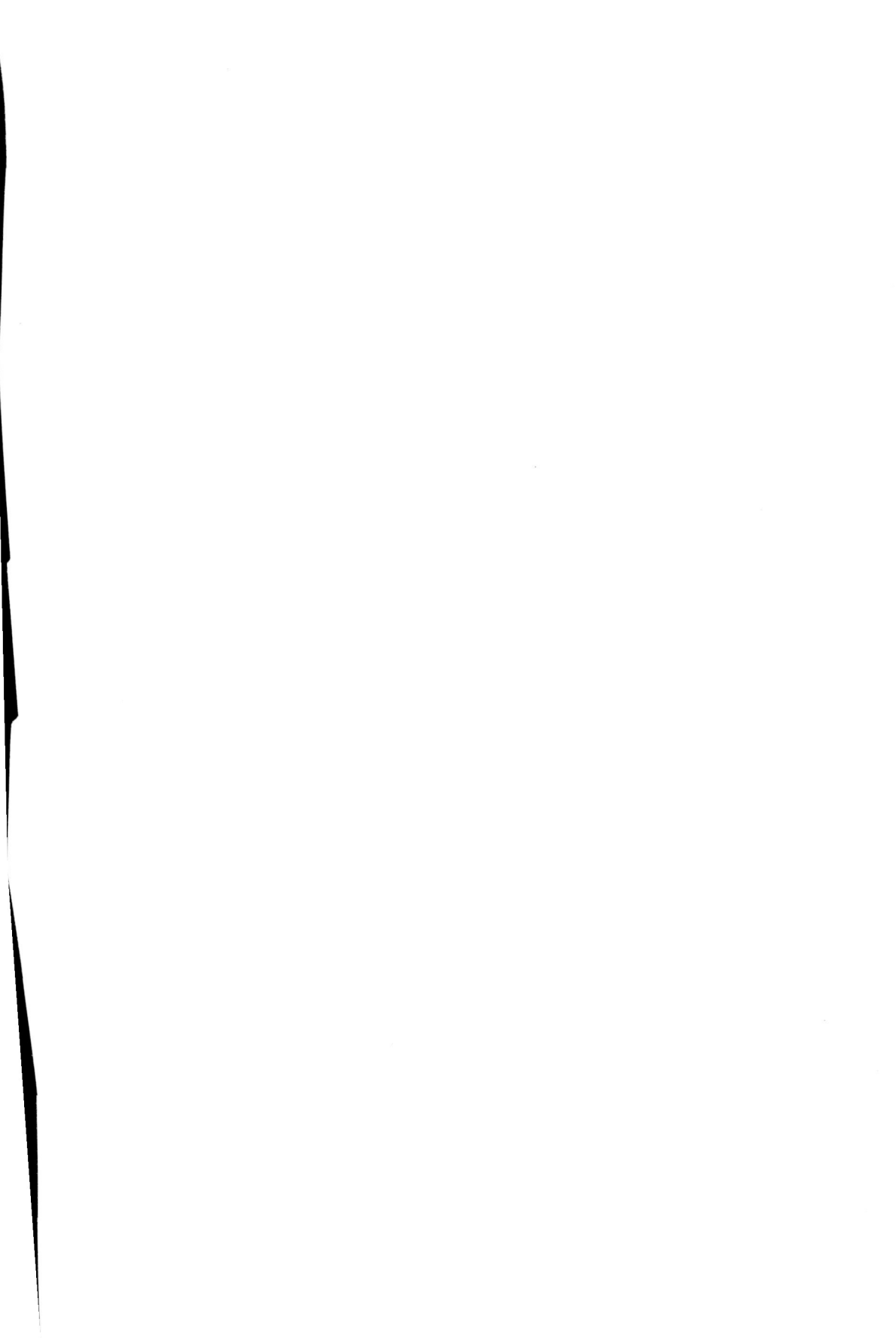